Nutrition and Health

Series Editors
Connie W. Bales, Duke University School of Medicine
Durham VA Medical Center, Durham, USA

Crystal Karakochuk, University of British Columbia
Vancouver, BC, Canada

The Nutrition and Health series has an overriding mission in providing health professionals with texts that are considered essential since each is edited by the leading researchers in their respective fields. Each volume includes: 1) a synthesis of the state of the science, 2) timely, in-depth reviews, 3) extensive, up-to-date fully annotated reference lists, 4) a detailed index, 5) relevant tables and figures, 6) identification of paradigm shifts and consequences, 7) virtually no overlap of information between chapters, but targeted, inter-chapter referrals, 8) suggestions of areas for future research and 9) balanced, data driven answers to patient/health professionals questions which are based upon the totality of evidence rather than the findings of a single study.

Nutrition and Health is a major resource of relevant, clinically based nutrition volumes for the professional that serve as a reliable source of data-driven reviews and practice guidelines.

Amal K. Mitra • Divya Vanoh

Editors

Essentials of Clinical and Public Health Nutrition

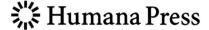 Humana Press

Editors
Amal K. Mitra 🆔
Department of Public Health
Julia Jones Matthews School of Population
and Public Health Texas Tech University
Health Sciences Center
Abilene, TX, USA

Divya Vanoh 🆔
Dietetics Programme,
School of Health Sciences
Universiti Sains Malaysia
Kubang Kerian, Kelantan, Malaysia

ISSN 2628-197X   ISSN 2628-1961   (electronic)
Nutrition and Health
ISBN 978-3-031-95372-9   ISBN 978-3-031-95373-6   (eBook)
https://doi.org/10.1007/978-3-031-95373-6

This Humana imprint is published by the registered company Springer Nature Switzerland AG
The registered company address is: Gewerbestrasse 11, 6330 Cham, Switzerland

If disposing of this product, please recycle the paper.

To my beloved wife, Ratna, the cornerstone of my world, whose unwavering love, remarkable patience, and extraordinary wisdom have been the guiding light of my life's journey. Your compassion has been my solace, your strength my anchor, and your belief in me has transcended every challenge we've encountered.

To my cherished children, Amlan and Paromita, who have been more than just inspiration, you have been my living legacy, my greatest teachers, and my most profound source of joy. Your curiosity, resilience, and boundless spirit have continuously reminded me of the beauty of discovery and the importance of pursuing knowledge with passion and integrity.

This work is not merely an academic endeavor but also a shared narrative of our family's collective dream—a testament to the power of love, education, and perseverance. Your endless love has been the invisible ink between these lines, the unwritten chapter that makes this book possible.

Amal Mitra

To my beloved spouse, whose steadfast support and boundless encouragement have been my greatest sources of strength.

To my dear parents, whose profound wisdom, unconditional love, and selfless sacrifices have fundamentally shaped the person I am today.

This book stands as a testament to the shared commitment of dedicated professionals in clinical and public health nutrition. May it illuminate the path for future generations, inspiring their quest to improve health and well-being through the transformative power of nutrition.

With deepest gratitude and heartfelt appreciation,

Divya Vanoh

Foreword

Nutrition Science: A Holistic Approach to Understanding Human Health

In an era of rapid scientific advancement and growing complexity in human health, comprehensive understanding becomes paramount. This textbook emerges as a critical resource, meticulously bridging theoretical knowledge with practical applications across clinical, public health and community education, and emerging research domains of nutrition.

The landscape of nutritional sciences has transformed dramatically over the past decades. What was once considered a relatively straightforward discipline, primarily focused in early years on reducing nutritional deficiencies, has evolved into a multifaceted field intersecting biochemistry, epidemiology, genetics, molecular biology, and social sciences. This volume reflects that complexity, offering readers a nuanced, comprehensive exploration into the diverse facets of nutrition science that transcend traditional boundaries.

By structuring the content into three strategic sections—clinical nutrition, public health nutrition, and recent advances in nutrition research—the authors have created a systematic framework that allows for both depth and breadth in understanding. Readers will find themselves navigating from foundational clinical perspectives to broader population-level interventions and finally to the cutting-edge and emerging research that promises to reshape our understanding of nutritional science.

Trainees (graduate students, postdoctoral students, and medical or other professionals) will discover a rich scholarly resource that challenges existing paradigms. Practicing nutritionists and dietitians will find practical insights that can be immediately translated into clinical and community practice. Researchers will appreciate the comprehensive review of recent advances, providing a robust platform for future investigations.

The transdisciplinary nature of this textbook is its greatest strength. It does not merely present information but also invites critical thinking, encouraging readers to view nutrition as a dynamic, interconnected multidisciplinary system that influences individual and collective health outcomes.

As we continue to confront global health challenges such as obesity, malnutrition, chronic diseases, and emerging nutritional interventions, resources like this become invaluable. They are not just repositories of knowledge but also catalysts for innovation and improved human health. This textbook is more than an academic publication—it is a testament to the evolving science of nutrition and its profound impact on human well-being.

Executive Director, Institute for   Naïma Moustaïd-Moussa
One Health Innovation
Lubbock, TX, USA
Paul W. Horn Distinguished Professor
TTU Department of Nutritional Sciences
Lubbock, TX, USA
Professor, TTUHSC Department
of Cell Biology & Biochemistry
Lubbock, TX, USA
Founding Director, Obesity Research Institute
Lubbock, TX, USA
President-elect, the American Society
for Nutrition (ASN)
Rockville, MD, USA

Preface

My journey in public health nutrition began in 1982 at a rural field hospital in Matlab, Bangladesh, operated by the International Center for Diarrheal Diseases Research, Bangladesh (Icddr,b). As a medical officer, I witnessed hundreds of children admitted daily for illnesses such as diarrhea, pneumonia, and shigellosis—most distressingly, the vast majority suffering from undernutrition.

The challenges I encountered were profound. Mothers from underserved families lacked basic health education, and communities were steeped in cultural myths and stigmas. Illnesses were often attributed to divine will or evil spirits, with villagers relying on unqualified practitioners for treatment. I vividly remember young mothers arriving with terminally ill babies, some practicing desperate rituals like "bloodletting" in misguided attempts to cure their children.

These experiences were not just personal trials but also microcosms of broader public health challenges. Consider the historical parallels: scurvy decimating sailors until James Lind's groundbreaking clinical trial or pellagra being misunderstood until Joseph Goldberger's nutritional research. Each discovery represented a triumph of scientific understanding over prevailing misconceptions.

My own research journey included confronting complex community resistance. During Dr. John Clemens's oral cholera vaccine field trial in 1985, I personally engaged with community leaders who believed that scientists were spreading disease. By leveraging trust and patient communication, we gradually overcame deep-seated skepticism.

Over 28 years of teaching public health, I have continuously evolved my pedagogical approach. The goal has always been to present clinical and public health nutrition concepts in an intuitive, accessible manner that engages and enlightens students.

Essentials of Public Health and Clinical Nutrition represents the culmination of these experiences. Designed for students, educators, researchers, dieticians, and clinicians, this textbook offers a comprehensive, practical guide to nutritional management.

Abilene, Texas, United States   Amal K. Mitra

Preface

We have meticulously organized the contents into three key sections:

1. *Clinical nutrition* explores critical areas from gut microflora to specialized dietary interventions.
2. *Public health nutrition* addresses nutritional needs across different life stages and societal contexts.
3. *Recent advances in nutrition research* presents cutting-edge insights into emerging nutritional science.

What distinguishes this textbook is the experience of its contributors. Each chapter reflects personal insights from managing nutritional challenges in hospital settings and diverse populations. From prenatal development to geriatric care, our authors bring real-world perspectives to theoretical knowledge.

To enhance learning, each chapter concludes with suggested further reading and a question-and-answer (Q&A) section, designed to reinforce key concepts and stimulate critical thinking. We have intentionally balanced scientific rigor with approachable, engaging narrative.

As you embark on this nutritional journey, we invite you to not just read but also reflect, question, and ultimately transform your understanding of human nutrition. We welcome your feedback and perspectives, which will be invaluable in shaping future editions of this book.

Kelantan, Malaysia   Divya Vanoh

Series Editor Bios

Adrianne Bendich has served as the Nutrition and Health Series editor for more than 25 years and has provided leadership and guidance to more than 200 editors who have developed the 95 well-respected and highly recommended volumes in this series.

1. *Essentials of Clinical and Public Health Nutrition*, edited by Amal K. Mitra and Divya Vanoh, 2025
2. *Nutrition, Fitness, and Mindfulness, An Evidence-Based Guide for Clinicians*, 2nd Edition, edited by Jaime Uribarri and Joseph A. Vassalotti, 2024
3. Nutritional Health, 4th Edition, edited by Norman J. Temple, Ted Wilson, David R. Jacobs, Jr. and George A. Bray, 2023
4. Nutritional Anemia, edited by Crystal Karakochuk, Michael B. Zimmermann, Diego Moretti, and Klaus Kraemer, 2023
5. Nutrition Guide for Physicians and Related Healthcare Professions, Third Edition, edited by Ted Wilson, Norman J. Temple, and George A. Bray, 2022
6. Nutrition and Infectious Diseases: Shifting the Clinical Paradigm, edited by Debbie Humphries, Marilyn Scott, and Sten H. Vermund, 2020
7. Nutritional and Medical Management of Kidney Stones, edited by Haewook Han, Walter Mutter, and Samer Nasser, 2019
8. Vitamin E in Human Health, edited by Peter Weber, Marc Birringer, Jeffrey B. Blumberg, Manfred Eggersdorfer, and Jan Frank, 2019
9. Handbook of Nutrition and Pregnancy, Second Edition, edited by Carol J. Lammi-Keefe, Sarah C. Couch, and John P. Kirwan, 2019
10. Dietary Patterns and Whole Plant Foods in Aging and Disease, edited and written by Mark L. Dreher, 2018
11. Dietary Fiber in Health and Disease, edited and written by Mark L. Dreher, 2017
12. Clinical Aspects of Natural and Added Phosphorus in Foods, edited by Orlando M. Gutiérrez, Kamyar Kalantar-Zadeh, and Rajnish Mehrotra, 2017
13. Nutrition and Fetal Programming, edited by Rajendram Rajkumar, Victor R. Preedy, and Vinood B. Patel, 2017

14. Nutrition and Diet in Maternal Diabetes, edited by Rajendram Rajkumar, Victor R. Preedy, and Vinood B. Patel, 2017
15. Nitrite and Nitrate in Human Health and Disease, Second Edition, edited by Nathan S. Bryan and Joseph Loscalzo, 2017
16. Nutrition in Lifestyle Medicine, edited by James M. Rippe, 2017
17. Nutrition Guide for Physicians and Related Healthcare Professionals, Second Edition, edited by Norman J. Temple, Ted Wilson, and George A. Bray, 2016
18. Clinical Aspects of Natural and Added Phosphorus in Foods, edited by Orlando M. Gutiérrez, Kamyar Kalantar-Zadeh, and Rajnish Mehrotra, 2016
19. L-Arginine in Clinical Nutrition, edited by Vinood B. Patel, Victor R. Preedy, and Rajkumar Rajendram, 2016
20. *Mediterranean Diet: Impact on Health and Disease*, edited by Donato F. Romagnolo and Ornella Selmin, 2016

Earlier books included *Alcohol, Nutrition and Health Consequences*, edited by Dr. Ronald Ross Watson, Dr. Victor R. Preedy, and Dr. Sherma Zibadi; *Nutritional Health, Strategies for Disease Prevention, Third Edition*, edited by Norman J. Temple, Ted Wilson, and David R. Jacobs, Jr.; *Chocolate in Health and Nutrition*, edited by Dr. Ronald Ross Watson, Dr. Victor R. Preedy, and Dr. Sherma Zibadi; *Iron Physiology and Pathophysiology in Humans*, edited by Dr. Gregory J. Anderson and Dr. Gordon D. McLaren; *Vitamin D, Second Edition*, edited by Dr. Michael Holick; *Dietary Components and Immune Function*, edited by Dr. Ronald Ross Watson, Dr. Sherma Zibadi, and Dr. Victor R. Preedy; *Bioactive Compounds and Cancer*, edited by Dr. John A. Milner and Dr. Donato F. Romagnolo; *Modern Dietary Fat Intakes in Disease Promotion*, edited by Dr. Fabien De Meester, Dr. Sherma Zibadi, and Dr. Ronald Ross Watson; *Iron Deficiency and Overload*, edited by Dr. Shlomo Yehuda and Dr. David Mostofsky; *Nutrition Guide for Physicians*, edited by Dr. Edward Wilson, Dr. George A. Bray, Dr. Norman Temple, and Dr. Mary Struble; *Nutrition and Metabolism*, edited by Dr. Christos Mantzoros; and *Fluid and Electrolytes in Pediatrics*, edited by Leonard Feld and Dr. Frederick Kaskel.

Recent volumes include *Handbook of Drug-Nutrient Interactions*, edited by Dr. Joseph Boullata and Dr. Vincent Armenti; *Probiotics in Pediatric Medicine*, edited by Dr. Sonia Michail and Dr. Philip Sherman; *Handbook of Nutrition and Pregnancy*, edited by Dr. Carol Lammi-Keefe, Dr. Sarah Couch, and Dr. Elliot Philipson; *Nutrition and Rheumatic Disease*, edited by Dr. Laura Coleman; *Nutrition and Kidney Disease*, edited by Dr. Laura Byham-Grey, Dr. Jerrilynn Burrowes, and Dr. Glenn Chertow; *Nutrition and Health in Developing Countries*, edited by Dr. Richard Semba and Dr. Martin Bloem; *Calcium in Human Health*, edited by Dr. Robert Heaney and Dr. Connie Weaver; and *Nutrition and Bone Health*, edited by Dr. Michael Holick and Dr. Bess Dawson-Hughes; *Diet and Human Immune Function*, edited by David A. Hughes, L. Gail Darlington, and Adrianne Bendich, 2004; *Beverages in Nutrition and Health*, edited by Ted Wilson and Norman J. Temple, 2004; *Handbook of Clinical Nutrition and Aging*, edited by Connie Watkins Bales and Christine Seel Ritchie, 2004; *Fatty Acids: Physiological and*

Behavioral Functions, edited by David I. Mostofsky, Shlomo Yehuda, and Norman Salem, Jr., 2001; *Nutrition and Health in Developing Countries*, edited by Richard D. Semba and Martin W. Bloem, 2001; *Preventive Nutrition: The Comprehensive Guide for Health Professionals, Second Edition*, edited by Adrianne Bendich and Richard J. Deckelbaum, 2001; *Nutritional Health: Strategies for Disease Prevention*, edited by Ted Wilson and Norman J. Temple, 2001; *Clinical Nutrition of the Essential Trace Elements and Minerals: The Guide for Health Professionals*, edited by John D. Bogden and Leslie M. Klevay, 2000; *Primary and Secondary Preventive Nutrition*, edited by Adrianne Bendich and Richard J. Deckelbaum, 2000; *The Management of Eating Disorders and Obesity*, edited by David J. Goldstein, 1999, *Vitamin D: Physiology, Molecular Biology, and Clinical Applications*, edited by Michael F. Holick, 1999; and *Preventive Nutrition: The Comprehensive Guide for Health Professionals*, edited by Adrianne Bendich and Richard J. Deckelbaum, 1997.

Dr. Bendich served as president of consultants for Consumer Healthcare LLC and has edited ten books, including *Preventive Nutrition: The Comprehensive Guide for Health Professionals, Fifth Edition*, coedited with Dr. Richard Deckelbaum (www.springer.com/series/7659). Dr. Bendich serves on the editorial boards of the *Journal of Nutrition in Gerontology and Geriatrics* and *Antioxidants* and has served as an associate editor for the international journal *Nutrition*, served on the editorial board of the *Journal of Women's Health and Gender-Based Medicine*, and served on the board of directors of the American College of Nutrition.

Dr. Bendich was the director of medical affairs at GlaxoSmithKline (GSK) Consumer Healthcare and provided medical leadership for many well-known brands, including TUMS and Os-Cal. Dr. Bendich had primary responsibility for GSK's support for the Women's Health Initiative (WHI) intervention study. Prior to joining GSK, Dr. Bendich was at Roche Vitamins Inc. and was involved in the groundbreaking clinical studies showing that folic acid–containing multivitamins significantly reduce major classes of birth defects. Dr. Bendich has coauthored over 100 major clinical research studies in the area of preventive nutrition. She is recognized as a leading authority on antioxidants, nutrition, and immunity in pregnancy outcomes, vitamin safety, and the cost-effectiveness of vitamin/mineral supplementation. She continues to serve on the editorial board of the journal *Antioxidants*, which she has done since its inception in 2010.

Dr. Bendich received the Roche Research Award, is a Tribute to Women and Industry awardee, and was a recipient of the Burroughs Welcome Visiting Professorship in Basic Medical Sciences. Dr. Bendich was given the Council for Responsible Nutrition (CRN) Apple Award in recognition of her many contributions to the scientific understanding of dietary supplements. In 2012, she was recognized for her contributions to the field of clinical nutrition by the American Society for Nutrition and was elected a fellow of ASN (FASN). Dr. Bendich served as an adjunct professor at Rutgers University. She is listed in *Who's Who in American Women*. Dr. Adrianne Bendich was included in Stanford University's list of the world's top 2% of most widely cited scientists, published in 2022. Dr. Bendich retired as series editor in 2024.

Connie W. Bales recently joined as coseries editor of the Nutrition and Health Series. Dr. Bales is a widely recognized expert in the field of nutrition, chronic disease, function, and aging. Over the past three decades, her laboratory at the Duke School of Medicine has explored many aspects of diet and physical activity as determinants of health during the latter half of the adult life course. She has also studied direct nutritional influences on the aging process and collaborated on a number of large, randomized National Institutes of Health (NIH) trials of key significance in the nutrition arena, including the DASH trial, the STRRIDE-PreDiabetes trial, and the CALERIE trial. Her current research focuses on the impact of higher protein intake during obesity reduction on muscle quality and cardiometabolic risk in functionally limited older adults, as well as racial differences in these responses. Another new work is examining the influence of dietary bioactives on a variety of health attributes in older adults. Dr. Bales has served on National Institutes of Health (NIH), United States Department of Veterans Affairs (VA), and United States Department of Agriculture (USDA) grant review panels and is the editor-in-chief of the *Journal of Nutrition in Gerontology and Geriatrics*. She has edited three editions of the *Handbook of Clinical Nutrition in Aging* in the Nutrition and Health Series and has editorial roles with two other journals, namely *Current Developments in Nutrition* and *Cogent Gerontology*.

Crystal Karakochuk is an associate professor in human nutrition in the Department of Food, Nutrition, and Health at the University of British Columbia (UBC), an investigator at the BC Children's Hospital Research and Women's Health Research Institutes, and a Canada Research Chair Tier 2 in micronutrients and human health. Dr. Karakochuk's research program focuses on micronutrients and human health. She evaluates programs and policies for anemia prevention and treatment and risk–benefit analyses of micronutrient interventions in children and pregnant people.

Series Editor

The Nutrition and Health Series, containing 95 volumes published over 30 years, has maintained a consistent overriding mission of providing health professionals and advanced-study students with texts that are essential because each includes the following: (1) a synthesis of the state of the science; (2) timely, in-depth reviews by the leading researchers and clinicians in their respective fields; (3) extensive, up-to-date, and fully annotated reference lists; (4) a detailed index; (5) relevant tables and figures; (6) the identification of paradigm shifts and their consequences; (7) virtually no overlap of information between chapters but targeted, interchapter referrals; (8) suggestions of areas for future research; and (9) balanced, data-driven answers to patient's and health professionals questions, which are based on the totality of evidence rather than the findings of any single study.

The series volumes are not the outcomes of a symposium. Rather, each editor has the potential to examine a chosen area with a broad perspective, both in subject matter and in the choice of chapter authors. The international perspective, especially regarding public health initiatives, is emphasized where appropriate. The editors, who are both research and practice oriented, have the opportunity to develop a primary objective for their book, define the scope and focus, and then invite the leading authorities from around the world to be part of their initiative. The authors are encouraged to provide an overview of the field, discuss their own research, and relate the research findings to potential human health consequences. Because each book is developed de novo, the chapters are coordinated so that the resulting volume imparts greater knowledge than the sum of the information contained in the individual chapters.

The newest volume in the series *Essentials of Clinical and Public Health Nutrition*, edited by Amal K. Mitra and Divya Vanoh, provides readers with 19 chapters that constitute a comprehensive, practical guide to the nutritional management of patients and population groups across the lifespan. The volume is designed to provide well-accepted findings covering core topics for students, educators, researchers, dieticians, and clinicians alike. Also included are new topics and the latest nutrition research areas. Because these chapters were written prior to the US November 2024 election and subsequent alterations to US federal programs and funding, the relevant chapters do not reflect these changes.

The editors of this volume are highly recognized professors with both research and diverse clinical experiences involving nutritional interventions and have expertise in public health interventions using nutritional research findings. Dr. Amal Mitra, MBBS, DIH, MPH, DrPH, a professor of the Department of Public Health at the Julia Jones Matthews School *of* Population *and* Public Health at Texas Tech University Health Sciences Center in Abilene, Texas. Dr. Mitra has authored over 120 publications and a book titled *Epidemiology for Dummies*, published by Wiley in 2023, and edited a textbook titled *Statistical Approaches for Epidemiology: From Concept to Application*, published by Springer Nature in 2024. Dr. Mitra is an internationally recognized scientist and a leader in public health, with over 40 years of research and 28 years of teaching. Dr. Mitra has received many awards and recognition, including, but not limited to, the Young Scientist Award from the American Society for Nutrition, the John Snow Award from the American Public Health Association, the US Fulbright-Nehru Academic and Professional Excellence Award, a Lifetime Achievement Award from the University of Southern Mississippi, Mississippi's Health Care Hero, and the U.S. Fulbright Scholar Award. Additionally, Dr. Mitra has been awarded significant research funding from the National Institutes of Health (NIH), the Centers for Disease Control and Prevention (CDC), the Environmental Protection Agency (EPA), the World Health Organization (WHO), and UNICEF. A dedicated mentor, he has guided numerous graduate students in public health research, both domestically and internationally.

Dr. Divya Vanoh was a lecturer in the Dietetics Program, School of Health Sciences at Universiti Sains Malaysia. Currently, she is the chair of the Dietetics Program at the *Universiti Sains Malaysia* (USM). Dr. Divya is a registered dietitian who is involved in managing pediatric patients with feeding issues at the USM Specialist Hospital. She is also a visiting lecturer in the Faculty of Medicine and the Faculty of Public Health, Universitas Andalas in Padang, Indonesia. She has also been appointed to one of the technical working group committees for establishing the Malaysian Dietary Guidelines for Older Persons by the Ministry of Health Malaysia. Dr. Vanoh teaches nutrition-related subjects such as dietetic skills, medical nutrition therapy, therapeutic diet preparation, nutrition and disease, the clinical dietetic practicum, and the community dietetic practicum. She is actively conducting research in the field of geriatric nutrition, focusing on sarcopenia, frailty, cognitive function, dietary patterns, and diet quality. She has developed a health information system known as WESIHAT 2.0, which consists of various recommendations for lowering the risk of memory impairment, healthy but simple recipes that can be prepared by older adults, and shopping tips. This is a web-based application that can be used by a large group of older adults in Malaysia. Currently, WESIHAT 2.0 has been used in various research studies involving older adults and has been translated into languages other than Malay to reach a wider community of older adults.

In Chapter 1, editors begin their volume with an in-depth review and update on the critical functions of the gut microbiome throughout the lifespan. Prebiotics and probiotics are discussed, including many of the nutritional functions of the microbiome. This chapter includes relevant figures and tables as well as 49 recent references.

The next four chapters investigate several of the major chronic diseases that are linked to positive nutritional interventions. Chapter 2 examines the spectrum of health effects seen with obesity and the potential for dietary intervention to treat obesity. Chapter 2 reviews the newest weight-loss approaches, including pharmaco-therapy and surgical procedures, and discusses their mechanisms, benefits, and potential risks. It includes tables and figures as well as over 100 references. Chapter 3 provides a comprehensive review of the types of diabetes, including gestational diabetes mellitus, that can be positively affected by dietary interventions and food choices and a review of the diabetic interactions seen in obese patients and other major health consequences of diabetes. It also includes eight relevant tables and two figures as well as 39 references. Chapter 4 examines the potential of dietary inter-ventions to stabilize chronic kidney disease (CKD) patients. It features a discussion of the evolution of CKD, its effects in the aging population, dialysis, and transplant; the importance of reducing protein and salt intakes are emphasized. Several risk factors for CKD are reviewed, including diabetes and obesity. This patient-focused chapter includes eight tables and four figures as well as 55 references. Another clini-cal condition that affects the aging population is sarcopenia—that is, the loss of muscle mass and strength. Chapter 5 reviews the metabolic factors that have been associated with sarcopenia, including cellular oxidation and the importance of anti-oxidant nutrients in balancing the adverse effects of free radicals in muscle. Particular emphasis is given to flavonoids. It features five tables, including one that reviews the current clinical trials in sarcopenic patients, and 69 references.

Chapter 6 provides a detailed description of the facets of oral health that are linked to dietary factors throughout the lifespan. The role of poor oral health in the development of most chronic diseases, including diabetes, cardiovascular disease, and cancer, are reviewed. The macro- and micronutrients that are key to optimal oral health are tabulated. Chapter 6 includes 99 references. The following chapter, Chapter 7, also related to oral health, discusses the consequences of post-stroke dysphagia. Chronic dysphagia, involving difficulty swallowing and an increased risk for the aspiration of food into the trachea, among other factors, is seen in half of all stroke patients. We learn that dysphagia is divided into two types according to the anatomical site: esophageal dysphagia and oropharyngeal dysphagia. The first affects the movement of food from the esophagus into the stomach, and the second affects the ability to swallow food and move the food from the mouth to the esopha-gus. The seven detailed tables and 118 references in Chapter 7 provide valuable information to those treating patients with dysphagia.

Chapter 8 reviews the essential micronutrients and provides information about the function of each; the current requirement for all ages and stages, including preg-nancy and lactation; content in foods; and deficiency signs. The fat-soluble and water-soluble vitamins and essential minerals are reviewed. It features seven helpful tables and one figure as well as 41 references.

The next chapter, Chapter 9, looks at the effects of nutritional status during the first 1000 days of life (i.e., from conception to the end of the second year of life for a newborn). The nutritional status of a woman who does not know that she is preg-nant on day one of conception greatly affects the growth and health of the embryo, fetus, newborn, and infant stages, and the nutrients provided to the infant during the first two years of life have health and development consequences throughout their life. As well, the maternal periconceptional and pregnancy nutritional status and her post-pregnancy recovery and lactation success are dependent on her nutritional status. Chapter 9 focuses on data from countries where undernutrition prior to pregnancy is often found, and the chapter provides several tables that outline the programs used by the WHO and other international organizations to enhance maternal diets and during breast feeding for the optimal growth of the newborn. It also features a discussion of the addition of solid foods to the toddler diet. Chapter 9 contains three detailed tables that review the nutritional needs during pregnancy, infant nutrition, and other interventions to improve nutritional outcomes. It contains two other valuable tables that review essential nutrient requirements and 15 targeted references.

Chapter 10 reviews two important topics: adolescent dietary needs and nutritional requirements in adults over 60 years of age. Chapter 10 begins with a discussion on the recommended intakes of foods during the adolescent years, between 10 and 19, and examines the changes in the recommendations that occur during adolescence due to sexual maturity. In addition to tabulating the requirements, Chapter 10 discusses eating disorders that are often seen during adolescence. It contains two tables that concern healthy eating habits during adolescence. The section concerning nutrition and aging includes a table of aging statistics, a discussion on the physiology of aging, common nutrition-related issues for older adults, and strategies for maintaining optimal nutrient intake in older adulthood. Older adults (aged 60 and older) have nutritional requirements that differ in many ways from those of younger adults, and these are tabulated. Sarcopenia is reviewed, as is the daily increased need for consuming adequate liquids. In addition to the 46 references, Chapter 11 provides a helpful glossary of relevant terms. Chapter 11 covers the topic of maternal nutrition and includes information about periconceptional nutrition, early pregnancy, and lactation and post-lactation nutritional concerns for both the mother and the neonate. It emphasizes key nutrients and dietary advice. Public health initiatives are also included. Chapter 11 features informative tables and figures as well as 65 references.

Chapter 12 provides the reader with a detailed discussion on the regulatory process of developing a food label and the growing functions of the label, from describing the contents to providing recommendations about the health and disease-related functions of specific nutrients. It contains five detailed figures that show the complexity of interactions that occur in the development of food label components. Chapter 12 includes 65 references. Chapter 13 provides a historical perspective on the evolution of school lunch programs in the United States and the current status of those programs across the globe. Its five figures provide information about the development of menus and ways to help children understand the nutritional value of meals. The review includes qualitative and quantitative studies, case studies, and meta-analyses. Studies have shown that children participating in school meal programs have a better dietary intake and are more likely to consume fruits, vegetables, and whole grains. Additionally, children who participate are more alert and focused and can better concentrate in class. Chapter 13 includes 33 references.

Chapter 14 extends the data linking food, nutrition, and health by examining the term *food insecurity*. Food security occurs when households have consistent, dependable access at all times to enough food for an active, healthy life. In contrast, a household is food insecure when any of its members does not have the resources needed to routinely take in adequate amounts of nutritious food. Chapter 14 includes a global perspective on the prevalence of food insecurity and the critical populations, such as pregnant people and young children, who may be the first to suffer from hunger and malnutrition, key signs of food insecurity. Figures in this chapter illustrate the public health Sustainable Development Goals, the social determinants of health, and the UNICEF goals for maternal and child nutrition. This informative chapter contains 49 references.

Chapter 15 reviews the relatively new area of ultra-processed foods (UPFs). UPFs are characterized by their high energy density, low nutrient content, and extensive use of additives. Chapter 15 includes two informative tables that define the NOVA categories of food processing and a second table that describes the nutritional composition of UPFs. Currently, few well-controlled clinical intervention studies have been carried out on UPFs, but survey data have shown associations between the consumption of UPFs and an increased risk of many chronic diseases. Chapter 15 examines the mechanisms through which UPFs may contribute to obesity, cardiometabolic disorders, cancer, and mental health issues. It contains 80 references. Chrononutrition is another relatively new area of investigation that examines the interaction of internal circadian rhythms with food intake, metabolism, and meal timing. Chapter 16 reviews the studies that show the impact of circadian body rhythm regularity, frequency, and timing on the degree of food intake and their effects on obesity and cardiovascular functions, including blood pressure. The authors emphasize that chrononutrition is a rapidly emerging field in nutrition, and compared to many other topics in health and nutrition, it still has considerable knowledge gaps. Chapter 16 contains 44 relevant references.

Chapter 17 also looks at the new fields of metabolomics and proteomics with respect to cancer prevention. Metabolomics investigates endogenous and exogenous metabolites in biological specimens that are associated with nutritional deficiency, metabolic imbalance, and the composition of the gut microbiome and can quantify pathways associated with cellular metabolism, mitochondrial function, and markers of oxidative stress. Metabolomics is complementary to new areas of investigation, including proteomics and genomics. Proteomics technologies are being used to examine the molecular mechanisms underlying cancer initiation and progression and cancer's responses to treatment. Nutriproteomics utilizes proteomic technologies to investigate the wide range of bioactive proteins and peptides in food and their effects on health and illness. Chapter 17 features a detailed discussion on the biochemical analysis tools used in this new field and the finding of several food-based molecules that appear to have anticancer activities in cell cultures. Chapter 17 contains 55 references.

Chapter 18, a clinically relevant chapter, reviews the current nutritional procedures to ensure patient recovery from surgery. Both presurgical nutrition and enhanced recovery after surgery (ERAS) protocols are reviewed. Chapter 18 focuses on the guidelines and surgery types that are most impactful on patient nutritional status. Additionally, it provides guidelines for assessing whether patients are malnourished prior to surgery and recommends that the baseline nutritional status be improved preoperatively through nutrition supplementation. The protocols for surgeries that affect the oral cavity, esophagus, and stomach are described. Chapter 18 reports that ERAS has developed 27 protocols. Immunonutrition for avoiding infection and improving recovery is also described. Two major manufacturers of immunonutrition products are used in the hospital setting, including the IMPACT enteral immunonutrition formula from Nestlé and the Abbott formula for the Ensure Surgery Immunonutrition Shake. Both companies offer oral and enteral nutrition formulations of their immunonutrition products. Chapter 18 contains informative tables and figures and 53 references. Chapter 19, also a highly clinically based chapter, provides a concise overview of enteral and parenteral nutrition in clinical and public health settings. It features a discussion of the types of enteral feeding methods, including nasogastric, nasojejunal, and percutaneous endoscopic gastrostomy (PEG) tubes. The indications for enteral nutrition, such as dysphagia, are enumerated. An analysis of enteral feeding formulas and common complications associated with enteral feeding are reviewed. Parenteral nutrition requirements and examples of nutritional compositions are also included in this comprehensive chapter. Chapter 19 has several helpful tables and 11 references.

The above description of the volume's 19 chapters attests to the depth of information provided by the widely recognized and well-respected editors and chapter authors. Each chapter includes complete definitions of terms with the abbreviations fully defined for the reader and the consistent use of terms between chapters. Key features of the comprehensive volume include detailed tables and informative figures, an extensive, detailed index and up-to-date references that provide the reader with excellent sources of worthwhile information. Each chapter includes an abstract, keywords, learning objectives, and review questions and answers.

In conclusion, *Essentials of Clinical and Public Health Nutrition*, edited by Amal K. Mitra and Divya Vanoh, provides health professionals in many areas of research and practice with up-to-date, well-referenced sources on the importance of nutrition and healthy food sources for the maintenance of overall health and reducing disease risk. This volume will serve the reader as the benchmark in this complex area of interrelationships between individual dietary intake and public health measures for population well-being. The editors are applauded for their efforts in developing the most authoritative and unique resource on clinical medicine, novel nutritional research areas, and public health innovations. This excellent text is a very welcome addition to the Nutrition and Health Series.

Adrianne Bendich

Contents

Editors and Contributors

About the Editors

Amal K. Mitra is an internationally recognized scientist and leader in public health, with over 40 years of research and 28 years of teaching experience. He currently serves as a professor of the Department of Public Health at the Julia Jones Matthews School *of* Population *and* Public Health at Texas Tech University Health Sciences Center (TTUHSC) in Abilene, Texas.

Dr. Mitra has held professorial positions in epidemiology and biostatistics at several prestigious institutions, including the University of Southern Mississippi, Kuwait University, and Jackson State University. His scholarly contributions are extensive, comprising more than 120 publications, including two seminal books on epidemiology. His doctoral research focused on the mechanism of vitamin A loss in urine during acute infections, with groundbreaking results published in leading journals such as the *Lancet* and the *American Journal of Clinical Nutrition*. Early in his public health nutrition research, Dr. Mitra received the Young Scientist Award from the American Society for Nutrition in 1997.

Throughout his distinguished career, Dr. Mitra has been recognized with numerous prestigious awards, including the John Snow Award (2024) from the American Public Health Association, the US Fulbright-Nehru Academic and Professional Excellence Award (2022–2023), a Lifetime Achievement Award (2013) from the University of Southern Mississippi, Mississippi's Health Care Hero (2011), and the U.S. Fulbright Scholar Award (2007–2008), among many others.

Dr. Mitra has secured significant research funding from leading organizations, including the National Institutes of Health (NIH), the Centers for Disease Control and Prevention (CDC), the Environmental Protection Agency (EPA), the World Health Organization (WHO), and UNICEF. A dedicated mentor, he has guided numerous graduate students in public health research, both domestically and internationally.

Divya Vanoh joined as a lecturer of the Dietetics Program, School of Health Sciences at the Universiti Sains Malaysia (USM) in 2018. Currently, she is the chair of the Dietetics Program at USM.

Dr. Vanoh teaches nutrition-related subjects such as dietetic skills, medical nutrition therapy, therapeutic diet preparation, nutrition and disease, the clinical dietetic practicum, and the community dietetic practicum. She is actively conducting research in the field of geriatric nutrition, focusing on sarcopenia, frailty, cognitive function, dietary patterns, and diet quality. Dr. Divya has developed a screening tool known as TUA-WELLNESS for screening the risk of mild cognitive impairment. This is a simple tool with 10 short questions that are able to predict the risk of memory impairment among older people. She has developed a health information system known as WESIHAT 2.0, which consists of various recommendations for lowering the risk of memory impairment, healthy but simple recipes that can be prepared by older adults, and shopping tips. This is a web-based application that can be used by a large group of older adults in Malaysia. Currently, WESIHAT 2.0 has been used in various research involving older adults and has been translated into languages other than Malay to reach a wider community of older adults.

Dr. Divya is a registered dietitian who is involved in managing pediatric patients with feeding issues at the USM Specialist Hospital. She is also a visiting lecturer in the Faculty of Medicine and Faculty of Public Health, Universitas Andalas in Padang, Indonesia. She has also been appointed to one of the technical working group committees for establishing the Malaysian Dietary Guideline for Older Persons by the Ministry of Health Malaysia.

About the Contributors

Harit Agroia is an adjunct professor of public health at San Jose State University, where she teaches public health courses to undergraduate and graduate students. Having more than a decade of experience in higher education and government health agencies, her research focuses on food and nutrition, including the laws governing food labeling, maternal and child nutrition, and digitalization in agricultural practices. In 2024, she earned an International Award for Excellence in Research and Practice at the International Conference on Business Innovation and Technology Start-ups. In 2023, she was awarded the International Award for Excellence alongside her coauthors for their contributions to the *International Journal for Health, Wellness, and Society*.

Madiha Ajaz has over five years of clinical experience and has spent around two years as a lecturer. Currently pursuing a PhD at Griffith University, she is actively contributing to academic leadership as an Habilitation to Supervise Research (HDR) and as a Health Group Board member. Additionally, she is serving as a Board of Studies member at Ziauddin University, shaping the future of nutrition education.

Misbah Ajaz is currently working as a lecturer at the College of Human Nutrition and Dietetics, Ziauddin University, Karachi, Pakistan. She is working over 8 years as a dietitian in tertiary care hospitals. She holds a bachelor of science in nutrition and dietetics and a master of science in public health, specializing in nutritional sciences. Her research interests focus on maternal and child nutrition and dietary practices and on their effects on health outcomes.

Sanowber Ajaz is a PhD researcher in the Nutrition and Aging Lab at the University of Waterloo. Her research focuses on nutrition risk assessment and intervention among South Asian immigrants, with a particular interest in older individuals with dementia and their caregivers. As a registered dietitian and a former lecturer, she aims to bridge cultural gaps in nutrition care for aging populations.

Mohammad Altamimi has been an associate professor at An-Najah National University, Nablus, Palestine, since 2013. He teaches food science, food microbiology, food biotechnology, functional food, food safety, general microbiology, and food preservation. His research interests include functional foods and the effect of bioactive ingredients of food on health and disease. More specifically, his research investigates the production of probiotics and prebiotics, gut models, microorganism and cell-line interactions, dietary patternss and gut microbiota.

Minoo Bagheri is an assistant professor of precision nutrition in the Department of Biomedical Informatics, Division of Cardiovascular Medicine, Vanderbilt University Medical Center. Her background is in nutritional epidemiology and big data analysis. During her graduate training at the Tehran University of Medical Sciences and the Harvard School of Public Health, she gained extensive experience in the identification of metabolomic biomarkers of diet and diseases.

Anna Dysart is a registered dietitian and an assistant professor of nutrition and dietetics at Western Carolina University. As a dietitian, she specializes in gerontology and metabolic support. Additionally, she earned the Virginia Cooperative Extension State Excellence Award in 2021 for her work in community health.

Francesca De Filippis is an associate professor of microbiology at the University of Naples Federico II, Italy, Department of Agricultural Sciences. She is an expert in bacterial metagenomic analysis, with a special interest in gut microbiota. More specifically, she studies the effects of diet and lifestyles on gut microbiota. In addition, she was listed as the world's top scientist in 2019 on the basis of the PLoS Biology ranking, with an h-index of 46.

Aliyar Cyrus Fouladkhah is a graduate of the Yale School of Public Health with a degree in applied biostatistics and epidemiology and has a graduate certification in food and drug regulatory affairs and a certificate in climate change and human health. He is currently a tenured associate professor at Tennessee State University and the founding director of the Public Health Microbiology Foundation in Nashville. He is the recipient of the 2024 Catherine Cowel Award from the Food and Nutrition Section of the American Public Health Association.

Tahniyah Haq is an associate professor in the Department of Endocrinology at Bangabandhu Sheikh Mujib Medical University (BSMMU), Dhaka, Bangladesh. She also serves as an assistant editor for the *BSMMU Journal* and is a working group member for the development of the National Diabetes Guideline under the Noncommunicable Disease (NCD) Control Program, Directorate General of Health. Additionally, she coordinates the Obesity Task Force of the Bangladesh Endocrine Society, contributing to national efforts in endocrinology and metabolic health.

Holly Huye is a registered dietitian and professor in the School of Kinesiology and Nutrition at the University of Southern Mississippi. She teaches undergraduate courses in service-learning as well as graduate courses. Dr. Huye's research focuses on community engagement, and she was awarded the 2025 Outstanding Faculty Contributions to Service-Learning in Higher Education for Research by the Gulf-South Summit on Service-Learning and Civic Engagement through Higher Education.

Ayah Ibrahim is the head of nutritionists at Nablus Speciality Hospital with a master's degree in nutrition and food technology from An-Najah National University, Palestine. Her research interest is in clinical nutrition, focusing on the role of diet in disease prevention and management. Her research explores the impact of medical nutrition therapy on patient outcomes, the relationship between dietary patterns and chronic diseases, and the integration of evidence-based nutrition practices in healthcare settings.

Santhia Ireen is a public health nutrition expert with research and program experiences in public health nutrition interventions and development programs. Currently, she is working as the deputy director of education and research at the BRAC James P. Grant School of Public Health, BRAC University, Bangladesh. Her areas of expertise are child nutrition with a focus on micronutrient research, infant and young child feeding, health system strengthening, social and behavioral change, and implementation research.

Mohammad Jahidul Islam is a distinguished teacher, investigator, and pharmacologist with a strong academic and clinical background, with which Dr. Islam serves as a medical instructor and a researcher in drug development and cancer pharmacology.

Kamyar Kalantar-Zadeh is a professor of medicine and epidemiology at the University of California–Los Angeles (UCLA). He was trained at the State University of New York–Brooklyn and the University of California–San Francisco (UCSF) medical schools and is triple board certified and recertified in internal medicine, nephrology, and pediatrics and a United Network for Organ Sharing (UNOS)–certified transplant physician. Dr. Kalantar has authored more than 1100 peer-reviewed papers and has led numerous NIH and VA–funded studies in chronic kidney disease (CKD), dialysis, and transplanted patients. He serves as

Harbor-UCLA Nephrology chief and medicine vice chair for research and innovation and as the chair of the Los Angeles County Kidney Health Workgroup. He has been named among the nation's top physicians by several US best doctors lists. Dr. Kalantar is the president of the National Forum of ESRD Networks.

Fatin Hanani Mazri is a senior lecturer in the Dietetics Program and a researcher at the Center for Healthy Ageing & Wellness (H-CARE), Faculty of Health Sciences, Universiti Kebangsaan Malaysia. Her research interests include chrononutrition, sleep, chronobiology, obesity, and weight management. She is actively involved in research exploring the relationship between chrononutrition and sleep across diverse populations.

Erin M. McKinley is the current director of dietetics and graduate studies in nutrition and food science and an associate professor at Louisiana State University. She has been a dietitian since 2013 and is also a certified lactation counselor and master certified health education specialist. She received her master of science in food and nutrition and her PhD in health education and health promotion from the University of Alabama. Her research focuses on survey instrument development in various areas, including infant feeding, medicinal plant supplements, and higher education quality improvement elements.

Amal K. Mitra is a professor of the Department of Public Health at Julia Jones Matthews School *of* Population *and* Public Health, Texas Tech University Health Sciences Center in Abilene, Texas. He is the author of two epidemiology books, namely *Statistical Approaches for Epidemiology: From Concept to Application* (Springer Nature 2024) and *Epidemiology for Dummies* (Wiley 2023). He has published more than 120 peer-reviewed research articles. He was the recipient of the prestigious John Snow Award in 2024 from the epidemiology section of American Public Health Association, the Fulbright-Nehru Academic and Professional Excellence Award in 2022–2023 (India), and the U.S. Fulbright Scholar Award in 2007–2008 (Bangladesh), among many others. His current research interests include cancer, the mental health of adolescents, and micronutrients.

Malay Kanti Mridha is a professor at the BRAC James P. Grant School of Public Health, BRAC University. He is also the founding director of a research center for excellence in noncommunicable diseases and nutrition research in Bangladesh. His research interests include public health nutrition, nutritional and noncommunicable disease epidemiology, and implementation research. He is an internationally recognized scientist in public health nutrition and noncommunicable diseases.

Mogana Das Murtey is a senior lecturer at the School of Dental Sciences, Universiti Sains Malaysia (USM), specializing in cancer biology. His research focuses on natural product–based therapies, particularly the anticancer effects of paddy husk extracts. He has secured multiple research grants and published extensively in high-impact journals and book chapters. Dr. Mogana has received several awards, including gold medals at international exhibitions, for his innovative research. He is actively involved in postgraduate supervision, journal reviewing, and academic consultancy. He is a fellow of the Royal Microscopy Society (UK) and a member of multiple professional organizations.

Kritee Niroula holds a PhD in human nutrition from Louisiana State University and is currently a postdoctoral researcher at the Institute for Collaboration on Health, Intervention, and Policy (INCHIP) at the University of Connecticut. Her research focuses on the food environment and its impact on food insecurity, exploring how access to nutritious food influences public health outcomes. With a passion for understanding the intersection between community health and nutrition, she aims to contribute valuable insights that will promote healthier, more-equitable food systems. She is dedicated to advancing research that can inform policy and improve food security for underserved populations.

Melissa D. Porter is a senior resident at Meharry Medical College in the Pediatric Dentistry Program, where she is passionate about enhancing preventive dental education to reduce the prevalence of oral diseases among pediatric populations. She completed her postgraduate training at Meharry Medical College, where she earned a master's degree in science and a doctorate in dental surgery, in addition to general practice residency. With nearly a decade of experience serving underrepresented populations, she has received numerous accolades. Dr. Porter has a special interest in promoting preventive care, merging dental public health and pediatric dentistry as well as educating future pediatric dentists.

Nila Pradhananga is a PhD candidate in human nutrition at the School of Nutrition and Food Sciences, Louisiana State University. She worked as a clinical nutrition staff member at Baptist Health South Florida prior this position. Nila is trained in nutrition and has experience in extension related fieldwork in Louisiana with research interests in understanding the influence of healthy eating and active living policies on the environment. As a graduate research assistant, she has worked in mixed methods and implementation science projects to inform policy, systems, and environmental change strategies to improve public health.

Sabuktagin Rahman is an associate professor at the American International University–Bangladesh. His areas of interest include micronutrients, anemia, dietary assessment, and child and maternal nutrition. His research led to the development of the National Micronutrient Deficiency Control Strategy of Bangladesh.

Desiree Ratcliffe registered dietitian-nutritionist, works as an instructor at the School of Kinesiology and Nutrition at the University of Southern Mississippi (USM), teaching medical nutrition therapy, food service management, and community nutrition courses and as a consultant dietitian for Diet with Desi, LLC. She is also an instructor and proctor for the National Restaurant Association's ServSafe food protection program. In 2023, Mrs. Ratcliffe was chosen as USM's Outstanding Visiting Faculty for the College of Education and Human Sciences.

Nurul Fatin Malek Rivan is a senior lecturer in the Nutritional Science Program and a researcher at the Center for Healthy Ageing & Wellness (H-CARE), Faculty of Health Sciences, Universiti Kebangsaan Malaysia. Her expertise includes nutritional neuroscience, frailty, mild cognitive impairment, cognitive frailty, salt taste perception, and sarcopenia. She is actively involved in research on healthy aging and cognitive health. Dr. Nurul Fatin has contributed to various academic and community-based initiatives to promote well-being among older adults.

Jylana L. Sheats is a public health scholar and behavioral scientist specializing in food-related behaviors, food insecurity, and citizen science to improve food access in underserved communities. She is a clinical associate professor at the Tulane University Celia Scott Weatherhead School of Public Health and Tropical Medicine. A former civic science fellow (2021–2023) with the Aspen Institute's Science & Society Program, she received the Tony A. Mobley International Distinguished Alumni Award from Indiana University Bloomington's School of Public Health and a 2016 National Institutes of Health Building Interdisciplinary Research Careers in Women's Health Career Development Award. Sheats works across sectors to bridge public health, science, and community-based approaches. Her research informs strategies to improve health behaviors and advance health outcomes.

Ekamol Tantisattamo is a transplant nephrologist and associate clinical professor of medicine at the Division of Nephrology, Hypertension and Kidney Transplantation, Department of Medicine, University of California Irvine School of Medicine in Orange County, California, United States. He is a founder and director of the American Heart Association Comprehensive Hypertension Center at the University of California Irvine Medical Center. In 2021, he was inducted into the Delta Omega Public Health Honorary Society, Alpha Chapter, Johns Hopkins University Bloomberg School of Public Health.

Kehinde Tom-Ayegunle is a clinical trial research associate at the Johns Hopkins School of Public Health, Baltimore, MD, USA. His research focuses on cardiovascular medicine, clinical trials in neuroscience devices, and quantitative epidemiological research in health disparities. He holds a doctor of medicine (honors) from People's Friendship University, Russia (2020), and a master's in public health in quantitative epidemiology and biostatistics (honors) from Johns Hopkins University (2024). A recipient of the Delta Omega Award and the African Impactful Leadership Award (2024), he has also won multiple Best Scientific Report awards at Science4Health Conferences. He serves as a data analyst, clinical trial researcher, and scientific reviewer for the American Heart Association.

Divya Vanoh is the chair of the Dietetics Program at Universiti Sains Malaysia. Her research interests are sarcopenia, frailty, cognitive impairment, and geriatrics nutrition. She developed a screening tool for memory impairment known as TUA-WELLNESS. Following that, she developed a health information system, WESIHAT 2.0, for educating older adults on strategies to lower their risk of memory impairment. Dr. Divya is on one of the technical working group committees for establishing the Malaysian Dietary Guideline for Older Person.

Jody L. Vogelzang works as the editor-in-chief for the journal *Hunger and Environmental Nutrition*, published by Taylor & Francis. Vogelzang has been bestowed the Medallion Award from the Academy of Nutrition and Dietetics for her service to the profession and has also received national awards for her work in public health nutrition by both the academy and the American Public Health Association.

Teresa Walker-Cartwright with 20 years of experience as a registered dietitian, Teresa Walker-Cartwright is a senior lecturer at the School of Kinesiology and Nutrition, University of Southern Mississippi. She teaches medical nutrition therapy, communication techniques, life-cycle nutrition, and food preparation and management courses. Mrs. Cartwright was named an outstanding educator twice in the past 10 years by the Mississippi Academy of Nutrition and Dietetics.

Elizabeth Wall-Bassett is a professor of nutrition and dietetics in the School of Health Sciences at Western Carolina University. She has continually assembled and integrated public and private resources to assess disease risk, nutritional status, and the nutrition needs of various populations to mitigate food insecurity and contribute to policy and program decisions that benefit society. Elizabeth has been recognized through numerous community engagement awards and presented and published with interdisciplinary teams around food issues throughout her career.

Contributors

Harit Agroia San Jose State University, San Jose, CA, USA

Madiha Ajaz School of Pharmacy and Medical Sciences, Griffith University, Gold Coast, QLD, Australia

Misbah Ajaz College of Human Nutrition and Dietetics – Allied Health Sciences, Ziauddin University, Karachi, Pakistan

Sanowber Ajaz Nutrition and Aging Lab, University of Waterloo, Ontario, Canada

Mohammad Altamimi Department of Nutrition and Food Technology, Faculty of Veterinary Medicine and Agriculture Engineering, An-Najah National University, Nablus, Palestine

Minoo Bagheri Department of Biomedical Informatics, Precision Nutrition Laboratory, Vanderbilt University Medical Center, Nashville, TN, USA

Anna Dysart Western Carolina University, Cullowhee, NC, USA

Francesca De Filippis Division of Microbiology, Department of Agricultural Sciences, University of Naples Federico II, Portici, NA, Italy

Aliyar Cyrus Fouladkhah Public Health Microbiology Laboratory, Tennessee State University, Nashville, TN, USA

Public Health Microbiology Foundation, Franklin, TN, USA

Tahniyah Haq Department of Endocrinology, Bangladesh Medical University, Dhaka, Bangladesh

Holly Huye School of Kinesiology and Nutrition, The University of Southern Mississippi, Hattiesburg, MS, USA

Ayah Ibrahim Department of Nutrition and Food Technology, Faculty of Veterinary Medicine and Agriculture Engineering, An-Najah National University, Nablus, Palestine

Santhia Ireen James P. Grant School of Public Health, Brac University, Dhaka, Bangladesh

Mohammad Jahidul Islam Department of Pharmacology, Faculty of Basic Science and Para Clinical Science, Bangbandhu Sheikh Mujib Medical University (BSMMU), Dhaka, Bangladesh

Kamyar Kalantar-Zadeh American Heart Association Comprehensive Hypertension Center at the University of California Irvine Medical Center, Division of Nephrology, Hypertension and Kidney Transplantation, Department of Medicine, University of California Irvine School of Medicine, Orange, CA, USA

Nephrology Section, Department of Medicine, Tibor Rubin Veterans Affairs Medical Center, Veterans Affairs Long Beach Healthcare System, Long Beach, CA, USA

Lundquist Biomedical Research Institute at Harbor-UCLA Medical Center, Torrance, CA, USA

Fatin Hanani Mazri Dietetics Programme and Centre for Healthy Ageing and Wellness (H-CARE), Faculty of Health Sciences, Universiti Kebangsaan Malaysia, Jalan Raja Muda Abdul Aziz, Kuala Lumpur, Malaysia

Erin M. McKinley School of Nutrition & Food Sciences, Louisiana State University, Baton Rouge, LA, USA

Amal K. Mitra Department of Public Health, Julia Jones Matthews School of Population and Public Health, Texas Tech University Health Sciences Center, Abilene, TX, USA

Malay Kanti Mridha BRAC James P. Grant School of Public Health, BRAC University, Dhaka, Bangladesh

Mogana Das Murtey School of Dental Sciences, Health Campus, Universiti Sains Malaysia, Kubang Kerian, Kelantan, Malaysia

Kritee Niroula Institute for Collaboration on Health, Intervention, and Policy (InCHIP), University of Connecticut, Storrs, CT, USA

Melissa D. Porter Meharry Medical College, Department of Pediatric Dentistry, Nashville, TN, USA

Nila Pradhananga Department of Nutritional Sciences, College of Education and Human Sciences, Oklahoma State University, Stillwater, OK, USA

Sabuktagin Rahman Department of Public Health, Faculty of Arts and Social Sciences, American International University-Bangladesh, Dhaka, Bangladesh

Desiree Ratcliffe School of Kinesiology and Nutrition, The University of Southern Mississippi, Hattiesburg, MS, USA

Nurul Fatin Malek Rivan Nutritional Sciences Programme and Centre for Healthy Ageing and Wellness (H-CARE), Faculty of Health Sciences, Universiti Kebangsaan Malaysia, Jalan Raja Muda Abdul Aziz, Kuala Lumpur, Malaysia

Jylana L. Sheats Tulane University Celia Scott Weatherhead School of Public Health & Tropical Medicine, New Orleans, LA, USA

Ekamol Tantisattamo American Heart Association Comprehensive Hypertension Center at the University of California Irvine Medical Center, Division of Nephrology, Hypertension and Kidney Transplantation, Department of Medicine, University of California Irvine School of Medicine, Orange, CA, USA

Nephrology Section, Department of Medicine, Tibor Rubin Veterans Affairs Medical Center, Veterans Affairs Long Beach Healthcare System, Long Beach, CA, USA

Multi-Organ Transplant Center, Section of Nephrology, Department of Internal Medicine, Corewell Health William Beaumont University Hospital, Oakland University William Beaumont School of Medicine, Royal Oak, MI, USA

Pacific Northwest University of Health Sciences, Yakima, WA, USA

Excellent Center for Organ Transplantation, Faculty of Medicine Ramathibodi Hospital, Mahidol University, Bangkok, Thailand

Kehinde Tom-Ayegunle Department of Epidemiology & Biostatistics, Bloomberg School of Public Health, Johns Hopkins University, Baltimore, MD, USA

Divya Vanoh Dietetics Programme, School of Health Sciences, Universiti Sains Malaysia, Kubang Kerian, Kelantan, Malaysia

Jody L. Vogelzang Grand Valley State University, Allendale, MI, USA

Teresa Walker-Cartwright School of Kinesiology and Nutrition, The University of Southern Mississippi, Hattiesburg, MS, USA

Elizabeth Wall-Bassett Western Carolina University, School of Health Science, Nutrition and Dietetics Program, Cullowhee, NC, USA

Abbreviations

ADA	American Diabetes Association
ADL	Activities of daily living
AHA	American Heart Association
AI	Adequate intake
AKF	American Kidney Fund
ARDS	Acute respiratory distress syndrome
ASN	American Society of Nephrology
AST	American Society of Transplantation
AWGS	Asian Working Group for Sarcopenia
BATB	Breakfast after the Bell
BIC	Breakfast in the Classroom
BMI	Body mass index
CACFP	Child and Adult Care Food Program
CDC	Centers for Disease Control and Prevention
CE-MS	Capillary electrophoresis-mass spectrometry
CHO	Carbohydrate
CHW	Community health workers
CKD	Chronic kidney disease
CMS	Centers for Medicare and Medicaid Services
CNCD	Chronic noncommunicable diseases
CSFP	Commodity Supplemental Food Program
DASH	Dietary Approach to Stop Hypertension
DGA	Dietary guidelines for Americans
DM	Diabetes mellitus
DOHaD	Developmental Origins of Health and Disease
DXA	Dual energy X-ray absorptiometry
EAA	Essential amino acid
EGCG	Epigallocathechin-3-gallate
eGFR	Estimated glomerular filtration rate
EN	Enteral nutrition
ERAS	Enhanced recovery after surgery
ERIC	Expert Recommendations for Implementing Change
ESKD	End stage kidney disease
ESRD	End-state renal disease

EVOO	Extra virgin olive oil
EWGSOP	European Working Group on Sarcopenia in Older People
FDA	US Food and Drug Administration
FDPIR	Food Distribution Program on Indian Reservations
FFA	Free fatty acid
FFQ	Food Frequency Questionnaire
FMLFPP	Farmers Market and Local Food Promotion Program
FNIH	Foundation for the National Institutes of Health
FOP	Front of pack
GAD	Glutamic acid decarboxylase
GC-MS	Gas chromatography–mass spectrometry
GCNF	Global Child Nutrition Foundation
GDA	Guideline daily amounts
GDM	Gestational diabetes mellitus
GI	Gastrointestinal tract
GI	Glycemic index
HDL	High density lipoprotein
HEI	Healthy eating index
HFFI	Healthy Food Financing Initiative
HHFK	Healthy Hunger-Free Kids Act
HHS	Health and human services
HMP	Human microbiome project
HPA	Hypothalamic pituitary adrenal
IADPSG	International Association of Diabetes and Pregnancy Study Groups
IBD	Inflammatory bowel disease
ICDDR,B	International Center for Diarrheal Disease Research, Bangladesh
IDA	Iron-deficiency anemia
IDDSI	International Dysphagia Diet Standardization Initiative
IDF	International Diabetic Federation
IGF-1	Insulin-like growth factor 1
IGT	Impaired glucose tolerance
IFG	Impaired fasting glucose
IH	Intermediate hyperglycemia
INCHIP	Institute for Collaboration on Health, Intervention, and Policy
INEP	Integrative Nutrition Education Program
IPM	Integrated pest management
IRLM	Implementation Research Logic Model
ISDA	Infectious Diseases Society of America
IUGR	Intrauterine growth retardation
KHD	Kidney healthy diet
LBW	Low birth weight
LC-MS	Liquid chromatography–mass spectrometry
LDL	Low-density lipoprotein

LPL	Lipoprotein lipase
MET	Metabolic equivalent of task
MNT	Medical nutrition therapy
MSG	Monosodium glutamate
NAFLD	Non-alcoholic fatty liver disease
NEAA	Nonessential amino acids
NEC	Necrotizing enterocolitis
NG	Nasogastric tube
NHLBI	National Heart, Lung, and Blood Institute
NIH	National Institutes of Health
NKF	National Kidney Foundation
NMR	Nuclear magnetic resonance
NSBP	National School Breakfast Program
NSL	No-school lunches
NSLP	National School Lunch Program
OBS	Oxidative balance score
OUT	Operational taxonomic unit
PAI-1	Plasminogen activator inhibitor 1
PBMA	Plant-based milk alternatives
PEG	Percutaneous endoscopic gastrostomy
PEJ	Percutaneous endoscopic jejunostomy
PEM	Protein energy malnutrition
PICC	Peripherally inserted central catheter
PKT	Patient with kidney diseases and transplantation
PLADO	Plant-dominant low-protein diet
PN	Parenteral nutrition
PSD	Post-stroke dysphagia
RAE	Retinol activity equivalent
RDA	Recommended dietary allowance
RDN	Registered dietitian-nutritionist
RE-AIM	Reach, Effectiveness, Adoption, Implementation, and Maintenance
SCN	Suprachiasmatic nucleus
SDG	Sustainable Development Goals
SDOH	Social determinants of health
SFMNP	Senior Farmers' Market Nutrition Program
SFSP	Summer Food Service Program
SKL	Skipping lunch
SMI	Skeletal muscle index
SNAP	Supplemental Nutrition Assistance Program
SOI	Standards of identity
SPPB	Short physical performance battery
SUN	Scaling Up Nutrition
TEFAP	The Emergency Food Assistance Program

TNF-α	Tumor necrosis factor-α
UCLA	University of California - Los Angeles
UCSF	University of California - San Francisco
UNOS	United Network for Organ Sharing
UPF	Ultra-processed food
USDA	United States Department of Agriculture
UTI	Urinary tract infection
VLBW	Very low birth weight
VLCKD	Very-low-carbohydrate ketogenic diet
WHO	World Health Organization
WIC	Women, infants, and children

Part I

Clinical Nutrition

Gut Harmony: Nourishing the Microbiome for Optimal Health and Well-being

1

Mohammad Altamimi, Ayah Ibrahim, and Francesca De Filippis

Learning Objectives

After completing this chapter, you will be able to

- Understand the role of different microbial communities in the gut in health and disease
- Comprehend the importance of microbial diversity in the gut
- Compare the different therapies for gut dysbiosis
- Apply personalized nutrition on the basis of the gut microbiome

Introduction

Most gut microorganisms are either harmless or helpful to the host. The gut microbiota (GM) aids in appropriate immunological function, in shielding against enteropathogens, and in harvesting minerals and energy from our food. Dysbiosis, a disturbance of the typical equilibrium in the host's gut microbiome, is widely believed to be linked to several diseases, including neurological conditions, cancer, obesity, and inflammatory bowel disease (IBD) [1–3]. Therefore, understanding how the gut microbiota interacts with the host and contributes to metabolic activities remains complex.

M. Altamimi (✉) · A. Ibrahim
Department of Nutrition and Food Technology, Faculty of Veterinary Medicine and
Agriculture Engineering, An-Najah National University, Nablus, Palestine
e-mail: m.altamimi@najah.edu

F. De Filippis
Division of Microbiology, Department of Agricultural Sciences, University of Naples
Federico II, Portici, NA, Italy

© The Author(s), under exclusive license to Springer Nature
Switzerland AG 2025
A. K. Mitra, D. Vanoh (eds.), *Essentials of Clinical and Public Health Nutrition*,
Nutrition and Health, https://doi.org/10.1007/978-3-031-95373-6_1

3

Characterizing the fundamentally healthy microbiota and any variations linked to illness is the first step toward comprehending the symbiotic interactions that gut bacteria have with their hosts. Significant advancements have been achieved by large-scale initiatives, such as the Human Microbiome Project (HMP) and the metagenomics of the human intestinal tract (in short, MetaHIT). Once the intended functional and compositional aspects of the gut microbiota have been understood, we can identify the characteristics of various microbiota that are supposedly linked to illnesses. Nevertheless, the intricacy of the microbiota, together with intra- and inter-individual diversity, presents a challenge to defining the "desired" condition for a particular group or individual [3, 4].

Microbial Diversity: The Key Player

Taxonomic Diversity

Research using culture-dependent techniques suggests that most gut bacterial species are shared among all healthy individuals, forming a core microbiota. However, this concept has been consistently challenged by the results of culture-independent sequencing experiments, which have revealed a vast microbial diversity that varies significantly over time and among human populations. Each population is estimated to harbor more than 1000 species-level phylotypes, which are groups of sequences displaying similar diversity in their small subunit rRNA genes to those observed in formally classified species. Most of these phylotypes belong to only a few phyla. Among them, Bacteroidetes (which exhibit proinflammatory properties) and Firmicutes (which exhibit anti-inflammatory effects) often predominate. Meanwhile, Actinobacteria, Proteobacteria, and Verrucomicrobia represent minor components of microbiota in adults [2, 3, 5].

Gut health relies on the diversity of the microbiome. Through the process of microbiological repair and rehabilitation, gut health solutions aim to restore normal gut function by limiting the growth of harmful bacteria and forming a protective barrier in the gut with beneficial microorganisms. The Firmicutes, a major bacterial family in the gut that is primarily Gram-positive, can become overly abundant when dysbiosis occurs. Although this group includes many beneficial bacteria, such as Lactobacillus and Clostridium species, an excessive growth of beneficial bacteria can be harmful. A common consequence of this imbalance is increased intestinal permeability, often referred to as "leaky gut," which allows toxic compounds to enter the bloodstream and trigger immune responses. Therapeutic approaches to dysbiosis focus on introducing beneficial microorganisms into the gut lining to create a protective barrier and restore microbial balance. Because a healthy microbiome is essential for immune function, digestion, and even mental health, its restoration is critical for maintaining overall health [2, 5].

Methanogenic archaea (primarily *Methanobrevibacter smithii*), eukarya (mainly yeasts), and viruses (particularly bacteriophages), are also components of the human gut microbiome. Although these key elements are consistently present, the specific species and their relative abundances vary significantly between individuals. Efforts to identify a core set of species-level phylotypes in the adult gut microbiota have highlighted several "major players," including *Bacteroides uniformis*, *Roseburia intestinalis*, and *Faecalibacterium prausnitzii*. However, these species can have relative abundances of less than 0.5% in some individuals. The notion of a core group of common species in the human gut microbiota has been further challenged by research that includes populations from underdeveloped nations and spans a wide age range—from infancy to the ninth and tenth decades of life [5].

Functional Diversity

Understanding the function of a microbial community is not always possible when based solely on its composition. Functional insights can be gained through the study of cultivated isolates with well-characterized genomes and ex vivo behaviors, as well as community DNA sequencing. Shotgun metagenomics enables functional screening by sequencing DNA from an entire microbial community, including uncultured species, and comparing these sequences to databases of known functional genes [2, 3]. Although functional capacities can be predicted by identifying genes involved in specific metabolic pathways, these predictions are based largely on conjecture rather than direct evidence from mRNA, protein, or metabolite profiling. However, as more human gut microbial genomes are sequenced and annotated and as additional supplementary "omics" datasets become available, the accuracy of this reference-mapping process continues to improve [1, 3, 6].

Functionality gene patterns are quite comparable among people, even though their gut microbiome compositions range greatly. This concept was initially seen in 18 women who shared > 93% of functional groups at the "enzyme" level but few phylotypes at the "genus" level. The HMP and MetaHIT validated this finding in considerably larger populations. The metabolism of carbohydrates and amino acids and other key metabolic pathways found in the gut are among the primary roles played by the gut microbiota. But not every route is represented in the core, and putting genes into broad functional categories might also mask important changes in function across individuals that happen at smaller scales. Variable activities that are specific to a species or strain, including motility, nutrient transporters, and vitamin and drug catabolism, which are pathogenicity islands, are interesting targets for customized diets and treatment approaches [6, 7].

Certain circumstances are necessary for the expression of many genes. Measurements of mRNA levels (known as "metatranscriptomics") or proteomics (known as "metaproteomics") using shotgun sequencing techniques may reveal functional variation associated with illness, nutrition, or other variables that are missed by DNA investigations. For instance, larger levels of protein expression than expected from metagenome data were seen for genes involved in energy production and glucose metabolism, indicating the importance of these activities in the gut [6, 7].

Studies on the core microbiome have generally shown that although we humans do not share a core microbiota, we do share a functional core microbiome. This concept can be illustrated with an analogy to macroecosystems. For example, although rainforests worldwide exhibit similar functional and visual characteristics, they are composed of distinct species that have evolved independently. A major challenge in ecological studies of the gut is understanding functional redundancy—that is, identifying community members with similar functional roles who can compensate for one another. Although taxonomic gene composition is much more variable than functional gene composition (at least at a general process level), numerous studies have demonstrated a connection between the two [1–3].

High microbial diversity, characterized by many distinct species evenly distributed within the gut microbiome, is crucial for maintaining a robust, healthy gut. This diversity not only aids in digestion and the absorption and synthesis of essential nutrients but also plays a critical role in regulating immune, metabolic, and neurological functions. Consequently, greater diversity in gut flora enhances their ability to support these vital processes [1]. The gut microbiota is continuously exposed to a variety of obstacles during life, such as viruses, harmful diets, drugs, alcohol, and intense physical activity, to mention a few. Reduced capacity to withstand these difficulties or swiftly and completely recover from the prechallenge condition may result in dysbiosis and a new equilibrium, which may hasten the onset of chronic noncommunicable diseases (CNCDs). Human participants treated with antibiotics showed a decreased capacity of their microbiota to return to baseline and create a new equilibrium. Therefore, taking action to keep the microbiota robust might be a way to postpone or stop the emergence of microbiota-related CNCDs [1].

Although limited evidence supports this intriguing concept, a connection between microbial resilience and health has been observed. In a human study, high species richness and strong inter–operational taxonomic unit (OTU) correlations were used as parameters to characterize microbiota resilience. Following ileocolic resection, the researchers found that microbiota resilience was positively correlated with Crohn's disease remission [1].

Microbiota from Infancy to Aging

Genetic makeup, food, exposure to illness and the environment, and life stage all affect the quantity and variety of gut microbiota microorganisms. These elements influence each person's unique microbiota growth from birth [8] (Fig. 1.1). Importantly, though, elements that may cause notable changes in certain populations have not yet been identified. In this sense, the diversity of the microbiome expands during the first few years of life, begins to decline at age three, and then stabilizes at age five (attaching the gut microbiota complexity observed in adults). However, the gut microbiota composition will be affected as people age because it loses diversity and abundance. On the other hand, a decreased Bacteroides population and decreased microbial abundance have been linked to elevated survival chances [9, 10].

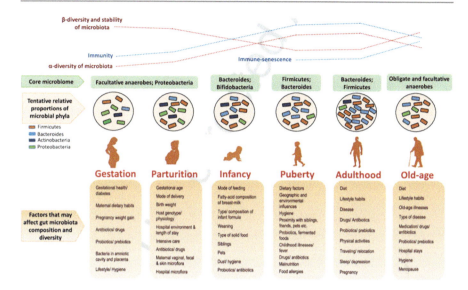

Fig. 1.1 Microbiota from infancy to aging [12]

Strangely, the gut microbiota of preterm infants who were fed with formula milk and delivered via cesarean section has been shown to be more likely to develop obesity, necrotizing enterocolitis, and other illnesses. This is most likely because of the nature of gut microbiota that interacts with the immune system and energy metabolism [8]. An individual's eating pattern during infancy and adulthood influences the composition and traits of genetically modified organisms (GMOs). People have developed obesogenic lifestyles since industrialization, which has affected gut microbiota composition. For example, compared to their lean and overweight counterparts, individuals who are obese have a higher rate of Firmicute than Bacteroidetes. Additionally, research has shown that patients with obesity have larger proportions of Bacteroides, whereas lean individuals have higher proportions of Firmicutes phylum species, such as *Blautia hydrogenotrophic*, *Coprococcus catus*, *Eubacterium ventriosum*, *Ruminococcus bromii*, and *Ruminococcus obeum* [11]. The gut microbiome of adolescents does not yet mirror that of an adult, but it does exhibit a change toward a general decline in the frequency of aerobes and facultative anaerobes, along with concomitant increases in anaerobic species, according to the research [8].

Microbial Therapy

One of the objectives in neonatal practice should be the creation of a healthy gut microbiome, which includes a balanced and diversified population of good bacteria. Protecting the innate microbiota by restricting therapy known to induce changes, like antibiotics, and by promoting therapies known to be beneficial, like breast milk feeding, is one strategy to sustain a healthy bacterial population. Clinical research has shown that the number of days that a newborn receives first empirical antibiotics increases the risk of necrotizing enterocolitis (NEC), whereas the amount of mother's milk given to the newborn as a proportion of all feeds during the first two weeks of life decreases the incidence of NEC [13].

Prebiotics

In the colon of mammals, *prebiotics* are defined as "nondigestible food ingredients that selectively stimulate the growth or activity of anaerobic/microaerophilic flora Bifidobacterium/Lactobacillus." Prebiotics aid in the development of bacteria that are already present in the digestive system rather than adding new organisms to the mix. The most common prebiotics are oligosaccharides, which are found in human milk. Other common prebiotics include lactoferrin and lactalbumin, which are milk proteins that are known as "bifidogenic factors" because they specifically encourage the growth of *Bifidobacteria* [13, 14].

Prebiotics may enhance intestinal motility and stomach-emptying times, which may enhance feeding tolerance in preterm infant populations, according to additional research. Indrio et al. conducted experiments wherein formula-fed infants receiving prebiotics of oligosaccharides showed enhanced motility and stomach-emptying times compared to breastfed infants; these findings were in contrast to formula-fed infants receiving sham treatments. Evidence has shown that prebiotics such as inulin, lactulose, fructo-oligosaccharides, or galacto-oligosaccharides increase the number of *Bifidobacteria* in fecal samples and improve intestinal motility, but no evidence has shown that these prebiotics lower the incidence of NEC or shorten the time required to reach full feeds [13, 14]. Prebiotics provide benefits such as simplifying taking them orally and encouraging the growth of good bacteria that are already in the gastrointestinal system. They are progressively added to baby formulae and are naturally present in human milk. Large evaluations, however, indicate that although prebiotic supplements seem safe in terms of growth and side effects for healthy newborns, routine usage is not advised, due to inadequate data. Additionally, research hasn't definitively demonstrated that prebiotics enhance clinical outcomes or development in premature newborns fed formula [14].

Prebiotic therapy can have gastrointestinal side effects, such as bloating, diarrhea, and flatulence, although these normally go away when the treatment is stopped. Serious side effects have not been associated with prebiotic therapy. Inulin, lactulose, short-chain fructo-oligosaccharides, and galacto-oligosaccharides are examples of prebiotics that have not been thoroughly studied in newborn and preterm patients [13].

> **Box 1.1: Benefits of Prebiotics**
> - Prebiotics, such as oligosaccharides, may improve intestinal motility and stomach emptying in preterm infants, enhancing feeding tolerance.
> - Formula-fed infants receiving prebiotics showed better motility and stomach-emptying times than infants receiving sham treatments or breastfed infants.
> - Prebiotics, including inulin, lactulose, fructo-oligosaccharides, and galacto-oligosaccharides, can increase *Bifidobacteria* in fecal samples and improve intestinal motility but have not been proven to lower the incidence of necrotizing enterocolitis (NEC) or shorten the time to full feeds.

Probiotics

Supplements containing living microorganisms, known as probiotics, have the potential to positively impact the host's microbiome and provide health benefits. Probiotics have the potential to foster a more robust gut microbiota in preterm newborns, who frequently lack certain beneficial microorganisms. Probiotics that are often utilized include lactobacilli and *Bifidobacteria*; they are usually given within the first week of life and kept up for a month or until the patient is released from the neonatal intensive care unit (NICU) [13, 14].

Probiotics work in several ways, including lowering inflammation, strengthening the intestinal barrier, creating bacteriocins, and competing with pathogenic microorganisms. They have been researched for promoting development, facilitating enteral feeding, and treating feeding-related problems in preterm newborns, such as reflux and colic. The ability of probiotics to prevent necrotizing enterocolitis (NEC), a dangerous gastrointestinal ailment with a high morbidity and death rate, is, however, their most important potential advantage in this population [13, 14]. Probiotics can reduce the incidence of severe NEC and death in preterm newborns, according to recent evaluations; however, their efficacy may vary depending on the probiotic administered and the infant's baseline risk of NEC. Probiotics seem to be safe overall and have the potential to prevent NEC and improve outcomes for preterm newborns [13, 14].

The effectiveness and safety of probiotic use throughout the neonatal stage, however, are still up for debate. Studies vary widely in every way, including the probiotic strain(s) used, the dosages given, and the inclusion and exclusion criteria used for enlisting research participants. To assess the safety of probiotic medication concerning potential dangers, such as sepsis, no research has been sufficiently conducted. When the host's defenses are weakened, whether by disease or immunological deficiencies, live probiotic microorganisms have the potential to turn dangerous [13, 14]. Premature newborns are thought to be relatively immunocompromised, and the use of live bacteria in them has been questioned given that research shows higher infant mortality in probiotic-treated animal models. If intestinal maturation is incomplete, even the introduction of "beneficial" probiotic bacteria may have detrimental effects on the infant's gut [13, 14].

No research has tracked long-term results. Probiotics are given to the growing child's microbiome during a period when long-term impacts are probably in store. Given the growing acknowledgment of the microbiome as the basis for immune system development and long-term consequences, any modification of the microbiome must first be understood to determine how it will affect long-term consequences before it can be deemed safe. A population's baseline NEC rate has a significant impact on the benefits of probiotic supplementation. The baseline rate of NEC in the most recent probiotic studies was extremely low, suggesting that the statistical decrease in NEC may not be clinically meaningful or adequate to offset other concerns [13, 14].

Dysbiotic microbiota may have a role in the development of cancer, inflammation, and obesity. Probiotics and prebiotics can be given to alter the composition of the microbiome and improve disease symptoms (Fig. 1.2) [15].

Fecal Microbial Transplantation (FMT)

Fecal samples from donors—whether related or unrelated—that have undergone thorough screening for infectious illnesses are used in FMT procedures. Donors must not be obese and should be free from gastrointestinal disorders, autoimmune or allergic diseases, and conditions that can be transmitted through feces or blood. Additionally, they must not have recently received antibiotic therapy [13, 14]. FMT administered via nasogastric or nasojejunal tubes offers the advantages of being cost-effective and less invasive. However, this method has limitations, such as a

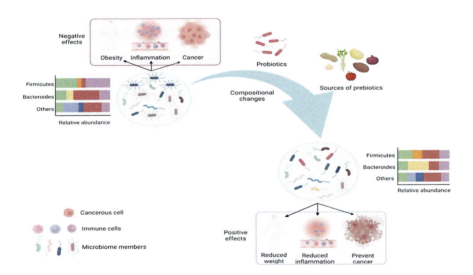

Fig. 1.2 Probiotics and prebiotics altering the composition of the microbiome

higher risk of aspiration events, vomiting, and patient discomfort. In contrast, upper gastrointestinal tract endoscopy, while more invasive, involves anesthesia and incurs higher medical costs but may reduce the risk of aspiration and vomiting. Administering oral capsules containing fecal samples is an inexpensive and noninvasive option, though further research is required to confirm their efficacy [13, 14].

Standardizing the makeup of the feces microbiota that is transplanted after each treatment is practically hard because the microbiota fluctuates over time and between persons. Unlike probiotics, which introduce only a single or small number of species into the intestinal tract, an FMT has the distinct advantage of quickly restoring a diverse makeup to the recipient's digestive microbiome, in contrast to the other modalities of the microbiome modulation that have been discussed [13, 14]. The procedure's usage as a therapy method in *Clostridioides difficile* infection (CDI) is very recent, which limits the quantity of long-term evidence available, despite the procedure's modest side effects. Several gastrointestinal symptoms, such as nausea, vomiting, diarrhea, bloating, flatulence, and stomach discomfort, are examples of minor, transient adverse effects. Allergic responses, the introduction of infectious agents like viruses or fungus, and the possible transmission of microbiota that may aid in the development of disorders like inflammatory bowel disease, irritable bowel syndrome, colorectal malignancies, type-II diabetes, or metabolic syndrome are additional concerns [13, 14].

Fiber-Rich Diets and the Mediterranean Diet: Nourishing Gut Bacteria for Digestive Health

What we eat serves as nourishment for our gut bacteria. Dietary fiber evades human digestion because our enzymatic system lacks the necessary activity for its breakdown. Once it reaches the colon, fiber is digested by our microbes through anaerobic fermentation, producing several metabolites, including short-chain fatty acids (SCFAs), primarily acetate, propionate, and butyrate, which are normally produced at a ratio of 3:1:1. As a result, terms such as *microbiota-accessible carbohydrates* (MACs) have been proposed to define *fiber*. However, importantly, fiber is not a single substance but rather a heterogeneous group of compounds, each with different end products and biological effects.

The production of SCFAs usually involves a complex network of microbial interactions, with cross-feeding cooperation among different taxa. From fiber breakdown, primary fiber degraders release into the gut to partially break down products (e.g., mono- and oligosaccharides) and fermentation metabolites (e.g., pyruvate), which can be used by the secondary fiber degraders and SCFA producers. Indeed, some studies have demonstrated that SCFA production is enhanced in vitro by the co-cultivation of different species. For example, *Roseburia hominis*, a well-known butyrate producer, is unable to grow on most polysaccharides in vitro. However, when co-cultured with *Bifidobacterium adolescentis* on fructo-oligosaccharides or starch, it was able to grow and produce butyrate [16]. Consistently, when inoculated in a fermenter with a fecal inoculum, therefore in the presence of a complex microbial community, *R. hominis* was able to proliferate on different polysaccharide sources [17]. The enzymes that act on carbohydrates are known as carbohydrate-active enzymes (CAZymes), including glycoside hydrolases, glycosyltransferases, polysaccharide lyases, and carbohydrate esterases. In the gut microbiome, a wide pattern of CAZymes classes has been identified, with differences among species [18].

Several interventions with dietary fiber are present in the literature, demonstrating a reshaping of the gut microbiome composition and functions, with the production of beneficial SCFAs. A recent trial with resistant starch (RS) demonstrated that *Bifidobacterium adolescentis*, *Bif. longum*, and *Ruminococcus bromii* increased after 8 weeks compared with placebo. These changes were associated with weight loss, a reduction in inflammation through the restoration of the intestinal barrier, the inhibition of lipid absorption, and an improvement in insulin sensitivity [19]. Consistently, another trial of 3 months on type-II diabetes patients demonstrated an improvement in glucose homeostasis, mediated by the enrichment in the gut microbiome of SCFA-producing taxa [20]. In addition, the authors also carried out a fecal transplant in mice, using fecal samples of subjects before and after the intervention. Interestingly, they could reproduce the metabolic effects in the animal model, demonstrating a causative role of the gut microbiome in glucose control, modulated by dietary fiber [20].

Although dietary interventions often cause a shift in the gut microbiome composition, several trials have suggested its resilience and shown that it usually tends to go back to the baseline composition [21]. Indeed, habitual and long-term diet seems to play a major role. Comparing the gut microbiome of Western subjects with that of non-Western populations from South America and Africa yields a clear difference [22]. Traditional, non-Western diets, usually featuring a much higher level of the consumption of complex polysaccharides from vegetables, tubers, and roots, boost the abundance of fiber-degrading taxa in the gut, such as *Prevotella*, *Treponema*, and *Succinivibrio* [23, 24]. On the contrary, Westernized diets and lifestyles progressively led to a loss of microbial diversity and the disappearance of some taxa in the Westernized gut microbiome [25–27]. However, also in Westernized countries, different dietary patterns can be identified (e.g., vegetarian, vegan, and Mediterranean diets). Generally, a long-term diet rich in complex carbohydrates of plant origin (such as vegan or vegetarian) enriches *Prevotella*, *Lachnospira*, *Roseburia*, *Faecalibacterium*, and other fiber-degrading Clostridia. On the contrary, the habitual consumption of a diet rich in fats and proteins selects for *Bacteroides*, *Alistipes*, and *Bilophila* [28]. Consistently, vegans or vegetarians show higher fecal levels of SCFAs [28].

The Mediterranean diet (MD) is an omnivore dietary pattern traditionally consumed in Southern European countries. It is characterized by a high consumption of fruit, vegetables, legumes, whole grain cereals, and nuts; a moderate consumption of fish, poultry, eggs, and dairy products; olive oil as a major source of fat; and low amounts of red and processed meats. Significant evidence has been reported on the benefits of the MD on health, and adherence to this dietary regimen has been associated with a reduction in the incidence of cardiovascular diseases, diabetes, metabolic syndrome, and neurodegenerative disorders (e.g. Alzheimer's disease) [29]. Long-term adherence to the MD promotes an abundance of microbial signatures consistent with those observed in vegetarians and vegans, in addition to higher levels of SCFAs and a lower urinary concentration of trimethylamine oxide (TMAO), coming from the microbial degradation of choline and subsequent oxidation in the liver [28–30]. TMAO was previously linked to cardiovascular disease risk.

Consistently, a large cohort study on the US population found that the MD adherence index was positively associated with several abundant fiber-metabolizing and C producers, including *Faecalibacterium prausnitzii*, *Eubacterium eligens*, and *Bacteroides cellulosilyticus*. On the contrary, there was a negative correlation with species such as *Ruminococcus torques* and *Clostridium leptum* [31]. Exploring the gut microbiome's functional potential, the same authors found an increased abundance of genes related to pectin and hemicellulose degradation in subjects with higher adherence, whereas those with low adherence showed an enrichment of the secondary bile acid biosynthesis potential [31]. Secondary bile acids, such as deoxycholate and lithocholate, have been identified as hepatotoxic and potentially carcinogenic [32].

The associations found between the MD and the gut microbiome have been confirmed by some ad hoc intervention studies. Meslier and colleagues (2020) [33] carried out a dietary intervention for 8 weeks among obese/overweight subjects with an isocaloric MD, designed for each subject to keep their habitual caloric intake but substitute nutrients typical of the Western diet (e.g., refined sugars, animal fats, and proteins) with those of the MD (whole grains, vegetable proteins from legumes, unsaturated fats from olive oil, and nuts). The MD intervention led to an increase in fiber-degrading taxa, such as *Faecalibacterium prausnitzii*, and in genes related to carbohydrate degradation. In addition, there was an increase in the urinary levels of urolithins in the MD group, a metabolite coming from the microbial metabolism of ellagitannins, a polyphenol class contained in nuts.

A longer trial (12 months) conducted among a population of older adults by Gosh et al. (2020) [6] suggests that changes in gut microbiome composition are positively associated with markers of frailty and cognitive function, as well as a reduction in inflammation. Although fiber is the dietary component most commonly studied for its impact on the gut microbiome, other nutrients and micronutrients may also be metabolized by the microbiome, releasing metabolites with either positive or negative health effects. For example, polyphenols—a diverse class of plant secondary metabolites—are found in fruits, vegetables, and cereals. This class includes a wide range of different molecules. The dietary intake of polyphenols is beneficial for human health in that they are reported to have antioxidant, anticarcinogenic, and anti-inflammatory effects [34]. As mentioned earlier, ellagitannins are metabolized by certain microbial species into various urolithins, such as urolithin A, B, and C, which exhibit antioxidant and anti-inflammatory properties. The soy isoflavone daidzein can be converted into equol, which has beneficial effects in cancer and cardiovascular disease prevention and in improving menopausal symptoms. Resveratrol can be metabolized into glucuronides and sulfates by microbial taxa such as *Slackia equolifaciens* and *Adlercreutzia equolifaciens*. These compounds may exhibit anti-inflammatory activity and appear to be linked to a reduction in cholesterol [35].

Unfortunately, most of the studies exploring the relationships of the gut microbiome with specific dietary patterns or nutrients have focused mainly on genus- or species-level composition. However, for several species, strain-level differences have been demonstrated [36, 37] in response to diet. Indeed, different *Prevotella copri* subtypes have shown different prevalences in Westernized and non-Westernized subjects. Evaluating their genomic potential, researchers highlighted that those strains from non-Western subjects have more genes related to complex fiber degradation, suggesting a strain-level selection driven by the diet [36]. Consistently, another study identified different strains of *Ruminococcus gnavus* in the gut microbiome of healthy and allergic children and suggested that strains linked to the allergic state have higher proinflammatory potential and a lower ability to produce SCFAs from fiber fermentation [38]. Therefore, when considering the complex interplay between the gut microbiome, diet, and human health, strain-level diversity should be also carefully taken into account.

Box 1.2: Benefits of the Mediterranean Diet
- Mediterranean diet (MD) benefits: The Mediterranean diet, rich in fruits, vegetables, whole grains, and healthy fats, has health benefits such as reducing the risk of cardiovascular diseases, diabetes, and neurodegenerative disorders.
- Adherence to MD enhances the abundance of microbes associated with vegan and vegetarian diets and increases short-chain fatty acid (SCFA) levels while lowering trimethylamine oxide (TMAO) concentrations, linked to cardiovascular risk.

The Role of Gut Bacteria in Inflammation and Chronic Disease Prevention

Microbiota and Personalized Nutrition

Not only can personalized nutrition be used to treat metabolic disorders, but it can also be used as prophylactic treatment for people at high risk of blood or lifestyle disorders, as well as additional treatment for autoimmune diseases, cancer, and neurological disorders. The general makeup and function of the gut microbiota are modulated by the diet, particularly by the types of polysaccharides ingested. Polysaccharides are an intriguing diet choice with good health qualities because of their low cost, availability, and relative safety; yet to enhance human health, an appropriate amount of individual polysaccharides or combinations must be found. Due to the great degree of compositional individuality, gut microbiota manipulation is not straightforward. Of the approximately three thousand individuals in the sample, 664 genera were identified; of these, only 14 were present in 95% of the participants [39]. Individual differences exist in the actual and relative numbers of species present in the microbiota and in its composition in the adult gut [40].

Both machine-learning and logical approaches can be useful in diet selection. Microbiome fingerprints along with their metabolic characteristics are determined for logical design. To achieve the intended effects, foods that are good for all types of microbiotas can be discovered once the microbial community has been characterized. According to Zeevi et al. (2015) [41], the machine-learning method works well for complex features and may be used for any measurable attribute because it doesn't require a prior understanding of complex mechanisms.

In one study, 800 participants' blood glucose levels were tracked by using a machine-learning technique to determine their postprandial glycemic reactions. Individuals' reactions to the meal that they were served were predicted and verified [41]. Individual differences in glucose metabolism have been found in reaction to dietary fiber. Those whose gut microbiota included a high concentration of the genus *Prevotella* had enhanced glucose tolerance [42]. These findings highlight the potential of these methods for selecting dietary interventions that can ameliorate pathological conditions in any individual or population. Individual differences in functional capacity are further reflected in variations in those species' overall abundance. Consequently, to increase an individual's genetically modified enzymatic pool, distinct genes or species must be introduced for each person.

Oligosaccharides produced through fermentation in the colon of porphyrin give both the host and the residing bacteria energy. But porphyrin is just another fiber to individuals who lack this particular bacterium. Compositional adjustments toward the higher abundance of the potent strains could be an alternative to improve the functional capacities of the resident or introduced bacteria. As a result, a customized strategy that screens each person's microbiome to identify the types and quantities of functions present enables a more accurate assessment of the requirements and thorough progression monitoring.

The fact that the effectiveness of strain engraftment or augmentation will rely on the individual gut microbiota (GM) setting is another reason to strive toward individualized modulation. Through priority effects, the highly individualized compositional "starting conditions" dictate how interventions turn out. Results from the procedure known as fecal material transplantation (FMT), which involves transplanting a donor's genetic material into a recipient's stomach, vary greatly. Some patients "accept" the donor GM to a certain extent, whereas others do not or eventually return to their original constellation. Depending on the microbiomes of the donor and recipient, FMT may or may not be able to (temporarily) treat the illness [43]. Although some investigations have suggested that some sort of "match" is necessary, these investigations have not yet yielded the principles for matchmaking. Dispersion methods such as FMT are likely to have different outcomes depending on a variety of criteria, including host selection and colonization resistance. Clinical researchers have determined that there is no one-size-fits-all approach to microbiome regulation. Therefore, tailoring the therapy to each patient is a good idea.

A person's genetic makeup and function significantly influence the effectiveness of microbial colonization. For instance, strains occupying the same nutritional niche will experience greater competition for resources, making steady colonization less likely. Similarly, prebiotic stimulation varies according to the presence and abundance of target bacteria, which can differ significantly between individuals and change over time [44]. In addition to conventional approaches, such as the use of probiotics, prebiotics, and synbiotics, following microbiome screening and assessment, other strategies may enable a more targeted and individualized modulation of the microbiome [45]. One promising approach involves using gut metabolites as modulators. Numerous studies have shown that adding lactate or acetate can promote the growth of butyrate-producing bacteria, while host mucus components may encourage the proliferation of mucus-degrading bacteria, such as *Akkermansia muciniphila*. Notably, the metabolites in the first example can be consumed by a wide range of bacteria.

Utilizing minerals is another option for microbiome modulation. Because most bacteria and other living organisms rely on minerals such as iron, magnesium, sodium, and calcium for survival, these elements may influence the composition of genetically modified organisms (GMOs). Research suggests that iron has a negative effect on the microbiome in that it reduces the production of butyrate and promotes the growth of pathogenic bacteria, potentially linked to siderophore production. Although there are some indications that other minerals, such as zinc, may also influence GMOs, knowledge in this area remains limited [46].

Microbiota and Inflammation

Clinical strategies for modifying gut microbiota often focus on reducing overabundant microorganisms or the overall microbial burden by using antibiotics, antifungal medications, dietary modifications, or live microbe supplementation (single or mixed species). Various therapeutic approaches have been proposed to target the gut microbiota, including dietary changes, probiotics, prebiotics, and TMAO-synthesis inhibitors. Fecal microbial transplantation (FMT) has also emerged as a promising intervention, showing encouraging results in treating a range of infectious, neurological, and gastrointestinal (GI) disorders [47, 48].

Although animal models have yielded promising results, showing the successful treatment of inflammatory conditions through gut microbiota modulation, data from human studies remain less conclusive. Recent research highlights that the composition of an individual's gut microbiota plays a critical role in determining an introduced microbe's ability to colonize the gut. This variability may explain differences observed between animal models and human trials, a factor often overlooked in microbiota-based clinical studies. For instance, treatment with a multispecies bacterial community has been shown to help patients with ulcerative colitis (UC) maintain remission, but it has not been effective in Crohn's disease (CD) patients [49].

Conclusions

The results of interventions involving live microbial supplementation have generally been promising. However, future research could significantly enhance efficacy by focusing on selecting microbial strains on the basis of their functional properties, optimizing the timing and duration of supplementation, and tailoring the supplemented organisms to the recipient's native gut microbiota. The goal of ongoing research is to understand the fundamentals of microbe–microbe interactions, enabling the identification of specific gut microbiomes that respond more effectively to targeted microbial therapies.

Further Practice

1. What is the major fat source in the Mediterranean diet?

    (a) Corn oil
    (b) Palm Oil
    (c) Butter
    (d) Olive Oil
    (e) Full cream milk

2. What does the term *gut microbiota imbalance* refer to?

    (a) Symbiosis
    (b) Dysbiosis
    (c) Parasite
    (d) Biotin
    (e) Biosis

3. The gut microbiota is beneficial in maintaining immune function.
       True or false

4. Which factor does not affect gut microbiota?

    (a) The composition of infant formula
    (b) Depression
    (c) Dietary factors
    (d) Antibiotics
    (e) Marital status

5. What is a prebiotic?

    (a) The digestible part of food
    (b) A nondigestible part of food that improves the growth of gut microbiota
    (c) Protein food that inhibits the growth of gut microbiota
    (d) The drug that inhibits the growth of gut microbiota
    (e) A type of fruit that inhibits the growth of gut microbiota

6. The following are examples of prebiotics except

   (a) Inulin
   (b) Lactulose
   (c) Fructooligosaccharide
   (d) Galacto-oligosaccharide
   (e) Glucose

7. Which of the following is a potential drawback of using nasogastric or nasojejunal tubes for fecal microbiota transplantation (FMT)?

   (a) High medical expenses due to the need for anesthesia
   (b) The risk of aspiration and vomiting
   (c) The requirement of donors with obesity
   (d) The inefficacy of the procedure compared to oral capsules
   (e) The need for invasive surgery

8. What is one drawback of using iron in microbiome modulation?

   (a) It promotes the growth of beneficial bacteria.
   (b) It reduces the production of lactic acid.
   (c) It decreases butyrate production and encourages pathogenic bacte-
       ria growth.
   (d) It enhances antibiotic resistance.
   (e) It inhibits prebiotic stimulation.

9. Which of the following bacteria is known to thrive in the presence of host
   mucus components?

   (a) *Escherichia coli*
   (b) *Lactobacillus acidophilus*
   (c) *Akkermansia muciniphila*
   (d) *Bifidobacterium breve*
   (e) *Clostridium difficile*

10. What role can gut metabolites such as lactate and acetate play in microbiome
    modulation?

    (a) They inhibit the growth of all bacteria.
    (b) They support the growth of pathogenic bacteria.
    (c) They promote the growth of butyrate-producing bacteria.
    (d) They eliminate mucus-degrading bacteria.
    (e) They suppress the production of siderophores.

11. What has recent research revealed about the factors that determine a microbe's
    ability to colonize the gut?

    (a) The type of treatment used plays the most significant role.
    (b) The composition of an individual's gut microbiota is a crucial factor.
    (c) The age of the individual is the primary determinant.

(d) Only prebiotic supplementation influences microbial colonization.

(e) Gut microbiota composition does not affect microbial colonization.

12. What is a key consideration for improving the efficacy of live microbial supplementation in future research?

(a) Using a single microbial strain without additional dietary interventions

(b) Tailoring the supplementation to the recipient's endogenous gut microbiome

(c) Increasing the amount of supplementation without considering strain variety

(d) Using probiotics for a short duration only

(e) Avoiding the customization of treatments based on individual microbiomes

13. Which of the following is a potential benefit of polyphenols?

(a) Polyphenols are linked primarily to weight gain.

(b) Polyphenols exhibit antioxidant, anticarcinogenic, and anti-inflammatory effects.

(c) Polyphenols increase the production of cholesterol.

(d) Polyphenols are found only in vegetables.

(e) Polyphenols decrease cognitive function.

14. Which of the following is **true** regarding dietary fiber?

(a) Fiber is fully digested by human enzymes in the digestive system.

(b) Dietary fiber produces only one type of metabolite, primarily butyrate.

(c) The fermentation of dietary fiber by gut microbes produces short-chain fatty acids (SCFAs) in a 3:1:1 ratio of acetate, propionate, and butyrate.

(d) Fiber is a single substance with uniform effects on the body.

(e) Microbiota-accessible carbohydrates (MACs) refer exclusively to proteins.

15. Which of the following is **true** regarding the differences between Western and non-Western diets and their effects on the gut microbiome?

(a) Both Western and non-Western diets promote the growth of the same microbial taxa.

(b) Non-Western diets, which are higher in complex polysaccharides, increase the abundance of fiber-degrading taxa in the gut, such as *Prevotella*, *Treponema*, and *Succinivibrio*.

(c) Westernized diets have been shown to improve gut microbiome diversity.

(d) Vegetarian and vegan diets tend to deplete the presence of fiber-degrading Clostridia in the gut.

(e) Western diets increase fecal levels of SCFAs in individuals who consume a high intake of fats and proteins.

Answer Key

1. (d)
2. (b)
3. True

4. (e)
5. (b)
6. (e)
7. (b)
8. (c)
9. (c)
10. (c)
11. (b)
12. (b)
13. (b)
14. (c)
15. (b)

References

1. Dogra SK, Doré J, Damak S. Gut microbiota resilience: definition, link to health and strategies for intervention. Front Microbiol. 2020;11(September):2014–21.
2. Huttenhower C, Gevers D, Knight R, Abubucker S, Badger JH, Chinwalla AT, et al. Structure, function, and diversity of the healthy human microbiome. Nature. 2012;486(7402):207–14.
3. Leroy N, Chirat C, Lachenal D, Robert D, Allison RW. Extended oxygen delignification. Part 2: multi-stage oxygen bleaching with intermediate hypochlorous acid stages. Appita J. 2004;57(3):224–7.
4. Shreiner AB, Kao JY, Young VB, Turnbaugh PJ, Ley RE, Mahowald MA, Magrini V, Mardis ER, Gordon JI, Wilson RC, Doudna JA. Dicer (E-7): sc-393328. Cell. 2015;69(1):393328.
5. Noh H, Jang HH, Kim G, Zouiouich S, Cho SY, Kim HJ, et al. Taxonomic composition and diversity of the gut microbiota in relation to habitual dietary intake in Korean adults. Nutrients. 2021;13(2):1–16.
6. Ghosh S, Pramanik S. Structural diversity, functional aspects and future therapeutic applications of human gut microbiome. Arch Microbiol. 2021;203(9):5281–308.
7. Johnson KVA. Gut microbiome composition and diversity are related to human personality traits. Hum Microb J. 2020;15:100069.
8. Ronan V, Yeasin R, Claud EC. Childhood development and the microbiome—the intestinal microbiota in maintenance of health and development of disease during childhood development. Gastroenterology. 2021;160(2):495–506.
9. Odamaki T, Kato K, Sugahara H, Hashikura N, Takahashi S, Xiao JZ, Abe F, Osawa R. Age-related changes in gut microbiota composition from newborn to centenarian: a cross-sectional study. BMC Microbiol. 2016;16(1):1–12.
10. Salazar J, Durán P, Díaz MP, Chacín M, Santeliz R, Mengual E, et al. Exploring the relationship between the gut microbiota and ageing: a possible age modulator. Int J Environ Res Public Health. 2023;20(10):5845.
11. Yao Y, Cai X, Ye Y, Wang F, Chen F, Zheng C. The role of microbiota in infant health: from early life to adulthood. Front Immunol. 2021;12(October):1–21.
12. Nagpal R, Mainali R, Ahmadi S, Wang S, Singh R, Kavanagh K, Kitzman DW, Kushugulova A, Marotta F, Yadav H. Gut microbiome and aging: physiological and mechanistic insights. Nutr Healthy Aging. 2018;4(4):267–85.
13. Yadav M, Chauhan NS. Microbiome therapeutics: exploring the present scenario and challenges. Gastroenterol Rep. 2022;10(September):1–19.
14. Teras LR. Microbial diversity – the key to gut health. Physiol Behav. 2017;176:139–48.

15. Aggarwal N, Kitano S, Puah GRY, Kittelmann S, Hwang IY, Chang MW. Microbiome and human health: current understanding, engineering, and enabling technologies. Chem Rev. 2023;123(1):31–72.
16. Belenguer A, Calder AG, Duncan SH, et al. Two routes of metabolic cross-feeding between Bifidobacterium adolescentis and butyrate-producing anaerobes from the human gut. Appl Environ Microbiol. 2006;72:3593–9.
17. Duncan SH, Scott KP, Ramsay AG, Harmsen HJM, Welling GW, Stewart CS, Flint HJ. Effects of alternative dietary substrates on competition between human colonic bacteria in an anaerobic fermentor system. Appl Environ Microbiol. 2003;69:1136–42.
18. Wardman JF, Bains RK, Rahfeld P, et al. Carbohydrate-active enzymes (CAZymes) in the gut microbiome. Nat Rev Microbiol. 2022;20:542–56.
19. Li H, Zhang L, Li J, et al. Resistant starch intake facilitates weight loss in humans by reshaping the gut microbiota. Nat Metab. 2024;6:578–97.
20. Zhao L, Zhang F, Ding X, Wu G, Lam YY, Wang X, et al. Gut bacteria selectively promoted by dietary fibers alleviate type 2 diabetes. Science. 2018;359(6380):1151–6.
21. Fragiadakis GK, Wastyk HC, Robinson JL, Sonnenburg ED, Sonnenburg JL, Gardner CD. Long-term dietary intervention reveals resilience of the gut microbiota despite changes in diet and weight. Am J Clin Nutr. 2020;111(6):1127–36.
22. Mancabelli L, Milani C, Lugli GA, et al. Meta-analysis of the human gut microbiome from urbanized and pre-agricultural populations. Environ Microbiol. 2017;19(4):1379–90.
23. Schnorr SL, Candela M, Rampelli S, Centanni M, Consolandi C, Basaglia G, et al. Gut microbiome of the Hadza hunter-gatherers. Nat Commun. 2014;5:3654.
24. Obregon-Tito AJ, Tito RY, Metcalf J, Sankaranarayanan K, Clemente JC, Ursell LK, et al. Subsistence strategies in traditional societies distinguish gut microbiomes. Nat Commun. 2015;6:6505.
25. Segata N. Gut microbiome: westernization and the disappearance of intestinal diversity. Curr Biol. 2015;25(14):R611–3.
26. Vangay P, Johnson AJ, Ward TL, Al-Ghalith GA, Shields-Cutler RR, Hillmann BM, et al. US immigration westernizes the human gut microbiome. Cell. 2018;175(4):962–972.e10.
27. Sonnenburg ED, Smits SA, Tikhonov M, Higginbottom SK, Wingreen NS, Sonnenburg JL. Diet-induced extinctions in the gut microbiota compound over generations. Nature. 2016;529(7585):212–5.
28. De Filippis F, Pellegrini N, Vannini L, Jeffery IB, La Storia A, Laghi L, et al. High-level adherence to a Mediterranean diet beneficially impacts the gut microbiota and associated metabolome. Gut. 2016;65(11):1812–21.
29. Guasch-Ferré M, Willett WC. The Mediterranean diet and health: a comprehensive overview. J Intern Med. 2021;290(3):549–66.
30. Latorre-Pérez A, Hernández M, Iglesias JR, et al. The Spanish gut microbiome reveals links between microorganisms and the Mediterranean diet. Sci Rep. 2021;11(1):21602.
31. Wang X, Chen L, Zhang C, Shi Q, Zhu L, Zhao S, Luo Z, Long Y. Effect of probiotics at different intervention times on glycemic control in patients with type 2 diabetes mellitus: a systematic review and meta-analysis. Front Endocrinol. 2024;15(July):1–10.
32. Wolf PG, Byrd DA, Cares K, Dai H, Odoms-Young A, Gaskins HR, et al. Bile acids, gut microbes, and the neighborhood food environment potential driver of colorectal cancer health disparities. mSystems. 2022;7(1):e0117421.
33. Meslier V, Laiola M, Roager HM, De Filippis F, Roume H, Quinquis B, et al. Mediterranean diet intervention in overweight and obese subjects lowers plasma cholesterol and causes changes in the gut microbiome and metabolome independently of energy intake. Gut. 2020;69(7):1258–68.
34. Rudrapal M, Khairnar SJ, Khan J, Dukhyil AB, Ansari MA, Alomary MN, et al. Dietary polyphenols and their role in oxidative stress-induced human diseases: insights into protective effects, antioxidant potentials and mechanism (s) of action. Front Pharmacol. 2022;13:806470.

35. Aravind S, Mithul, Chakkaravarthi S, Ramakrishnan S, Tsao R, Wichienchot S. Role of dietary polyphenols on gut microbiota, their metabolites and health benefits. Food Res Int. 2021;142:110189.
36. De Filippis F, Pasolli E, Tett A, Tarallo S, Naccarati A, De Angelis M, Neviani E, Cocolin L, Gobbetti M, Segata N, Ercolini D. Distinct genetic and functional traits of human intestinal Prevotella copri strains are associated with different habitual diets. Cell Host Microbe. 2019;25(3):444–453.e3.
37. Blanco-Míguez A, Gálvez EJC, Pasolli E, et al. Extension of the Segatella copri complex to 13 species with distinct large extrachromosomal elements and associations with host conditions. Cell Host Microbe. 2023;31(11):1804–1819.e9.
38. De Filippis F, Paparo L, Nocerino R, et al. Specific gut microbiome signatures and the associated pro-inflammatory functions are linked to pediatric allergy and the acquisition of immune tolerance. Nat Commun. 2021;12(1):5958.
39. Falony G, Joossens M, Vieira-Silva S, Wang J, Darzi Y, Faust K, et al. Population-level analysis of gut microbiome variation. Science. 2016;352:560–4.
40. Vandeputte D, Kathagen G, D'hoe K, Vieira-Silva S, Valles-Colomer M, Sabino J, et al. Quantitative microbiome profiling links gut community variation to microbial load. Nature. 2017;551:507–11.
41. Zeevi D, Korem T, Zmora N, Israeli D, Rothschild D, Weinberger A, et al. Personalized nutrition by prediction of glycemic responses. Cell. 2015;163(5):1079–94.
42. Kovatcheva-Datchary P, Anne N, Rozita A, Ying SL, Filipe VD, Tulika A, Anna H, Eric M, Inger B, Fredrik B. Dietary fiber-induced improvement in glucose metabolism is associated with increased abundance of Prevotella. Cell Metab. 2015;22(6):971–82.
43. Zheng L, Wen XL, Duan SL, Ji YY. Fecal microbiota transplantation in the metabolic diseases: current status and perspectives. World J Gastroenterol. 2022;28(23):2546–60.
44. Vandeputte D. Personalized nutrition through the gut microbiota: current insights and future perspectives. Nutr Rev. 2020;78:66–74.
45. Roy S, Dhaneshwar S. Role of prebiotics, probiotics, and synbiotics in management of inflammatory bowel disease: current perspectives. World J Gastroenterol. 2023;29(14):2078–100.
46. Yilmaz B, Li H. Gut microbiota and iron: the crucial actors in health and disease. Pharmaceuticals. 2018;11(4):1–20.
47. Durack J, Lynch SV. The gut microbiome: relationships with disease and opportunities for therapy. J Exp Med. 2019;216(1):20–40. https://doi.org/10.1084/jem.20180448.
48. Matzaras R, Nikopoulou A, Protonotariou E, Christaki E. Gut microbiota modulation and prevention of dyasbasis. 2022;95:479–94.
49. Hasan N, Yang H. Factors affecting the composition of the gut microbiota, and its modulation. PeerJ. 2019;2019(8):1–31.

A Holistic Guide to the Nutritional Management of Obesity

2

Kritee Niroula, Nila Pradhananga, and Erin M. McKinley

Learning Objectives

After completing the chapter, you will be able to

- Describe the associated risk factors contributing to obesity
- List the common health impacts associated with being obese
- Study the nutritional importance of each macronutrient
- Learn about the existing popular approaches to obesity management
- Discuss behavioral and lifestyle management techniques for weight loss and maintenance

Introduction to Obesity

The World Health Organization (WHO) states that obesity is the abnormal or excessive deposition of body fat that causes health risks. When categorizing obesity among adults, body mass index (BMI) over 30 is considered obese [92]. BMI is the body weight in kilograms divided by the square of height in meters. The Centers for

K. Niroula (✉)
Institute for Collaboration on Health, Intervention, and Policy (InCHIP), University of Connecticut, Storrs, CT, USA
e-mail: ubl24004@uconn.edu

N. Pradhananga
Department of Nutritional Sciences, College of Education and Human Sciences, Oklahoma State University, Stillwater, OK, USA
e-mail: nilapradhananga@outlook.com

E. M. McKinley
School of Nutrition & Food Sciences, Louisiana State University, Baton Rouge, LA, USA
e-mail: emckinley@agcenter.lsu.edu

© The Author(s), under exclusive license to Springer Nature Switzerland AG 2025
A. K. Mitra, D. Vanoh (eds.), *Essentials of Clinical and Public Health Nutrition*, Nutrition and Health, https://doi.org/10.1007/978-3-031-95373-6_2

Disease Control and Prevention (CDC) recognizes it as a reliable screening measure for body weight among populations—obesity, overweight, normal weight, and underweight [12]. Other measures for body fatness as suggested by CDC include bioelectrical impedance, skinfold-thickness-measuring calipers, and dual-energy X-ray absorptiometry [12]. Obesity is assessed differently among children. For children under five years, obesity is categorized when the weight-over-height is greater than three standard deviations above the WHO growth standard median, whereas for children aged five to 19 years, obesity is BMI-for-age greater than two standard deviations above the WHO growth reference median [93]. According to the WHO, in 2022, one in eight adults were experiencing obesity. The number of adults with obesity accounted for 890 million, and the number of children and adolescents with obesity was 160 million. Adult obesity prevalence was 16% in 2022, which has doubled since 1990 [93].

The WHO reports obesity as a multifactorial disease due to several intertwined factors collectively creating an obesogenic environment [93]. It tends to develop gradually over time when the consumption of calories exceeds their expenditure. Having a high calorie/energy imbalance causes fat storage in the body over time. Fats are stored predominantly as triglycerides in fat cells [55]. In general, the risk of developing obesity is determined mainly by the types and amount of food consumed and the level of daily physical activity [55].

Risk Factors of Obesity

1. Eating behavior: The consumption of excess calories is a major factor linked to obesity. The number of calories required by an individual is determined by age, sex, and daily physical activity level. Eating food high in saturated fat and refined sugar is the most common reason behind excess calorie intake [55].
2. Lack of physical activity: A modern sedentary lifestyle representing excessive screen time or most of one's time spent sitting either at home or in the office while being inactive also contributes to obesity [55].
3. Stress and a lack of sleep: Stress, in response to our daily activities, triggers stress hormones, especially cortisol, that regulate hunger cues and promote overeating. Similarly, a lack of sleep, less than the ideal 7–8 hours, also affects hormonal balance, which as a result increases daily food consumption [55].
4. Health and medication: Some medicines, predominantly antidepressants, beta-blockers, antipsychotics, and birth control pills, cause weight gain [55]. A few psychotropic drugs, such as chlorpromazine, clozapine, olanzapine, and antidepressants, namely amitriptyline and mirtazapine, have been shown to cause weight gain [70].
5. Genetics: The balance between energy intake and expenditure is modulated by genetics. At least 15 genes are responsible for influencing obesity [55]. Genetics increases the risk of obesity by influencing and regulating metabolic and neural pathways. Epigenetic variations are passed on to offspring, and they ultimately can have "intergenerational and transgenerational effects" [68].

Health Impacts of Obesity

Growing evidence tells us that obesity increases the incidence of diabetes, cardio-vascular disease, hypertension, depression, and anxiety [75]. An excessive amount of body fat introduces what researchers refer to as "a constellation of metabolic abnormalities and diseases." It encompasses high plasma triglyceride and low high-density lipoprotein (HDL) cholesterol, insulin resistance, and type-2 diabetes [36]. Some of them are discussed below.

1. Type-2 diabetes: It is caused by multiorgan insulin resistance, which is charac-terized predominantly by a decrease in b cell function. Researchers report that the worldwide increase in obesity contributes to a significant increase in the prevalence of type-2 diabetes. As a progressive disease, obesity gradually causes progression toward the development of the disease. People with fat deposits pre-dominantly in the abdominal area, pancreatic area, and upper body have a sig-nificantly higher risk of developing diabetes [36].
2. Nonalcoholic fatty liver disease (NAFLD): NAFLD is a condition characterized by the gradual development of fat in the liver. Obesity has been found to be the most important risk factor for NAFLD. About three-quarters of cases of obesity in humans are followed by fatty liver [1]. The incidence of NAFLD starts with the gradual accumulation of fat in the liver cells (hepatocytes) and is found to be associated with insulin resistance and altered fatty acid regulation. Upon not undergoing any treatment or not undertaking further prevention, it ultimately proceeds toward cirrhosis and fibrosis [62].
3. Cancer: Adiposity in the body promotes an increase in free fatty acids (FFAs), tumor necrosis factor α (TNF-α), and plasminogen activator inhibitor 1 (PAI-1). It then leads to the increased bioavailability of insulin-like growth factor 1 (IGF-1), which hampers apoptosis and promotes the proliferation of cells in the body [54]. The risk of colorectal cancer increases by 1.5-fold among individuals with obesity compared to those with a healthy weight [51]. It also increases the risk of gallbladder cancer by impacting lipid and hormone metabolism. Researchers claim that obesity might be related to a lower survival rate among obese patients with cancer [54].
4. Dyslipidemia: The term *dyslipidemia* typically denotes increased plasma triglyc-erides and FFAs and might be accompanied by decreased high-density lipopro-tein (HDL) and increased low-density lipoprotein (LDL). The lipolysis activity of lipoprotein lipase (LPL) is decreased in obesity due to its reduced mRNA expression levels [37]. Higher levels of LDL lead to a gradual accumulation of plaque in the inner lining of arteries, leading to atherosclerosis. On the contrary, the ability of HDL to aid in the removal of excess blood cholesterol is reduced [97].
5. Hypertension: Obesity can be lethal in terms of damaging the kidney structure with a loss of nephron function, renal dysfunction, and an increase in arterial pressure. Higher insulin levels and the impairment of glucose tolerance are evi-dent in central obesity; they have roles in disrupting the arterial function through

vasoconstriction. Insulin also influences kidney function by stimulating sodium reabsorption and volume overload, which increases blood pressure [2].

6. Cardiovascular disease: The excess fat deposit in adipose tissue increases the total blood volume, which results in increased cardiac output. The increased circulating blood volume causes the dilation of the atrium and gradually proceeds toward atrial fibrillation and heart failure. The infiltration of myocardial fibers due to fat deposition causes a change in structure and abnormal functioning. Thus, the development of cardiomyopathy also further increases the risk of cardiac arrhythmias and coronary heart disease [32].

Being overweight or obese also jeopardizes the mental health of individuals. Clinical evidence has shown that obese people are susceptible to a lack of confidence and self-esteem, perceived impaired body image, and having difficulty with interpersonal communication, which can further lead to stress eating and other eating disorders and ultimately exacerbate their health condition [71].

Understanding Obesity Through a Different Lens

As Fig. 2.1 shows, obesity is a complex, multifactorial condition that remains intertwined between individual factors, social factors, lifestyle, and behavioral and environmental factors. At the ground-root level, it is understood to be a health consequence that is a result of long-term energy imbalance characterized by excess energy consumption compared to energy expenditure. This energy imbalance is termed a *positive energy balance* [63, 84].

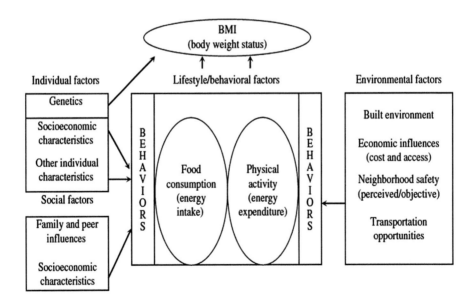

Fig. 2.1 The built environment and obesity [63]

Individual Factors The individual factors that influence obesity are age, sex, and even one's socioeconomic status. Genetics has been one of the influential individual factors contributing to obesity. The way that genes function in the human body alters the metabolic pathways and appetite centers. It is responsible for contributing to dyslipidemia, insulin resistance, and the deposition of fat in the liver, which are the well-known markers of obesity [68]. Furthermore, epigenetic changes have been found to pass down from the mother to the fetus, thus altering the fetal metabolism. Researchers have been studying this as the "fetal programming of body composition" [34].

Prenatal and Postnatal Factors Obesity, especially among children, is highly influenced by the pre- and postnatal environment. Having a high maternal BMI and high infant birth weight significantly increases the risk of obesity among infants and children [96]. The risk of developing obesity generally develops early in life and remains attached to adulthood, having a lifelong impact [93].

Social Factors Socioeconomic factors, including one's income, education level, and job status, also influence obesity. An individual's job/income influences their lifestyle, which affects the person's ability to consume healthy food and engage in physical activity [4]. People from low socioeconomic backgrounds are far less likely to indulge in sports and other physical activities [8]. Those people generally have been found to consume fewer fresh fruits and vegetables and more food high in fat and simple carbohydrates. Education is also another factor affecting people's ability to gain health information and put it into regular practice. This means that having a poor education might prevent them from making healthy food choices and behavioral and lifestyle changes [3].

Environmental Factors Environmental factors sum up the wide array of aspects ranging from our neighborhood and community, basically our surroundings, either natural or humanmade, and are external to the individual. The surroundings in which we exist have been known to significantly affect our health by fostering conditions that might promote a positive energy balance [30]. Some common environment-related influences might be the values attached to eating behavior and physical activity, existing trends in social networking, and support for community-related behavior such as the use of local parks, community spaces, and gyms [10]. The types of restaurants and food vendors available within a given community space are also indirectly related to the prevalence of obesity. Individuals living in a "high-density fast-food neighborhood" were found more likely to be obese when comparing the density of fast-food restaurants within the neighborhood [44].

Having access to safe areas such as parks and playgrounds is considered to influence physical activity, especially among children [63]. Neighborhoods that have walkable areas automatically reduce the incidence of obesity [15]. Other infrastructures, such as recreational facilities and safe sidewalks, have also been found to be equally beneficial [42]. Our work environment also plays a crucial role in our daily energy balance. We have clear evidence of decreased "work-related energy expenditure" and gaining weight over time [13]. Advancements in technology have further exacerbated this condition by saving labor through the use of machines and robots [13].

Holistic Management of Obesity

Energy balance is a state of equilibrium achieved when energy intake equals energy expenditure. Researchers often bring up this concept to explain the change in body weight that comes in response to our daily dietary intake and the energy expended for body metabolic processes and physical activity. When one has energy or calorie balance, body weight remains constant [26, 29]. The imbalance in the energy balance, especially a positive energy balance, is the excess energy consumption compared to energy expenditure, which over time causes weight gain. On the contrary, a negative energy balance occurs when energy expenditure exceeds energy intake, which results in weight gain [46].

Energy intake occurs through the food and drinks that we take in over the course of an entire day, whereas energy expenditure involves the energy used for the resting metabolic rate, the thermic effect of food, and daily physical activity. The resting metabolic rate is the energy we expend for our normal body functioning and maintaining homeostasis. It accounts for about 50–80% of the daily energy expenditure. The thermic effect of food is the energy required for the digestion of food and drinks, the absorption of nutrients, and transportation; also known as thermogenesis, it accounts for 5–10% of the daily energy expenditure. The energy required for daily physical activity adds up with the energy required for thermogenesis and resting metabolic rate to calculate our total daily energy expenditure [29].

The approaches to prevent or manage obesity have been studied under two classifications: The first is behavior oriented, which is based on the individual, and the second is environment oriented. Behavior-oriented interventions focus on bringing changes to individual lifestyles, which basically include increasing physical activity and controlling diet. On the contrary, environment-oriented approaches prioritize influencing health behavior through residential-, neighborhood-, and community-related interventions [41, 45, 88]. The main behavior-oriented approaches to managing obesity have been studied as nutritional management and having an active lifestyle. The treatment of obesity incorporates a multidisciplinary yet individualized approach depending on the other comorbidities, which typically aids in weight loss and maintenance. Lifestyle and behavior modifications with a special focus on negative energy balance and increased physical activity are called the "cornerstones" of treating obesity and associated conditions [7].

Dietary Approach

According to the Dietary Guidelines of Americans 2020–2025, the total number of calories necessary for an individual depends on the age, sex, height, weight, and physical activity of the individual or some other physiological status, such as pregnancy or lactation. The calorie requirements are lower for women and girls than for men and boys. In general, a woman between the ages of 19 and 30 years requires about 1800–2400 calories a day, whereas a man of the same age range requires 2400–3000 calories a day. Similarly, regarding the calorie requirements for adults aged 31–59 years, women require 1600–2200 calories a day, whereas men require 2200–3000 calories a day [80]. A negative energy balance through calorie deficit is a significant factor responsible for weight loss. A low-calorie diet with limited carbohydrate and fat content is recommended for calorie deficit [24].

Body adipose tissue and glycogen are the two main sources of body energy, which is derived and extracted in the form of kilocalories (kcal). Adipose tissue has high energy density, making it a better source of fuel, which is stored as triglycerides and produces approximately 9.3 kcal per gram upon oxidation, whereas glycogen generates about 4.1 kcal per gram [36]. A calorie deficit of about 500 calories a day is required for the weight loss of about one pound per week. It can be accomplished through the intake of 1200–1500 kcal a day in women and about 1500–1800 kcal a day in men. To maintain this daily reduction in energy intake, a proper modification of macronutrients is suggested, one that should be low in calories yet possess the necessary nutrition [72].

Carbohydrate A low-carbohydrate diet has been popularly used for weight loss and maintenance. For a healthy adult, carbohydrate intake is suggested to be maintained within 45–65% of the total calories [82]. In the case of individuals seeking weight reduction, carbohydrate intake ranging from 10% to 45% of the total intake is recommended [67]. In addition to the total carbohydrate intake, the type of carbohydrate that we eat also affects our metabolic profile. Simple carbohydrates, fructose, and sucrose, generally found in excessive amounts in cookies, soda, and candies, increase adiposity and weight gain. Fiber, a complex carbohydrate, is derived from whole grains, fruits, and vegetables and helps in promoting weight loss and insulin sensitivity [85]. The dietary fiber intake recommended is between 25 and 30 grams daily for adults aged 19–50 years [82]. The glycemic index (GI) is a measure of glycemic response when we consume food containing 50 grams of carbohydrates. Foods with a GI above 70, which are considered high-GI foods, spike blood glucose and insulin. Such a spike leads to insulin resistance and obesity in the long run [65]. On the other hand, the intake of low-GI foods has been related to the delayed return of hunger and slowing gastric emptying. These types of foods are known to have high fiber and to increase the secretion of the hormones ghrelin, glucagon, and cholecystokinin, which increases satiety [65].

Protein Dietary protein is necessary for the maintenance of body weight. This nutrient is known to exert higher satiating effects, which stimulate gut hormone secretion, thus limiting energy intake. The intake of protein also increases thermogenesis, which contributes to an increase in the total energy expenditure [43]. Further, a higher intake of protein favors a reduction in body fat and maintains a healthy body weight [94]. One's daily protein intake is suggested to be between 10% and 35% of one's total calories [82].

Fats Dietary fat is greatly responsible for a positive energy balance, resulting in increased total energy intake. It stimulates the hypothalamic gene, which increases calorie intake and adiposity [76]. A high-fat diet has been known to interfere with ghrelin secretion and promote abdominal fat accumulation. On the contrary, a low-fat diet reduces the fat taste threshold while increasing the fat taste sensitivity and boosting the satiety response. One's total fat intake should be between 20% and 35% of one's total calories, whereas saturated fat should be kept within the daily limit of 10% [82]. According to studies on the types of fats, replacing saturated fatty acids in the diet with polyunsaturated fatty acids lowers the risk of obesity. It aids in increasing the thermogenic effect and thus increases the total energy expenditure [17].

Healthy-Eating Approaches

Healthy-eating approaches encompass a range of strategies designed to promote overall well-being and prevent chronic diseases [11]. One fundamental aspect is maintaining a balanced diet, which includes a proper mix of macronutrients—carbohydrates, proteins, and fats—and micronutrients—vitamins and minerals. Macronutrients provide the energy required for daily activities and bodily functions, while micronutrients are essential for metabolic processes and preventing deficiencies [6]. A balanced diet ensures that individuals receive adequate amounts of these nutrients, supporting optimal physical and mental health [56]. Consuming a variety of foods from all food groups—fruits, vegetables, grains, proteins, and dairy—ensures nutrient diversity and helps prevent the risk of nutrient deficiencies or excesses that can lead to health issues.

Dietary Assessment and Meal Planning

A dietary intake assessment systematically evaluates a person's food and nutrient intake, offering insights into their eating habits and nutritional status. This process aids in designing a balanced diet that includes the right proportions of macronutrients—carbohydrates, proteins, and fats—and micronutrients—vitamins and minerals—to satisfy the body's requirements. Common methods for assessing current intake include 24-hour recall, estimated food records, and weighed food records. Nutritional assessment methods rely on dietary analysis, laboratory-biochemical data, anthropometric measurements, and clinical observations [69].

Meal planning is a crucial component of healthy eating that helps individuals manage their food intake and maintain a balanced diet. Meal planning involves preparing meals ahead of time, ensuring a consistent intake of nutritious foods and reducing the likelihood of making unhealthy food choices due to time constraints or convenience [18].

Portion control helps individuals regulate their calorie intake, preventing overeating and promoting a healthy weight. Using visual aids, such as dividing a plate into sections for different food groups, can make portion control more manageable [66].

Available Resources on Healthy Eating

Dietary guidelines provide a foundation for making informed food choices that promote health and reduce the risk of chronic diseases. These guidelines, typically issued by health organizations and governments, offer evidence-based recommendations on the types and quantities of foods to consume. They emphasize the importance of consuming a variety of nutrient-dense foods while limiting the intake of added sugars, saturated fats, and sodium. Understanding and adhering to these guidelines can help individuals make healthier food choices that align with their nutritional needs and lifestyle. For example, the Dietary Guidelines for Americans suggests focusing on whole fruits, varied vegetables, whole grains, lean proteins, and low-fat dairy products while limiting sugar-sweetened beverages and processed foods [80].

MyPlate, developed by the United States Department of Agriculture (USDA), is an example of portion control and a guide for creating balanced meals. It divides a plate into sections: half for fruits and vegetables, a quarter for grains (preferably whole grains), and a quarter for protein, with an additional serving of dairy on the side. MyPlate encourages individuals to fill half their plate with fruits and vegetables, a quarter with grains (preferably whole grains), and the remaining quarter with protein. The accompanying dairy portion highlights the importance of including low-fat or fat-free dairy products in the diet. This simple visual approach helps people easily understand and implement portion control and balanced eating in their daily lives [81] (Fig. 2.2).

> **Box 2.1**
> - Meal planning helps individuals manage their food intake, promotes balance, and reduces the temptation of making unhealthy food choices.
> - Sectioned plates can help individuals manage their calorie intake and can promote healthy weight by preventing overeating.
> - MyPlate helps individuals create balanced meals by dividing a plate into sections for fruits, vegetables, grains, protein, and dairy.

Additionally, special dietary considerations, such as food allergies, intolerances, and specific health conditions, require tailored meal plans to meet individual needs. For example, individuals with diabetes may need to closely monitor their carbohydrate intake, and those with celiac disease must avoid gluten-containing foods. Addressing these unique dietary needs is essential for maintaining health and preventing adverse reactions [81].

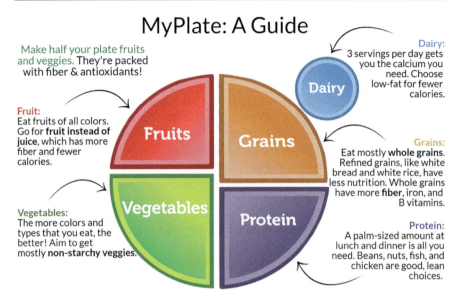

Fig. 2.2 MyPlate visual aid. (*Source*: https://www.snap4ct.org/myplate.html)

Popular Dietary Approaches

A nutritious diet is essential for overall well-being and good health. Modifying dietary habits can significantly impact health by improving various health markers. Eating healthily offers numerous benefits, including better mood, improved organ function, and a reduced risk of chronic illnesses like cancer, diabetes, and heart disease. A healthy-eating plan involves selecting foods rich in nutrients instead of those high in trans fats, added salt, and sugar, and this practice focuses on key dietary factors and their influences on health. A report by Harvard University suggests that over 160 million Americans are on a diet at any given time, spending more than USD 70 billion annually on commercial weight-loss plans, supplements, and other methods. Success in these dietary changes hinges on two key factors: first, finding a method tailored to individuals and, second, making individuals feel good and motivated [27].

The paleo, keto, and Mediterranean diets are three popular dietary approaches that emphasize different eating patterns to promote health and well-being. Each of these diets offers unique benefits and can be tailored to individual health goals and preferences.

1. The paleo diet, also known as the paleolithic diet, is based on the idea of eating like our ancient ancestors [31]. It focuses on whole foods that could be hunted or gathered, such as meat, fish, fruits, vegetables, nuts, and seeds. The diet excludes processed foods, grains, legumes, and dairy, aiming to improve health by reducing the intake of modern industrialized food products [31]. The idea of the paleolithic diet originated in the 1970s and gained significant popularity following

Loren Cordain's 2002 book *The Paleo Diet: Lose Weight and Get Healthy by Eating the Foods You Were Designed to Eat* [14]. Since its publication, the public has shown considerable interest in this diet, also known as the "caveman diet" or "Stone Age diet." The health benefits of this diet include potential weight loss, improved blood lipids, and better management of autoimmune conditions [5].

2. The keto, or ketogenic, diet is a low-carbohydrate, high-fat diet designed to put the body into a state of ketosis. In ketosis, the body burns fat for fuel instead of carbohydrates [33]. This diet involves a significant reduction in carbohydrate intake and a higher consumption of fats (compared to other diets), with moderate protein [89]. Foods commonly eaten on the keto diet include meat, fatty fish, butter, eggs, nuts, and low-carbohydrate vegetables, whereas high-carb foods like bread, pasta, and sugar are avoided [52]. The ketogenic diet, originally developed to reduce the frequency of epileptic seizures in children, has also been explored as a weight-loss method [79]. When carbohydrate intake is restricted to under 50 grams per day, the body depletes its accessible blood sugar within 3 to 4 days, subsequently breaking down protein and fat for energy in a process known as ketosis [60]. This can lead to weight loss; however, the ketogenic diet should be used as a short-term strategy to initiate weight reduction rather than as a long-term approach for overall health benefits. Health benefits may include a reduced risk of type-2 diabetes [87], improved cognitive function, and potentially therapeutic effects on epilepsy and neurodegenerative diseases [90].

3. The Mediterranean diet is inspired by the traditional eating habits of people living in the Mediterranean region. It emphasizes plant-based foods, such as fruits, vegetables, whole grains, legumes, and nuts. Olive oil is the primary source of fat, and a moderate consumption of fish, poultry, and dairy is encouraged, whereas red meat and sweets are limited [16]. The diet also promotes a balanced lifestyle that includes regular physical activity and social interactions [95]. Health benefits include a lower risk of heart disease, stroke [23], and certain cancers [50] and improved cognitive function and overall well-being [48].

Nutritional Components and Potential Challenges

Each of the paleo, keto, and Mediterranean diets offers distinct nutritional components and potential challenges for lifestyle integration and sustainability. The paleo diet emphasizes lean meats, fish, fruits, vegetables, nuts, and seeds while excluding grains, legumes, and dairy. Challenges include its restrictive nature, high costs due to quality food choices, and potential social difficulties [38]. The keto diet features high fat, moderate protein, and very low carbohydrate intake to induce ketosis, promoting rapid weight loss and improved insulin sensitivity [61]. Challenges include the initial side effects, nutrient deficiencies from limited fruit and vegetable intake, and the difficulty of long-term adherence [35]. In contrast, the Mediterranean diet focuses on plant-based foods, healthy fats like olive oil, and a moderate consumption of fish and dairy, promoting heart health and longevity. Challenges include access to fresh produce and seafood, adaptation from traditional eating habits, and varying costs. Each diet offers unique nutritional benefits and requires considering the practical challenges for sustained integration into daily life [40].

Resources and Success Stories

A case study report on one of the numerous randomized controlled trials (RCTs) is showcased in Table 2.1, reporting on multiple positive nutritional changes through a detailed and comprehensive analysis.

Table 2.1 Study trials on paleo, keto, and Mediterranean diets

Diets	Paleo	Keto	Mediterranean
Study	Benefits of a paleolithic diet with and without supervised exercise on fat mass, insulin sensitivity, and glycemic control: a randomized controlled trial in individuals with type-2 diabetes.	Very low-carbohydrate ketogenic diet vs. low-fat diet for long-term weight loss: a meta-analysis of randomized controlled trials.	The Mediterranean diet improves high-density lipoprotein function in high-cardiovascular-risk individuals: a randomized controlled trial.
Objective	To have subjects with type-2 diabetes consume a paleolithic diet for 12 weeks, with or without supervised aerobic exercise and resistance training.	To determine whether overweight and obese individuals assigned to a very low-carbohydrate ketogenic diet (VLCKD) achieve greater weight loss and manage cardiovascular risk factors more effectively.	To explore the long-term consumption of a traditional Mediterranean diets, enriched with virgin olive oil or nuts, which was able to improve different HDL functional properties.
RCT Design/ Objective	Randomized groups (paleo diet and paleo diet-exercise) were introduced to the paleolithic diet after baseline examinations and were instructed to follow the diet until all study measurements were completed.	Individuals older than 18 years who were assigned to a low-fat diet (i.e., a restricted-energy diet with less than 30% of energy from fat) or to a VLCKD (i.e., a diet with no more than 50 g carbohydrates or 10% of daily energy from carbohydrates).	A random selection of individuals with biological samples at baseline and after 1 year of dietary intervention of a Mediterranean diet enriched with nuts (Mediterranean diet with nuts; $n = 100$) and a low-fat control diet.
Results/ Takeaways	12 weeks on a paleolithic diet improved fat mass and metabolic balance, including insulin sensitivity, glycemic control, and leptin, among individuals with type-2 diabetes [59].	Individuals assigned to a VLCKD achieved greater weight loss than those assigned to a low-fat diet, in the long term [9].	Individuals adhering to a Mediterranean diet, especially when enriched with virgin olive oil, induced beneficial changes by improving HDL oxidative status and composition [28].

Resources such as ThePaleoDiet.com and DietDoctor.com provide comprehensive guides, recipes, and meal plans tailored to these diets. Books like *The Paleo Solution*, by Robb Wolf; *The Keto Diet*, by Leanne Vogel; and *The Complete Mediterranean Cookbook*, by America's Test Kitchen offer detailed insights and practical advice for adopting these lifestyles. Websites like OldwaysPT.org and MayoClinic.org are among the resources to help understand the Mediterranean diet, emphasizing its focus on plant-based foods and healthy fats.

Fad Diets

A fad diet is a popular eating regimen that promises quick results with minimal effort. These diets often become popular rapidly, typically claiming to offer a quick fix by following specific, often restrictive, eating patterns [58]. Common types of fad diets include low-carb diets like juice cleanses, detox diets, and meal-replacement shake plans, the majority of which lack scientific backing and can be nutritionally unbalanced, leading to potential health risks [58]. Additionally, the restrictive nature of fad diets can promote unhealthy relationships with food and disordered eating behaviors. Adverse effects could lead to nutrient deficiencies, muscle loss, metabolic slowdown, and the possibility of a higher likelihood of regaining lost weight in the long run [77].

Adjunct Approaches

Pharmacotherapy

Pharmacotherapy is another approach aiding in weight loss among obese patients who generally do not see any significant changes with lifestyle modification and healthy eating. Researchers talk about six medicines that have been approved by the US Food and Drug Administration (FDA) and are referred to as antiobesity medications. People who have a BMI above and equal to 30 kg/m^2 and or above and equal to 27 kg/m^2 along with comorbidities are considered eligible to get the medication, and the treatment is combined with lifestyle modification [78].

These treatments are generally known to act on the neurohormonal dysregulation that alters the hormonal response in relation to diet-induced weight loss. Those hormones are leptin and ghrelin [39]. Those medications approved by the FDA for long-term weight loss are orlistat, phentermine-topiramate, bupropion-naltrexone, liraglutide, Gelesis100, setmelanotide, and semaglutide. Orlistat acts as a lipase inhibitor, which reduces the absorption of fat from the gastrointestinal tract, whereas others decrease appetite and increase satiety.

On the other hand, the discontinuation of these medications has been found to lead to regaining the lost weight, and thus, patients are supposed to follow the treatment process lifelong [39]. Along with that, these medications may have mild-to-moderate side effects. Some of the symptoms of orlistat include fatty stool, frequent and inconsistent defecation, diarrhea, abdominal pain, and flatulence [19]. Phentermine increases acidosis and the risk of developing renal stones [22], and bupropion might cause vomiting, dizziness, nausea, insomnia, and constipation [20]. Crucially, all these cited researchers state that polypharmacotherapy can be an effective treatment to address the growing problem of obesity.

FDA-approved tirzepatide (Mounjaro and Zepbound) and semaglutide (Ozempic, Wegovy, and Rybelsus) injections are used for the management of type-2 diabetes and for weight loss. Weight-loss injections work by regulating appetite, enhancing metabolism, and promoting fat loss via interaction with the body's natural hormonal pathways.

Bariatric Surgery

Bariatric surgery has been deemed appropriate for individuals with a BMI higher than 40 kg/m^2 or a BMI between 35 and 40 along with the presence of comorbidities [21]. In the past, the surgical procedure was associated with reducing the size of the gastric pouch, which led to the malabsorption of nutrients and ultimately caused weight loss. Modern bariatric surgery is categorized into a few types of procedures. Roux-en-Y gastric bypass involves stomach transection, in which the gastric pouch with an approximate 30 mL (1-ounce) capacity is created: "The vagal trunks are not disturbed but a variable number of branches to the body of the stomach are divided in the process of dividing the stomach." The vertical sleeve gastrectomy procedure is associated with the removal of about 80% of the stomach and the creation of a tubular stomach body. Biliopancreatic diversion with duodenal switch is the anastomosis between the proximal duodenum and the bypassed intestine, resulting in impaired nutrient absorption. In addition to surgical procedures are other implantation devices, namely adjustable gastric banding and intermittent vagal blockade, that would basically constrict the size of the gastric pouch. Weight loss occurs due to reduced appetite and early satiety [74].

However, several long-term and short-term complications have been reported, which are not limited to gallstones, ventral hernias, intestinal obstruction, and ulcers. Hypoglycemia and several vitamin and mineral deficiencies have been documented so far, including iron, calcium, vitamin D, and vitamin B12 [25]. In the long term, these deficiencies lead to osteoporosis, neuropathy, xeropthalmia, and anemia [83]. Along with these health complications, patients also have an increased risk of weight regain, especially after the second year of the surgery and thereafter [73]. Researchers suggest that patients have a regular dietetic consultation to monitor weight change. Maintaining a low glycemic load with high protein and fiber intake is generally advised. Similarly, processed and refined foods are restricted, and patients are advised to focus on consuming whole grains, fruits, and vegetables [64].

Active-Living Approaches

Active-living approaches focus on integrating physical activity into daily routines to improve overall health and well-being. Regular physical activity is crucial for maintaining a healthy body weight, enhancing cardiovascular health, strengthening muscles and bones, and boosting mental health [86]. Health organizations, such as the WHO, recommend at least 150 minutes of moderate-intensity aerobic activity or 75 minutes of vigorous-intensity activity per week for adults, complemented by muscle-strengthening activities on 2 or more days a week [91]. Meeting these recommended levels of physical activity can significantly reduce the risk of chronic diseases such as heart disease, diabetes, and certain cancers.

Individuals can incorporate various types of physical activities into their lives to meet these guidelines. Aerobic exercises, such as walking, running, swimming, and

Table 2.2 Physical activity recommendations and examples obtained from the WHO and the US Department of Health and Human Services [91]

Type of activity	Examples	Recommended length of time
Moderate-Intensity Aerobic	Brisk walking, water aerobics, bicycling, dancing, gardening, recreational swimming, etc.	150–300 minutes per week
Vigorous-Intensity Aerobic	Running or jogging, swimming laps, aerobic dancing, soccer, jumping rope, etc.	75–150 minutes per week
Muscle Strengthening	Weightlifting, resistance-band exercises, yoga, climbing stairs, functional training, etc.	2 or more days per week (all major muscle groups)

cycling, are effective for improving cardiovascular health and endurance. Strength-training exercises, such as weightlifting and resistance-band workouts, help build and maintain muscle mass. Flexibility exercises, such as yoga and stretching routines, enhance one's range of motion and prevent injuries [57]. Additionally, lifestyle physical activities, such as gardening, household chores, and taking the stairs instead of the elevator, provide practical ways to integrate movement into daily routines. Adopting an active lifestyle through these diverse forms of physical activity can help individuals achieve and maintain optimal health [47, 53] (Table 2.2).

The metabolic equivalent of task (MET) measures the energy expenditure needed to perform a specific activity, where 1 MET represents the energy used while sitting at rest. This corresponds to an oxygen consumption of 3.5 milliliters per kilogram of body weight per minute [82]. Physical activities are often classified according to their intensity by using MET values. Moderate-intensity physical activity is defined, on an absolute scale, as the activity performed at 3.0 to 5.9 METs. Relative to an individual's personal capacity, it typically rates as a 5 or 6 on a scale of 0 to 10. Vigorous-intensity physical activity is defined, on an absolute scale, as any physical activity performed at 6.0 or more METs. When assessed relative to an individual's personal capacity, this level of activity typically starts at a 7 or 8 on a scale of 0 to 10 [49].

Physical activity and exercise are important for everyone; however, special considerations should be taken into account for older adults, people who are pregnant, and adults with chronic conditions such as hypertension, diabetes, or any other physical disabilities. Walking an extra kilometer, jogging, climbing stairs, and gardening are all examples of beneficial physical activities in everyday life [82].

Conclusion

The holistic management of obesity emphasizes comprehensive approaches beyond weight maintenance, addressing dietary habits, physical activity, and psychological and social factors to improve overall health. Important strategies involve habit formation and sustained behavior change, supported by personalized coaching. Embracing a holistic approach offers a sustainable path to health by integrating nutrition, activity, mental well-being, and social support. In general, the environment in which we live can increase the risk factors of obesity. Unhealthy food habits such as the frequent consumption of fast food loaded with saturated fat and high amounts of sugar contribute to obesity. On the contrary, having an open environment with ample access to community parks and sidewalks motivates people to be physically active. Studying the connections between the built environment and obesity across different age groups is crucial for gaining a better understanding of the need for long-term interventions to prevent and treat obesity. Given the role of individual, social, and environmental factors in influencing lifestyle and behavior, extensive research is required to understand the relationships and combine clinical, pharmacological, and behavior-intensive approaches to address the growing problem of obesity.

Further Practice

1. According to the WHO, which class of BMI indicates obesity?

   (a) BMI < 18.5
   (b) BMI 25–29.9
   (c) BMI of 30 or greater

2. According to the categories of BMI, if you have a BMI of 22.5, under which category do you fall?

   (a) Underweight
   (b) Normal
   (c) Overweight

3. How many kilocalories does a gram of fat provide when oxidized?

   (a) 4.1
   (b) 9.3
   (c) 6.5

4. Which lipoprotein that removes excess cholesterol from your body is called the "good" cholesterol?

   (a) High-density lipoprotein (HDL)
   (b) Low-density lipoprotein (LDL)
   (c) Very low-density lipoprotein (VLDL)

5. What does negative energy balance mean?

   (a) Energy input (calories in) > energy output (calories out)
   (b) Energy input (calories in) < energy output (calories out)
   (c) Energy input (calories in) = energy output (calories out)

6. In general, what contributes to the total calorie requirement of a person?

   (a) Resting metabolic rate
   (b) Thermogenesis
   (c) Physical activity
   (d) All of the above

7. According to the Dietary Guidelines of Americans 2020–2025, how many calories does a woman aged 31–59 years require on a daily basis?

   (a) 1800–2400 calories
   (b) 2400–3000 calories
   (c) 1600–2200 calories

8. What health condition is eligible for antiobesity medication?

   (a) BMI above and equal to 30 kg/m^2
   (b) BMI above and equal to 27 kg/m^2 with comorbidity
   (c) Both

9. What are the WHO's guidelines on physical activity and sedentary behavior for an adult?

   (a) At least 150–300 minutes of moderate-intensity aerobic activity per week
   (b) About 10–20 minutes of moderate-intensity aerobic activity per week
   (c) None

10. Which diet consists of plant-based foods, such as fruits, vegetables, whole grains, legumes, and nuts?

    (a) The ketogenic diet
    (b) The Mediterranean diet
    (c) The paleolithic diet

11. Which category of physical activity does jumping rope fall under?

    (a) Moderate-intensity aerobic
    (b) Vigorous-intensity aerobic
    (c) Muscle strengthening
    (d) None of the above

12. According to MyPlate guidelines, how should a plate be proportioned?

    (a) Half with protein, a quarter with grains, and the remaining quarter with fruits and vegetables.
    (b) Half with grains, a quarter with fruits and vegetables, and the remaining quarter with protein.
    (c) Half with fruits and vegetables, a quarter with grains, and the remaining quarter with protein.

13. How is vigorous-intensity physical activity defined in terms of METs and relative intensity?

   (a) 6.0 or more METs; 9 or 10 on a scale of 0 to 10
   (b) 3.0 to 5.9 METs; 5 or 6 on a scale of 0 to 10
   (c) 6.0 or more METs; 7 or 8 on a scale of 0 to 10

14. Which of the following BMI criteria are generally considered appropriate for bariatric surgery?

   (a) Greater than 30 kg/m^2
   (b) Greater than 35 kg/m^2
   (c) Greater than 40 kg/m^2
   (d) Greater than 25–30 kg/m^2

15. In general, what is the estimated daily calorie requirement for a woman aged 19–30 years?

   (a) 1200–1600 calories
   (b) 1800–2400 calories
   (c) 2400–3000 calories
   (d) 3000–36,000 calories

Answer Key

   1. (c)
   2. (b)
   3. (b)
   4. (a)
   5. (b)
   6. (d)
   7. (c)
   8. (c)
   9. (a)
  10. (b)
  11. (b)
  12. (c)
  13. (c)
  14. (c)
  15. (c)

References

1. Angulo P, Lindor KD. Non-alcoholic fatty liver disease. J Gastroenterol Hepatol. 2002;17:S186–90. https://doi.org/10.1046/j.1440-1746.17.s1.10.x.
2. Artunc F, Schleicher E, Weigert C, Fritsche A, Stefan N, Haring H-U. The impact of insulin resistance on the kidney and vasculature. Nat Rev Nephrol. 2016;12:721–37. https://doi.org/10.1038/nrneph.2016.145.
3. Ball K, Crawford D. Socio-economic factors in obesity: a case of slim chance in a fat world? Asia Pac J Clin Nutr. 2006;15:15–20. https://pubmed.ncbi.nlm.nih.gov/16928657/.
4. Ball K, Mishra G, Crawford D. Which aspects of socioeconomic status are related to obesity among men and women? Int J Obes. 2002;26(4):559–65. https://doi.org/10.1038/sj.ijo.0801960.
5. Ballantyne S. The paleo approach: reverse autoimmune disease and heal your body. Victory Belt Publishing; 2014.
6. Berdanier CD, Berdanier LA, Zempleni J. Advanced nutrition: macronutrients, micronutrients, and metabolism. CRC Press; 2008. https://doi.org/10.1201/9781420055559.
7. Bischoff SC, Boirie Y, Cederholm T, Chourdakis M, Cuerda C, Delzenne NM, Deutz NE, Fouque D, Genton L, Gil C, Koletzko B, Leon-Sanz M, Shamir R, Singer J, Singer P, Stroebele-Benschop N, Thorell A, Weimann A, Barazzoni R. Toward a multidisciplinary approach to understand and manage obesity and related diseases. Clin Nutr. 2017;36(4):917–38. https://doi.org/10.1016/j.clnu.2016.11.007.
8. Britton JA, Gammon MD, Kelsey JL, Brogan DJ, Coates RJ, Schoenberg JB, Potischman N, Swanson CA, Stanford JL, Brinton LA. Characteristics associated with recent recreational exercise among women 20 to 44 years of age. Women Health. 2000;31(2–3):81–96. https://doi.org/10.1300/j013v31n02_04.
9. Bueno NB, de Melo IS, de Oliveira SL, da Rocha Ataide T. Very-low-carbohydrate ketogenic diet v. low-fat diet for long-term weight loss: a meta-analysis of randomised controlled trials. Br J Nutr. 2013;110(7):1178–87. https://doi.org/10.1017/S0007114513000548.
10. Cagney KA. Neighborhood age structure and its implications for health. J Urban Health. 2006;83(5):827–34. https://doi.org/10.1007/s11524-006-9092-z.
11. Cena H, Calder PC. Defining a healthy diet: evidence for the role of contemporary dietary patterns in health and disease. Nutrients. 2020;12(2):334. https://doi.org/10.3390/nu12020334.
12. Centers for Disease Control and Prevention [CDC]. 2024. Body Mass Index (BMI). https://www.cdc.gov/healthyweight/assessing/bmi/index.html.
13. Church TS, Thomas DM, Tudor-Locke C, Katzmarzyk PT, Earnest CP, Rodarte RQ, Martin CK, Blair SN, Bouchard C. Trends over 5 decades in U.S. occupation-related physical activity and their associations with obesity. PLoS One. 2011;6(5):e19657. https://doi.org/10.1371/journal.pone.0019657.
14. Cordain L. The paleo diet revised: lose weight and get healthy by eating the foods you were designed to eat. John Wiley & Sons; 2012. https://books.google.gp/books?id=JIl19w3t8zAC&printsec=copyright#v=onepage&q&f=false.
15. Creatore MI, Glazier RH, Moineddin R, Fazli GS, Johns A, Gozdyra P, Matheson FI, Kaufman-Shriqui V, Rosella LC, Manuel DG, Booth GL. Association of neighborhood walkability with change in overweight, obesity, and diabetes. J Am Med Assoc. 2016;315(20):2211–20. https://doi.org/10.1001/jama.2016.5898.
16. Davis C, Bryan J, Hodgson J, Murphy K. Definition of the mediterranean diet: a literature review. Nutrients. 2015;7(11):9139–53. https://doi.org/10.3390/nu7115459.
17. DiNicolantonio JJ, O'Keefe JH. Good fats versus bad fats: a comparison of fatty acids in the promotion of insulin resistance, inflammation, and obesity. Mo Med. 2017;114(4):303–7. https://www.ncbi.nlm.nih.gov/pmc/articles/PMC6140086/.
18. Domingo L. How to make a meal plan, the ultimate guide. 2024. Available at: https://nutriadmin.com/blog/how-to-make-a-meal-plan/, accessed on 12 Apr 2025.
19. Elsevier. Orlistat. 2024. https://elsevier.health/en-US/preview/orlistat.

20. Food and Drug Administration [FDA]. CONTRAVE (naltrexone HCl and bupropion HCl). 2014. https://www.accessdata.fda.gov/drugsatfda_docs/label/2014/200063s000lbl.pdf.
21. Frühbeck G. Bariatric and metabolic surgery: a shift in eligibility and success criteria. Nat Rev Endocrinol. 2015;11(8):465–77. https://doi.org/10.1038/nrendo.2015.84.
22. Fujioka K. Safety and tolerability of medications approved for chronic weight management. Obesity. 2015;23(1):S7–11. https://doi.org/10.1002/oby.21094.
23. Fung TT, Rexrode KM, Mantzoros CS, Manson JE, Willett WC, Hu FB. Mediterranean diet and incidence of and mortality from coronary heart disease and stroke in women. Circulation. 2009;119(8):1093–100. https://doi.org/10.1161/CIRCULATIONAHA.108.816736.
24. Gardner CD, Trepanowski JF, Del Gobbo LC, Hauser ME, Rigdon J, Ioannidis JPA, Desai M, King AC. Effect of low-fat vs low-carbohydrate diet on 12-month weight loss in overweight adults and the association with genotype pattern or insulin secretion: the DIETFITS randomized clinical trial. J Am Med Assoc. 2018;319(7):667–79. https://doi.org/10.1001/jama.2018.0245.
25. Gletsu-Miller N, Wright BN. Mineral malnutrition following bariatric surgery. Adv Nutr. 2013;4(5):506–17. https://doi.org/10.3945/an.113.004341.
26. Hafekost K, Lawrence D, Mitrou F, O'Sullivan TA, Zubrick SR. Tackling overweight and obesity: does the public health message match the science? BMC Med. 2013;11(1):41. https://doi.org/10.1186/1741-7015-11-41.
27. Harvard Health Publishing. Diet & weight loss. 2024. https://www.health.harvard.edu/topics/diet-and-weight-loss.
28. Hernáez Á, Castañer O, Elosua R, Pintó X, Estruch R, Salas-Salvadó J, Corella D, Arós F, Serra-Majem L, Fiol M, Ortega-Calvo M, Ros E, Martínez-González MÁ, de la Torre R, López-Sabater MC, Fitó M. Mediterranean diet improves high-density lipoprotein function in high-cardiovascular-risk individuals: a randomized controlled trial. Circulation. 2017;135(7):633–43. https://doi.org/10.1161/CIRCULATIONAHA.116.023712.
29. Hill JO, Wyatt HR, Peters JC. Energy balance and obesity. Circulation. 2012;126(1):126–32. https://doi.org/10.1161/circulationaha.111.087213.
30. Hill JO, Wyatt HR, Reed GW, Peters JC. Obesity and the environment: where do we go from here? Science. 2003;299(5608):853–5. https://doi.org/10.1126/science.1079857.
31. Jew S, AbuMweis SS, Jones PJ. Evolution of the human diet: linking our ancestral diet to modern functional foods as a means of chronic disease prevention. J Med Food. 2009;12(5):925–34. https://doi.org/10.1089/jmf.2008.0268.
32. Kenchaiah S, Evans JC, Levy D, Wilson PWF, Benjamin EJ, Larson MG, Kannel WB, Vasan RS. Obesity and the risk of heart failure. N Engl J Med. 2002;347(5):305–13. https://doi.org/10.1056/NEJMoa020245.
33. Kennedy AR, Pissios P, Otu H, Roberson R, Xue B, Asakura K, Furukawa N, Marino FE, Liu FF, Kahn BB, Libermann TA, Maratos-Flier E. A high-fat, ketogenic diet induces a unique metabolic state in mice. Am J Physiol Endocrinol Metab. 2007;292(6):E1724–39. https://doi.org/10.1152/ajpendo.00717.2006.
34. Kensara OA, Wootton SA, Phillips DI, Patel M, Jackson AA, Elia M. Fetal programming of body composition: relation between birth weight and body composition measured with dual-energy X-ray absorptiometry and anthropometric methods in older Englishmen. Am J Clin Nutr. 2005;82(5):980–7. https://doi.org/10.1093/ajcn/82.5.980.
35. Kirkpatrick CF, Bolick JP, Kris-Etherton PM, Sikand G, Aspry KE, Soffer DE, Willard KE, Maki KC. Review of current evidence and clinical recommendations on the effects of low-carbohydrate and very-low-carbohydrate (including ketogenic) diets for the management of body weight and other cardiometabolic risk factors: a scientific statement from the National Lipid Association Nutrition and Lifestyle Task Force. J Clin Lipidol. 2019;13(5):689–711. https://doi.org/10.1016/j.jacl.2019.08.003.
36. Klein S, Gastaldelli A, Yki-Järvinen H, Scherer PE. Why does obesity cause diabetes? Cell Metab. 2022;34(1):11–20. https://doi.org/10.1016/j.cmet.2021.12.012.
37. Klop B, Elte JWF, Cabezas MC. Dyslipidemia in obesity: mechanisms and potential targets. Nutrients. 2013;5(4):1218–40. https://www.mdpi.com/2072-6643/5/4/1218.

38. Konner M, Eaton SB. Paleolithic nutrition: twenty-five years later. Nutr Clin Pract. 2010;25(6):594–602. https://doi.org/10.1177/0884533610385702.
39. Korner J, Aronne LJ. The emerging science of body weight regulation and its impact on obesity treatment. J Clin Invest. 2003;111(5):565–70. https://doi.org/10.1172/JCI17953.
40. Lăcătuşu CM, Grigorescu ED, Floria M, Onofriescu A, Mihai BM. The mediterranean diet: from an environment-driven food culture to an emerging medical prescription. Int J Environ Res Public Health. 2019;16(6):942. https://doi.org/10.3390/ijerph16060942.
41. Lange D, Wahrendorf M, Siegrist J, Plachta-Danielzik S, Landsberg B, Müller MJ. Associations between neighbourhood characteristics, body mass index and health-related behaviours of adolescents in the Kiel obesity prevention study: a multilevel analysis. Eur J Clin Nutr. 2011;65(6):711–9. https://doi.org/10.1038/ejcn.2011.21.
42. Lee AM, Cardel MI, Donahoo WT. Social and environmental factors influencing obesity. 2019. https://www.ncbi.nlm.nih.gov/books/NBK278977/#.
43. Lejeune MPGM, Westerterp KR, Adam TCM, Luscombe-Marsh ND, Westerterp-Plantenga MS. Ghrelin and glucagon-like peptide 1 concentrations, 24-h satiety, and energy and substrate metabolism during a high-protein diet and measured in a respiration chamber. Am J Clin Nutr. 2006;83(1):89–94. https://doi.org/10.1093/ajcn/83.1.89.
44. Li F, Harmer P, Cardinal BJ, Bosworth M, Johnson-Shelton D. Obesity and the built environment: does the density of neighborhood fast-food outlets matter? Am J Health Promot. 2009;23(3):203–9. https://doi.org/10.4278/ajhp.071214133.
45. Ludwig J, Sanbonmatsu L, Gennetian L, Adam E, Duncan GJ, Katz LF, Kessler RC, Kling JR, Lindau ST, Whitaker RC, McDade TW. Neighborhoods, obesity, and diabetes – a randomized social experiment. N Engl J Med. 2011;365(16):1509–19. https://doi.org/10.1056/NEJMsa1103216.
46. Lustig RH. The efferent arm of the energy balance regulatory pathway: neuroendocrinology and pathology. In: Donohoue PA, editor. Energy metabolism and obesity: research and clinical applications. Humana Press; 2007. p. 69–85. https://doi.org/10.1007/978-1-60327-139-4_5.
47. Machida D. Relationship between community or home gardening and health of the elderly: a web-based cross-sectional survey in Japan. Int J Environ Res Public Health. 2019;16(8):1389. https://doi.org/10.3390/ijerph16081389.
48. Martínez-Lapiscina EH, Clavero P, Toledo E, Estruch R, Salas-Salvadó J, San Julián B, Sanchez-Tainta A, Ros E, Valls-Pedret C, Martinez-Gonzalez MÁ. Mediterranean diet improves cognition: the PREDIMED-NAVARRA randomised trial. J Neurol Neurosurg Psychiatry. 2013;84(12):1318–25. https://doi.org/10.1136/jnnp-2012-304792.
49. Mendes MDA, da Silva I, Ramires V, Reichert F, Martins R, Ferreira R, Tomasi E. Metabolic equivalent of task (METs) thresholds as an indicator of physical activity intensity. PLoS One. 2018;13(7):e0200701. https://doi.org/10.1371/journal.pone.0200701.
50. Mentella MC, Scaldaferri F, Ricci C, Gasbarrini A, Miggiano GAD. Cancer and mediterranean diet: a review. Nutrients. 2019;11(9):2059. https://doi.org/10.3390/nu11092059.
51. Mizoue T, Inoue M, Wakai K, Nagata C, Shimazu T, Tsuji I, Otani T, Tanaka K, Matsuo K, Tamakoshi A, Sasazuki S, Tsugane S. Alcohol drinking and colorectal cancer in Japanese: a pooled analysis of results from five cohort studies. Am J Epidemiol. 2008;167(12):1397–406. https://doi.org/10.1093/aje/kwn073.
52. Moore J. Real food keto: applying nutritional therapy to your low-carb, high-fat diet. Victory Belt Publishing; 2018.
53. Murphy MH, Donnelly P, Breslin G, Shibli S, Nevill AM. Does doing housework keep you healthy? The contribution of domestic physical activity to meeting current recommendations for health. BMC Public Health. 2013;13:966. https://doi.org/10.1186/1471-2458-13-966.
54. Nam SY. Obesity-related digestive diseases and their pathophysiology. Gut Liver. 2017;11(3):323–34. https://doi.org/10.5009/gnl15557.
55. National Heart, Lung, and Blood Institute. Overweight and Obesity. 2024. https://www.nhlbi.nih.gov/health/overweight-and-obesity/causes.

56. National Institute of Environmental Health Sciences. Nutrition, health and your environment. 2024. https://www.niehs.nih.gov/health/topics/nutrition.
57. National Institute on Aging. Four types of exercise can improve your health and physical ability. 2024. https://www.nia.nih.gov/health/exercise-and-physical-activity/four-types-exercise-can-improve-your-health-and-physical.
58. Obert J, Pearlman M, Obert L, Chapin S. Popular weight loss strategies: a review of four weight loss techniques. Curr Gastroenterol Rep. 2017;19(12):61. https://doi.org/10.1007/s11894-017-0603-8.
59. Otten J, Stomby A, Waling M, Isaksson A, Tellström A, Lundin-Olsson L, Brage S, Ryberg M, Svensson M, Olsson T. Benefits of a Paleolithic diet with and without supervised exercise on fat mass, insulin sensitivity, and glycemic control: a randomized controlled trial in individuals with type 2 diabetes. Diabetes Metab Res Rev. 2017;33(1) https://doi.org/10.1002/dmrr.2828.
60. Paoli A, Bosco G, Camporesi EM, Mangar D. Ketosis, ketogenic diet and food intake control: a complex relationship. Front Psychol. 2015;6:104339. https://doi.org/10.3389/fpsyg.2015.00027.
61. Paoli A, Rubini A, Volek JS, Grimaldi KA. Beyond weight loss: a review of the therapeutic uses of very-low-carbohydrate (ketogenic) diets. Eur J Clin Nutr. 2013;67(8):789–96. https://doi.org/10.1038/ejcn.2013.116.
62. Papandreou D, Rousso I, Mavromichalis I. Update on non-alcoholic fatty liver disease in children. Clin Nutr. 2007;26(4):409–15. https://doi.org/10.1016/j.clnu.2007.02.002.
63. Papas M, Alberg A, Ewing R, Helzlsouer K, Gary-Webb T, Klassen A. The built environment and obesity. Epidemiol Rev. 2007;29:129–43. https://doi.org/10.1093/epirev/mxm009.
64. Pawlak DB, Ebbeling CB, Ludwig DS. Should obese patients be counselled to follow a low-glycaemic index diet? Yes. Obes Rev. 2008;3(4):235–43. https://doi.org/10.1046/j.1467-789X.2002.00079.x.
65. Radulian G, Rusu E, Dragomir A, Posea M. Metabolic effects of low glycaemic index diets. Nutr J. 2009;8(1):5. https://doi.org/10.1186/1475-2891-8-5.
66. Rolls BJ. What is the role of portion control in weight management? Int J Obes. 2014;38(1):S1–8. https://doi.org/10.1038/ijo.2014.82.
67. Sackner-Bernstein J, Kanter D, Kaul S. Dietary intervention for overweight and obese adults: comparison of low-carbohydrate and low-fat diets. A meta-analysis. PLoS One. 2015;10(10):e0139817. https://doi.org/10.1371/journal.pone.0139817.
68. Sanghera DK, Bejar C, Sharma S, Gupta R, Blackett PR. Obesity genetics and cardiometabolic health: potential for risk prediction. Diabetes Obes Metab. 2019;21(5):1088–100. https://doi.org/10.1111/dom.13641.
69. Schoeller DA, Westerterp M. Advances in the assessment of dietary intake. CRC Press; 2017. https://doi.org/10.1201/9781315152288.
70. Schwartz TL, Nihalani N, Virk S, Jindal S, Chilton M. Psychiatric medication-induced obesity: treatment options. Obes Rev. 2004;5(4):233–8. https://doi.org/10.1111/j.1467-789X.2004.00149.x.
71. Scott KM, Bruffaerts R, Simon GE, Alonso J, Angermeyer M, de Girolamo G, Demyttenaere K, Gasquet I, Haro JM, Karam E, Kessler RC, Levinson D, Medina Mora ME, Oakley Browne MA, Ormel J, Villa JP, Uda H, Von Korff M. Obesity and mental disorders in the general population: results from the world mental health surveys. Int J Obes. 2008;32(1):192–200. https://doi.org/10.1038/sj.ijo.0803701.
72. Seo MH, Lee WY, Kim SS, Kang JH, Kang JH, Kim KK, Kim BY, Kim YH, Kim WJ, Kim EM, Kim HS, Shin YA, Shin HJ, Lee KR, Lee KY, Lee SY, Lee SK, Lee JH, Lee CB, et al. 2018 Korean Society for the study of obesity guideline for the management of obesity in Korea. J Obes Metab Syndr. 2019;28(1):40–5. https://doi.org/10.7570/jomes.2019.28.1.40.
73. Shah M, Simha V, Garg A. Long-term impact of bariatric surgery on body weight, comorbidities, and nutritional status. J Clin Endocrinol Metabol. 2006;91(11):4223–31. https://doi.org/10.1210/jc.2006-0557.

74. Shikora SA, Wolfe BM, Apovian CM, Anvari M, Sarwer DB, Gibbons RD, Ikramuddin S, Miller CJ, Knudson MB, Tweden KS, Sarr MG, Billington CJ. Sustained weight loss with vagal nerve blockade but not with sham: 18-month results of the ReCharge trial. J Obes. 2015;2015(1):365604. https://doi.org/10.1155/2015/365604.

75. Stunkard AJ, Faith MS, Allison KC. Depression and obesity. Biol Psychiatry. 2003;54(3):330–7. https://doi.org/10.1016/S0006-3223(03)00608-5.

76. Subramaniam A, Landstrom M, Luu A, Hayes KC. The Nile Rat (Arvicanthis niloticus) as a superior carbohydrate-sensitive model for type 2 diabetes mellitus (T2DM). Nutrients. 2018;10(2):235. https://www.mdpi.com/2072-6643/10/2/235.

77. Tahreem A, Rakha A, Rabail R, Nazir A, Socol CT, Maerescu CM, Aadil RM. Fad diets: facts and fiction. Front Nutr. 2022;9:960922. https://doi.org/10.3389/fnut.2022.960922.

78. Tchang BG, Aras M, Kumar RB, Aronne LJ. Pharmacologic treatment of overweight and obesity in adults. Endotext [Internet]. 2021; https://www.ncbi.nlm.nih.gov/books/NBK279038/.

79. Ułamek-Kozioł M, Czuczwar SJ, Januszewski S, Pluta R. Ketogenic diet and epilepsy. Nutrients. 2019;11(10):2510. https://doi.org/10.3390/nu11102510.

80. U.S. Department of Agriculture [USDA]. Dietary Guidelines for Americans, 2020–2025. 2020. https://www.dietaryguidelines.gov/sites/default/files/2021-03/Dietary_Guidelines_for_Americans-2020-2025.pdf.

81. U.S. Department of Agriculture [USDA]. MyPlate. 2024. https://www.myplate.gov/eat-healthy/what-is-myplate.

82. U.S. Department of Health and Human Services [USDHHS]. Nutrition & Physical Activity. 2024. https://health.gov/our-work/nutrition-physical-activity/dietary-guidelines/previous-dietary-guidelines/2015/advisory-report/appendix-e-3/appendix-e-31a4.

83. von Drygalski A, Andris DA. Anemia after bariatric surgery: more than just iron deficiency. Nutr Clin Pract. 2009;24(2):217–26. https://doi.org/10.1177/0884533609332174.

84. Wakefield J. Fighting obesity through the built environment. Environ Health Perspect. 2004;112(11):A616–8. https://doi.org/10.1289/ehp.112-a616.

85. Wali JA, Solon-Biet SM, Freire T, Brandon AE. Macronutrient determinants of obesity, insulin resistance and metabolic health. Biology. 2021;10(4):336. https://doi.org/10.3390/biology10040336.

86. Warburton DE, Nicol CW, Bredin SS. Health benefits of physical activity: the evidence. Can Med Assoc J. 2006;174(6):801–9. https://doi.org/10.1503/cmaj.051351.

87. Westman EC, Tondt J, Maguire E, Yancy WS Jr. Implementing a low-carbohydrate, ketogenic diet to manage type 2 diabetes mellitus. Expert Rev Endocrinol Metab. 2018;13(5):263–72. https://doi.org/10.1080/17446651.2018.1523713.

88. Weihrauch-Blüher S, Wiegand S. Risk factors and implications of childhood obesity. Curr Obes Rep. 2018;7(4):254–9. https://doi.org/10.1007/s13679-018-0320-0.

89. Wheless JW. History of the ketogenic diet. Epilepsia. 2008;49(8):3–5. https://doi.org/10.1111/j.1528-1167.2008.01821.x.

90. Włodarek D. Role of ketogenic diets in neurodegenerative diseases (Alzheimer's disease and Parkinson's disease). Nutrients. 2019;11(1):169. https://doi.org/10.3390/nu11010169.

91. World Health Organization [WHO]. WHO guidelines on physical activity and sedentary behaviour. 2020. https://www.who.int/publications/i/item/9789240015128.

92. World Health Organization [WHO]. Obesity. 2024. https://www.who.int/health-topics/obesity#tab=tab_1.

93. World Health Organization [WHO]. Obesity and overweight. 2024. https://www.who.int/news-room/fact-sheets/detail/obesity-and-overweight.

94. Wycherley TP, Moran LJ, Clifton PM, Noakes M, Brinkworth GD. Effects of energy-restricted high-protein, low-fat compared with standard-protein, low-fat diets: a meta-analysis of randomized controlled trials123. Am J Clin Nutr. 2012;96(6):1281–98. https://doi.org/10.3945/ajcn.112.044321.

95. Yannakoulia M, Kontogianni M, Scarmeas N. Cognitive health and Mediterranean diet: just diet or lifestyle pattern? Ageing Res Rev. 2015;20:74–8. https://doi.org/10.1016/j. arr.2014.10.003.
96. Yu Z, Han S, Zhu J, Sun X, Ji C, Guo X. Pre-pregnancy body mass index in relation to infant birth weight and offspring overweight/obesity: a systematic review and meta-analysis. PLoS One. 2013;8(4):e61627. https://doi.org/10.1371/journal.pone.0061627.
97. Zhang T, Chen J, Tang X, Luo Q, Xu D, Yu B. Interaction between adipocytes and high-density lipoprotein: new insights into the mechanism of obesity-induced dyslipidemia and atherosclerosis. Lipids Health Dis. 2019;18(1):223. https://doi.org/10.1186/s12944-019-1170-9.

Metabolic Harmony: Nourishing Solutions for Managing Diabetes Mellitus Through Nutrition

3

Amal K. Mitra ⓘ and Tahniyah Haq ⓘ

Learning Objectives

After completing this chapter, you will be able to

1. Identify the different types of diabetes and understand the importance of prediabetes
2. Learn the basic concept of nutrition and apply it to formulate a diet plan
3. Be familiar with the main principles of nutrition in a patient with diabetes mellitus, including gestational diabetes mellitus
4. Understand how to modify a diet for a patient with complications from diabetes, such as chronic kidney disease

An Overview of Prediabetes, Type 1-Diabetes, Type 2-Diabetes, and Gestational Diabetes

Diabetes mellitus is a metabolic disorder. There are several etiological types of diabetes mellitus, which are discussed below.

A. K. Mitra (✉)
Department of Public Health, Julia Jones Matthews School of Population and Public Health,
Texas Tech University Health Sciences Center, Abilene, TX, USA
e-mail: amal.mitra@ttuhsc.edu

T. Haq
Department of Endocrinology, Bangladesh Medical University,
Dhaka, Bangladesh
e-mail: tahniyah81@bsmmu.edu.bd

Prediabetes

Prediabetes encompasses the terms *impaired fasting glucose* (IFG) and *impaired glucose tolerance* (IGT). It is an intermediate state between healthy glucose tolerance and diabetes mellitus (DM), which increases the risk of developing diabetes by two- to threefold [1, 2]. Because not everyone with prediabetes develops diabetes, some prefer the term *intermediate hyperglycinemia* [3]. The diagnostic criteria for prediabetes are shown in Table 3.1 [1, 3, 4].

An intensive lifestyle intervention program reduced the incidence of diabetes by 58% [5]. Therefore, all patients with prediabetes should be treated with lifestyle intervention, controlling their cardiovascular risk factors, and annual screening for diabetes mellitus. Metformin is indicated in those with body mass index > 35 kg/m^2, age < 60 years, fasting plasma glucose ≥ 6.1 mmol/l, HbA1c $\geq 6\%$, or a history of gestational diabetes mellitus, as significant benefit was seen in these groups [5].

Type 2 Diabetes Mellitus (T2DM)

T2DM is the most common type of diabetes and accounts for 90–95% of cases. It is due to insulin resistance and relative insulin deficiency. Increasing age, obesity, a lack of physical activity, family history, and being of one among several ethnicities increase the risk of developing T2DM. Most patients with this form of diabetes are obese with other cardiometabolic complications, such as hypertension or dyslipidemias. The presentation is usually asymptomatic or with microvascular or macrovascular complications. Therapy comprises oral antidiabetic medication and insulin [6]. The diagnostic criteria for diabetes mellitus are given in Table 3.2 [6].

Table 3.1 Diagnostic criteria for prediabetes according to different expert bodies

	WHO 2006	ADA 2003	IDF 2024
Venous plasma glucose (mmol/l)			
Fasting (IFG)	6.1–6.9	5.6–6.9	
1 h after 75 g glucose load (IH)	–	–	8.6–11.5
2 h after 75 g glucose load (IGT)	7.8–11.0	7.8–11.0	–
HbA1c (%)	–	5.7–6.4	–

WHO World Health Organization, *ADA* American Diabetes Association, *IDF* International Diabetic Federation, *IFG* impaired fasting glucose, *IH* intermediate hyperglycemia, and *IGT* impaired glucose tolerance

Table 3.2 Diagnostic criteria for the diagnosis of diabetes mellitus

	WHO 2006	ADA 2003
Fasting venous plasma glucose (mmol/l)	≥7	≥7
Venous plasma glucose 2 h after 75 g glucose load (mmol/l)	≥11.1	≥11.1
*HbA1c (%)	–	≥6.5

WHO World Health Organization and *ADA* American Diabetes Association
DM is diagnosed if any one of the above criteria has been met
*NGSP certified laboratory and standardized to the Diabetes Control and Complications Trial (DCCT) assay

Type 1 Diabetes Mellitus (T1DM)

T1DM accounts for 5–10% of all diabetes mellitus cases. T1DM occurs due to the destruction of pancreatic beta cells, leading to absolute inulin deficiency, mostly due to an autoimmune process. The autoimmune markers of beta cell destruction, such as islet cell autoantibodies, autoantibodies to glutamic acid decarboxylase (GAD), insulin, tyrosine phosphatases islet antigen 2 (IA-2), and zinc transporter 8 (ZnT8), are found in 85–90% of patients at the time of diagnosis. T1DM has a strong association with human leukocyte antigen (HLA), especially with the DQB and DRB genes [6].

T1DM commonly occurs in young people (<35 years) but may occur at any age. Patients are usually not obese and have unintentional weight loss and osmotic symptoms. Ketoacidosis with plasma glucose > 20 mmol/l is a common presentation. These patients are more likely to have other autoimmune diseases. Insulin is required for treatment from the beginning. However, the diagnosis may not be straightforward, especially in adults, as T1DM can occur without the classical symptoms in obese individuals, who gradually progress to insulin therapy [6]. Features differentiating between the two main types of diabetes are shown in Box 3.1.

Box 3.1: Features Differentiating Between Type 1 and Type 2 Diabetes

	Type 1 diabetes mellitus	Type 2 diabetes mellitus
Age of diagnosis	Usually children (may present in adults)	Usually adults (may occur in children, especially in obese children during puberty)
Obesity	Usually thin (but may be obese)	Usually overweight or obese
Insulin dependent	Yes	No
Risk of diabetic ketoacidosis	High	Low
Family history of diabetes	Infrequent	Frequent (> 75%)
HLA association	Present	Absent
Insulin resistance	Absent	Present
C peptide	Low	High
Autoantibodies	Present	Absent

Table 3.3 Different diagnostic criteria for GDM

Criteria	Abnormal values for diagnosis	Fasting plasma glucose	1 h after load	2 h after load	Load	Time of testing
WHO (2013)	≥ 1	5.1	10	8.5	75 g	Any time in pregnancy
*ADA (2023)	≥ 1	5.1	10	8.5	75 g	24–28 weeks
IADPSG (2010)	≥ 1	5.1	10	8.5	75 g	24–28 weeks

WHO World Health Organization, *ADA* American Diabetes Association, and *IADPSG* International Association of Diabetes and Pregnancy Study Groups
GDM is diagnosed when any one of the plasma glucose values has been met and is performed with three-step 75 g OGTT, at any time (WHO) or at 24–28 weeks of pregnancy

Gestational Diabetes Mellitus (GDM)

Hyperglycemia in pregnancy includes pre-existing or pregestational diabetes (different types of diabetes diagnosed before pregnancy) and GDM. GDM is diagnosed with a three-step 75 g oral glucose tolerance test (OGTT). The diagnosis of GDM involves multiple criteria (Table 3.3) [6]. Maternal diabetes affects all aspects of pregnancy from conception to birth. Individuals with GDM have a tenfold increased risk of developing diabetes mellitus [7].

The principles of therapy are similar to the standard treatment of diabetes mellitus—that is, diet, exercise, and pharmacotherapy. However, the target blood glucose levels are more stringent. Most individuals with GDM can achieve target glucose levels with lifestyle modification alone. Pharmacotherapy is started only when glucose targets cannot be achieved with lifestyle interventions alone. Insulin is the treatment of choice in pregnancy [8].

Meal-Planning Strategies

Food is an integral part of our lives, and a balanced diet ensures good health. Nutrition therapy is the first-line measure in the treatment of metabolic diseases. The principles and components of nutrition therapy are described below. Table 3.4 shows some commonly used definitions in nutrition.

Goals of Medical Nutrition Therapy (MNT)

Nutrition therapy is advised as part of the treatment plan of diabetes mellitus with certain goals in mind. The most important goal of nutrition therapy is to support an eating habit that promotes overall health. The diet plan should improve glycemic control, blood pressure, blood lipids, and weight. It should also address the complications of diabetes mellitus, such as preventing hypoglycemia and hyperglycemic crisis and managing sick days, gastroparesis, and cardiovascular and renal disease. The diet should be designed according to an individual's choice and needs while including the pleasure of eating. Food choices should be limited only on the basis of scientific evidence [10]. Medical nutrition therapy reduced HbA1c by 0.3–1% in T1DM and 0.5–2% in T2DM [14, 15]. Controlling hypertension and dyslipidemias reduces cardiovascular risk [16, 17]. MNT designed to treat dyslipidemias lowered serum triglyceride levels by 11–31%, LDL cholesterol by 7–22%,

Table 3.4 Some commonly used definitions in nutrition

Nutrition therapy	This is the treatment of a disease or condition through the modification of nutrient or whole-food intake [9]
Medical nutrition therapy (MNT)	This is the process by which a registered dietitian-nutritionist (RDN) tailors a meal-planning approach specific to a patient's underlying condition and includes medical, lifestyle, and personal factors [10]
Eating pattern/ food pattern	This is the totality of all foods and beverages consumed over a given period of time. Examples are Mediterranean style, DASH, and low carbohydrate [10]
Eating/meal plan/diet	This is an individualized guide to help to plan when, what, and how much to eat daily, completed by the person with diabetes and the RDN [10]
Dietary approach	This is a method or strategy to individualize a desired eating pattern and provide a practical tool(s) for developing healthy eating patterns. Examples include the plate method, carbohydrate choice, carbohydrate counting [11]
Glycemic index	This is an in vivo measure of the relative impact of carbohydrate-containing foods on blood glucose. A particular food's glycemic index is determined by evaluating the incremental rise in blood glucose after the ingestion of a portion of the test food containing 50 g of carbohydrate, compared with the same amount of carbohydrate from a reference food [12]
Glycemic load	This is the product of the glycemic index value of a food and its total carbohydrate content [13]

DASH Dietary Approach to Stop Hypertension

and total cholesterol by 7–21% [18]. The Dietary Approach to Stop Hypertension (DASH) diet reduced systolic blood pressure by 5.2 mmHg, diastolic blood pressure by 2.6 mm Hg, total cholesterol by 0.20 mmol/l, and overall cardiovascular risk by 13% [19].

Components of MNT

A proper meal plan encompasses not only quantity but also quality and eating patterns. For these reasons, MNT has five components: a daily calorie requirement, the nutritional content of food, the timing and consistency of meals, and weight management strategies [10].

Daily Calorie Requirement
The basal metabolic rate can be calculated by using age, sex, height, and weight. Several formulas can be used to calculate the calories needed to maintain body weight. One such formula is given below [20].

$$662 - \left(9.53 \times age\left[year\right]\right) + physical\ activity\ coefficient$$
$$\times \left(15.91 \times weight\left[kg\right] + 539.6 \times height\left[m\right]\right) for\ men\ 354 - \left(6.91 \times age\left[year\right]\right)$$
$$+ physical\ activity\ coefficient \times \left(9.36 \times weight\left[kg\right] + 726 \times height\left[m\right]\right) for\ women$$

Physical activity coefficients for men are 1 (sedentary), 1.11 (low active), 1.25 (active), and 1.48 (very active). Those for women are 1 (sedentary), 1.12 (low active), 1.27 (active), and 1.45 (very active).

Example 3.1 Calculate the daily calorie requirement of a 42-year-old woman with a sedentary lifestyle. Her height is 1.52 m, and her weight is 60 kg.

$$354 - \left(6.91 \times 42\right) + 1 \times \left(9.36 \times 60 + 726 \times 1.52\right)$$
$$= 354 - \left(290.22\right) + 1 \times \left(561.6 + 1103.52\right)$$
$$= 354 - \left(290.22\right) + 1 \times \left(1665.12\right)$$
$$= 354 - \left(290.22\right) + 1665.12$$
$$= 1728.9\ kcal\ /\ day$$

Another simple working formula to calculate daily energy needs is

$$15\ kcal\ /\ lb\left(men\right) 13\ kcal\ /\ lb\left(women\right)$$

Nutritional Composition
There is no ideal portion of calories from carbohydrates, protein, or fat in diabetes mellitus. Therefore, macronutrients should be allocated on the basis of normal dietary guidelines, eating preferences, culture, and individualized health goals [10]. Although the amount of food consumed is important, emphasis has more recently

been placed on the quality of food as well. The carbohydrate content of a meal primarily determines the postprandial glucose response. Whole grains decrease post-meal blood glucose levels. Therefore, whole grains determine the quality of carbohydrates and should be consumed from natural sources [21]. Table 3.5 shows the daily recommended amounts and sources of nutrients for individuals with diabetes mellitus, which are based on various studies looking at the effects of food on health [10].

Eating Patterns

The Mediterranean diet emphasizes consuming vegetables, seafood, and olive oil as the main source of carbohydrate, protein, and fat, respectively. The DASH diet consists primarily of vegetables and fruits with no saturated fat, sugar, or sodium. The low-carbohydrate and very low-carbohydrate diets consist of 26–45% and < 26% of total calories derived from carbohydrate, respectively. In the low-fat and very

Table 3.5 Recommended amount and source of macronutrients

Type of nutrient	Recommended daily intake	Dietary source
Carbohydrate	45% of total calories	Vegetables, legumes, fruit, dairy (milk, yogurt), whole grains
Protein	15–20% of total calories	Animal: dairy products (milk, cheese, yogurt), eggs, meat, poultry, seafood (fish, shellfish) Plant based: legumes, nuts, tofu, seeds
Fat	< 30% of total calories	
Monounsaturated fatty acid	No limit	Canola, peanuts, olive oils, avocados, nuts (almonds, hazelnuts, pecans), seeds (pumpkin, sesame seeds)
Saturated fatty acid	< 10% of total calories	Whole milk, butter, cheese, ice cream, red meat, chocolate, coconut, coconut milk, coconut oil, palm oil
Trans fatty acid	< 1% of total calories	Some margarines, partially hydrogenated vegetable oil, deep-fried foods, fast foods, commercial baked goods, dairy products, beef, lamb
Cholesterol	300 mg/day 200 mg/day (for patients with high cardiovascular risk)	Egg, chicken, beef, lamb, cheese
Dietary fiber	Minimum 14 g/1000 kcal	Whole grains, nonstarchy vegetables, avocados, fruits, pulses (beans, peas, lentils), nuts
Salt **Sodium**	< 6 g/day < 2.3 g/day	

Boldface indicates an overarching category

low-fat diets, the total calories consumed from fat are ≤ 30% and ≤ 10%, respectively [10]. Although no clear recommendation has been reached on a specific eating pattern for diabetes mellitus, a network meta-analysis of 42 randomized controlled trials showed that the ketogenic, Mediterranean, moderate-carbohydrate, and low-glycemic-index diets were effective in improving HbA1c in individuals with diabetes [22].

The Dietary Approach

The Plate Model
This has replaced the food guide pyramids set by the Dietary Guidelines for Americans in 2011. In this model, a 9-inch plate is divided in to three parts, such that half contains vegetables or fruits, one-quarter contains lean meat, and one-quarter contains whole grains (Fig. 3.1). It is accompanied by a glass of low-fat milk. The plate model is an easy way to visually demonstrate meal planning and portion size [23].

Carbohydrate Counting
This is a simple tool that allows us to monitor the amount of carbohydrates consumed. Each unit or serving of carbohydrate equals 15 grams of carbohydrate. An average of 3–4 units (women) and 4–5 units (men) of carbohydrates are allocated for each meal. However, this may vary depending on obesity, pregnancy, and the

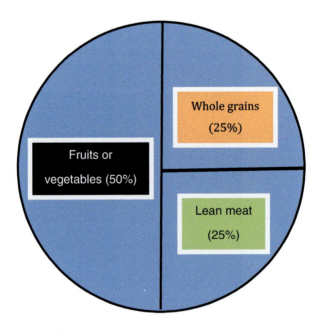

Fig. 3.1 The plate model

level of physical activity [24]. Carbohydrate counting is a simple method that helps individuals with diabetes to estimate mealtime insulin doses and thus improve their blood glucose control [25].

Exchange List Approach

This was designed by the American Diabetes Association and the Academy of Nutrition and Dietetics in 1950. Food is divided into three main categories: carbohydrates, protein, and fat. Each group contains a list of foods, each having the same calorie content (Table 3.6). Therefore, food can be exchanged within each group while maintaining the same number of calories. This allows more flexibility and diversity in meal planning [26]. Figure 3.2 shows some of the foods that can be consumed freely, those that can be consumed in moderation, and those that should be avoided.

Table 3.6 Exchange list of common nutrients

	Size of one serving	Amount of macronutrient
		Carbohydrate
Cereal, grain, pasta (cooked)	1/2 cup	15 g
Bread product	1 ounce	
Rice (white or brown cooked)	1/3 cup	
		Protein
Meat (chicken, beef, pork)	1 ounce	7 g
Fish (fresh, frozen)	1 ounce	
Milk (whole)	1 cup	
Egg white	3	
Cheese	1/4 cup	

1 cup = 125 ml

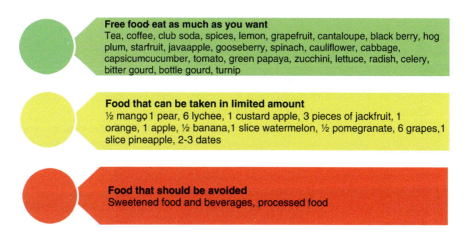

Fig. 3.2 A guide to which foods are acceptable in diabetes mellitus

Dietary Guidelines for Type 1 Diabetes, Type 2 Diabetes, and Gestational Diabetes Mellitus

Diet plays an integral part in the management of diabetes mellitus. The nutritional management of diabetes mellitus is aimed not only at achieving glycemic control but also at addressing the comorbidities and complications associated with the condition. Meal planning should be tailored to an individual's condition, preference, culture, availability, and cost. The main aspects of nutrition therapy in diabetes are shown in Box 3.2.

Box 3.2: Highlights of Dietary Recommendation for Diabetes Mellitus
- There is no specific eating pattern for diabetes mellitus.
- The diet in diabetes mellitus should be individualized.
- Both the quantity and the quality of food are important.
- Individuals with diabetes mellitus should consume food rich in dietary fibers.
- Food rich in sugar, salt, and saturated fat should be restricted.
- Meals/snacks should be evenly spaced throughout the day, such as every 3 h.
- The diet should be consistent from day to day.
- Medical nutrition therapy should be provided by a registered dietician-nutritionist.

Recommendations of Medical Nutrition Therapy (MNT) for T2DM

Certain recommendations are made for nutrition therapy in diabetes mellitus to achieve the treatment goals of medical nutrition therapy [10, 27]. The main focus in T2DM is the caloric content of food for the prevention of obesity.

1. Medical nutrition therapy should be provided by a registered dietician-nutritionist (RDN), preferably one who is experienced in diabetes care. The individual with diabetes should visit an RDN at diagnosis, three to six times in the first 6 months of diagnosis, once every year thereafter, and during times of change or upon the development of complications [28].
2. There is no specific eating pattern or eating plan for diabetes mellitus. Diet should therefore be based on principles of healthy nutrition, individual preferences, and treatment goals.
3. The overall theme is to increase the consumption of dietary fiber and reduce the consumption of refined and processed food rich in sugar, salt, and saturated fat.
4. A reduction in the total carbohydrate content has been shown to improve glycemic control.
5. High fiber sources of carbohydrate are preferred.

6. Water and low-/zero-calorie beverages should replace sugar-sweetened beverages.
7. Processed food with added sugar should be avoided.
8. Individuals should be aware of the glycemic impact of carbohydrates because it affects postprandial blood glucose levels.
9. The diet should be consistent from day to day .
10. The timing of meals should match fixed insulin regimens to avoid hypoglycemia. Three meals and three snacks every 3 h is a good option.
11. Protein-rich sources of carbohydrate should not be used in the treatment of hypoglycemia, because amino acids stimulate the release of insulin without increasing blood glucose levels.
12. Foods rich in monounsaturated, polyunsaturated, and long-chain fatty acids are preferred over foods containing saturated fatty acid because they improve the lipid profile and reduce cardiovascular risk.
13. Dietary supplementation with vitamins, minerals, herbs, and spices do not confer any glycemic or cardiovascular benefit and should not be taken.
14. Salt consumption should be limited.
15. Only a moderate use of non-nutritive sweeteners is acceptable to reduce calorie and sugar content.
16. Overweight and obese individuals should aim for a 5% reduction in body weight.

Example 3.2

A typical diet plan for a patient with diabetes mellitus requiring 1600 calories per day.

Breakfast	3 small slices of bread
	1 egg
	Any number of vegetables
Mid-morning snack	2 cups of puffed rice/1 cup of cereal/4 biscuits
Lunch	2¼ cups of rice/2¼ cups of pasta/4 slices of bread
	2 pieces of fish or meat
	Any number of vegetables
	½ cup of pulses
Evening snack	2 cups of puffed rice/1 cup of cereal/4 biscuits
Dinner	1½ cups of rice/1½ cups of pasta/3 slices of bread
	2 pieces of fish or meat
	Any number of vegetables
	½ cup of pulses
At bedtime	1 glass of milk

Amount of cooking oil = 20 ml

Recommendations of Medical Nutrition Therapy (MNT) for T1DM [10, 28]

The goal for type 1 diabetes is to achieve glycemic control without hypoglycemia. Therefore, consistency in timing and the amount of food eaten is vital [27]. Below are some recommendations.

1. The carbohydrate-counting approach is a recommended option for patients with T1DM because it improves glycemic control.
2. Carbohydrate counting cannot be used when mixed meals containing all three macronutrients are consumed. In that case, the insulin dose should be adjusted by monitoring blood glucose levels, either via a finger prick or continuous glucose monitoring.
3. The timing of meals is also important, especially if a fixed insulin regimen is prescribed. The timing of meals should match the type and regimen of insulin to reduce the risk of hypoglycemia.
4. Obesity worsens insulin resistance, glycemic control, and microvascular and macrovascular complications in T1DM. Furthermore, 50% of individuals with T1DM are now obese. Therefore, weight loss is recommended for overweight and obese individuals with T1DM.

Recommendations of Medical Nutrition Therapy (MNT) for GDM

MNT is the cornerstone in the management of GDM. The diet should be designed to achieve normoglycemia and to promote optimum gestational weight gain and fetal well-being. A diet plan should be provided by an RDN at diagnosis and reviewed in each trimester [29]. The calorie and nutrient requirements in GDM are similar to those of pregnant women with healthy glucose tolerance. The main emphasis in GDM is on the consumption of small-to-medium-size meals distributed throughout the day to maintain normoglycemia and avoid ketosis or hypoglycemia. Because carbohydrates are the main determinant of postprandial glucose levels, special attention should be paid to the type and amount of carbohydrate consumed. Nutrient-dense, high-quality carbohydrate is preferred over blunt postprandial glucose levels [29].

1. An ideal meal plan is three meals and three snacks. A bedtime snack should be encouraged to avoid fasting hypoglycemia and ketosis [29].
2. The calorie requirement depends on prepregnancy body weight and trimester (Table 3.7). It is the same as for women without GDM. For those of a healthy weight, the calorie requirement in the first trimester is the same as that before pregnancy. Calories should be increased by 340 and 452 cal/day in the second

Table 3.7 Recommended weight gain and calorie allocation in gestational diabetes mellitus

Prepregnancy BMI category	Weight gain (kg)	Calories (kcal/kg/day)	
		First trimester	Second and third trimester
Underweight	12.5–18	35	40
Healthy weight	11.5–16	30	35
Overweight	7–11.5	25	30
Obese	5–9	30% calorie restriction	

BMI body mass index

    and third trimester, respectively. In case of obesity, total calories should be restricted by 30% [30].
3. The daily recommended dietary reference intake of carbohydrate, protein, and fiber in pregnancy is 175 g, 71 g, and 28 g, respectively. Fat should be < 40% and saturated fat < 7% of total calories [31]. Diet should not include simple carbohydrates such as sweets or food rich in saturated fat.

Special Consideration for Diabetes and Coexisting Conditions

Diabetes mellitus is associated with several comorbidities and complications. Diet may need to be adjusted depending on these complications. Box 3.3 highlights the main considerations in such cases.

Box 3.3: Importance of Diet in Comorbidities Associated with Diabetes Mellitus
- A reduction in food rich in saturated fat and an increase in the consumption of food rich in unsaturated fat are recommended in patients with dyslipidemia.
- Limited salt consumption is recommended to control hypertension.
- A low-calorie balanced diet is recommended in cases of obesity.
- Small portions should be taken when patients experience gastroparesis.
- In cases of chronic kidney disease, protein requirement is the same as the daily recommended amount for healthy individuals.

Cardiovascular Diseases

A reduction in food rich in saturated fatty acid and an increase in the consumption of food rich in unsaturated fatty acid (e.g., eating fatty fish at least twice a week) reduce total and low-density lipoprotein cholesterol (LDL-C). Foods low in carbohydrate and high in fat improve glycaemia, triglycerides, and high-density lipoprotein cholesterol (HDL-C). This improvement in blood lipids confers an overall cardiovascular benefit. Consuming < 6 g/day of salt or < 2300 mg/day of sodium lowers blood pressure [10, 27].

Obesity

Weight loss confers a cardiometabolic benefit and improves quality of life. At least 5% weight loss is recommended for clinical benefit in diabetes patients with overweight or obesity [10]. Moreover, 7–10% weight loss delays the progression of prediabetes to diabetes [5]. Weight loss of 5–10% reduces HbA1c by 0.6% to 1%. Recent evidence suggests that 10–15% weight loss can lead to remission in type 2 diabetes [32]. The main determinants of a successful weight loss diet plan are calorie content and dietary adherence. Nutrient composition and eating pattern do not affect weight [33, 34]. The recommendation is to consume a balanced low-calorie diet. An overall reduction of 500 cal/day will lead to sustained weight loss. The diet should include five portions of fruit and vegetables a day. All high-calorie or sugar-containing beverages and processed foods containing sugar and saturated fat should be avoided. Other pieces of dietary advice that help reduce weight are portion control and self-monitoring. Adopting a healthy eating habit that can be followed for a long time increases adherence to maintaining weight loss [35].

Example 3.3

A typical meal plan of 1600 calories per day for an obese adult with diabetes mellitus

Breakfast	3 small slices of bread 1 egg Any number of vegetables
Mid-morning snack	Fruits (1 apple/pear/nashpati)/1 cup vegetable soup/mixed green salad/1 cup puffed rice/1 cup noodles/2–3 salty biscuits/1 cup cornflakes
Lunch	2¼ cups of rice 2 pieces of fish or meat Any number of vegetables ½ cup of lentil soup (dal)
Evening snack	Fruits (1 apple/pear/nashpati)/1 cup vegetable soup/mixed green salad/1 cup puffed rice/1 cup noodles/2–3 salty biscuits/1 cup cornflakes
Dinner	1½ cups of rice 2 pieces of fish or meat Any number of vegetables ½ cup of lentil soup (dal)

One glass of skimmed milk along with the above food

Gastroparesis

Consuming small amounts of food at each meal may help improve the symptoms of gastroparesis. Hyperglycemia causes delayed gastric emptying and should be corrected [10, 27].

Table 3.8 Recommended calories and nutrition for patients with chronic kidney disease

Type of nutrient	Recommended daily intake	Comments
Carbohydrate	30–35 kcal/kg/day	Should maintain a healthy BMI
Protein	0.8 g/kg/day 1–1.2 g/kg/day (preferably plant source)	For those not on dialysis For those on dialysis
Fat	< 30% of total calories	
Saturated fat	< 10% of total calories	
Sodium	< 2.3 g/day < 2 g/day	With hypertension/fluid overload/proteinuria
Potassium	Restricted	When eGFR < 30 ml/min/1.73 m²
Calcium	1000 mg/day	Not more than 500 mg from supplements
Phosphorus	0.8–1 g/day	Avoid highly processed food
Dietary fiber	25–38 g/day	

BMI body mass index and *eGFR* estimated glomerular filtration rate

Chronic Kidney Disease (CKD)

Individuals with CKD do not need to restrict their protein intake to less than the recommended amount, because this does not confer any benefit. However, protein intake > 1.3 g/kg body weight/day worsens albuminuria, renal function, and cardiovascular mortality [36]. Therefore, the recommended amount of protein in individuals with non-dialysis-dependent CKD is the recommended daily allowance [37]. However, this amount is increased in those on dialysis because protein energy malnutrition is a major problem in this group [38]. Table 3.8 shows the recommended nutrition for patients with CKD when their glomerular filtration rate (eGFR) is < 60 ml/min/1.73 m² [36].

Further Practice

1. Which of the following 2-h postglucose load plasma glucose value meets the diagnostic criteria for impaired glucose tolerance (IGT)?

   (a) 8.6 mmol/l
   (b) 7.9 mmol/l
   (c) 7.8 mmol/l
   (d) 6.1 mmol/l

2. How many components are in medical nutrition therapy?

   (a) 3
   (b) 5
   (c) 4
   (d) 7

3. The daily calorie requirement depends on

   (a) The basal metabolic rate and physical activity
   (b) Only the basal metabolic rate
   (c) Only physical activity
   (d) Body fat percentage

4. The postprandial glucose response is primarily due to

   (a) The protein content of food
   (b) The fat content of food
   (c) The carbohydrate content of food
   (d) Dietary fiber

5. The daily recommended amount of saturated fat in the diet should not exceed

   (a) 10% of total daily calories
   (b) 30% of total daily calories
   (c) 1% of total daily calories
   (d) 15% of total daily calories

6. The daily recommended amount of salt in the diet should not exceed

   (a) 6 g/day
   (b) 5 g/day
   (c) 2.3 g/day
   (d) 1.5 g/day

7. Which of the following statements is true?

   (a) There is no specific recommended eating pattern for diabetes mellitus.
   (b) The Mediterranean eating pattern is recommended for diabetes mellitus.
   (c) The DASH diet is recommended for diabetes mellitus.
   (d) A moderate-carbohydrate and low-glycemic-index diet is recommended for diabetes mellitus.

8. Which nutrient determines the quality of carbohydrates?

   (a) The amount of polysaccharides
   (b) The amount of monosaccharides
   (c) The amount of dietary fiber
   (d) The amount of sugar

9. Which of the following statements is true?

   (a) Dietary supplementation with vitamins and minerals confers a cardiometabolic benefit.
   (b) Foods rich in unsaturated fatty acid are preferred.

(c) Foods rich in saturated fatty acid are preferred.

(d) Artificially sweetened beverages should replace sugar-sweetened beverages.

10. Carbohydrates in a diabetic diet for a type 1 diabetes mellitus are

   (a) Divided into three meals and three snacks
   (b) Coordinated with the insulin schedule
   (c) a and b
   (d) Are consumed in a fixed ratio

11. The diet in gestational diabetes mellitus should

   (a) Consist of small-to-medium-size meals
   (b) Be distributed throughout the day
   (c) Be designed to prevent hypoglycemia
   (d) All of the above

12. The recommendation for weight loss is to

   (a) Emphasize nutrient composition
   (b) Emphasize eating patterns
   (c) Consume a balanced low-calorie diet
   (d) All of the above

13. The recommended protein intake in a patient with chronic kidney disease (CKD) is

   (a) 0.8 g/kg/day
   (b) 1.8 g/kg/day
   (c) 0.6 g/kg/day
   (d) None of the above

14. 7 g of protein is present in

   (a) 1 ounce of chicken
   (b) 1 cup of milk
   (c) Three egg whites
   (d) All of the above

15. Type 1 diabetes mellitus (T1DM) is characterized by

   (a) Autoantibodies
   (b) Insulin resistance
   (c) Low C peptide
   (d) a and c

Answer Key

1. (c)
2. (b)
3. (a)
4. (c)
5. (a)
6. (a)
7. (a)
8. (c)
9. (a)
10. (c)
11. (d)
12. (c)
13. (a)
14. (d)
15. (d)

References

1. Expert Committee on the Diagnosis and Classification of Diabetes Mellitus. Report of the expert committee on the diagnosis and classification of diabetes mellitus. Diabetes Care. 2003;26(Suppl 1):S5–20. https://doi.org/10.2337/diacare.26.2007.s5. PMID: 12502614.
2. Zhang X, Gregg EW, Williamson DF, Barker LE, Thomas W, Bullard KM, Imperatore G, Williams DE, Albright AL. A1C level and future risk of diabetes: a systematic review. Diabetes Care. 2010;33(7):1665–73. https://doi.org/10.2337/dc09-1939. PMID: 20587727; PMCID: PMC2890379.
3. World Health Organization (WHO) Consultation. Definition and diagnosis of diabetes mellitus and intermediate hyperglycemia. Geneva: WHO; 2006.
4. Bergman M, Manco M, Satman I, Chan J, Inês Schmidt M, Sesti G, et al. International diabetes federation position statement on the 1-hour post-load plasma glucose for the diagnosis of intermediate hyperglycaemia and type 2 diabetes. Diabetes Res Clin Pract. 2024;209:111589. https://doi.org/10.1016/j.diabres.2024.111589. Epub 2024 Mar 7. PMID: 38458916.
5. ElSayed NA, Aleppo G, Aroda VR, et al. On behalf of the American Diabetes Association. 3. Prevention or delay of type 2 diabetes and associated comorbidities: standards of care in diabetes–2023. Diabetes Care. 2023;46(suppl 1):S41–8. https://doi.org/10.2337/dc23-S003.
6. American Diabetes Association. Diagnosis and classification of diabetes mellitus. Diabetes Care. 2014;37(Supplement_1):S81–90. https://doi.org/10.2337/dc14-S081.
7. Vounzoulaki E, Khunti K, Abner SC, Tan BK, Davies MJ, Gillies CL. Progression to type 2 diabetes in women with a known history of gestational diabetes: systematic review and meta-analysis. BMJ. 2020;369:m1361. https://doi.org/10.1136/bmj.m1361. PMID: 32404325; PMCID: PMC7218708.
8. Society of Maternal-Fetal Medicine (SMFM) Publications Committee. Electronic address: pubs@smfm.org. SMFM statement: pharmacological treatment of gestational diabetes. Am J Obstet Gynecol. 2018;218(5):B2–4. https://doi.org/10.1016/j.ajog.2018.01.041. Epub 2018 Feb 2. PMID: 29409848.

9. Institute of Medicine. The Role of Nutrition in Maintaining Health in the Nation's Elderly: Evaluating Coverage of Nutrition Services for the Medicare Population [Internet], 1999. Available from https://www.nap.edu/catalog/9741/therole-of-nutrition-in-maintaining-health-in-thenations-elderly. Accessed 20 Mar 2024.

10. Evert AB, Dennison M, Gardner CD, Garvey WT, Lau KHK, MacLeod J, et al. Nutrition therapy for adults with diabetes or prediabetes: a consensus report. Diabetes Care. 2019;42(5):731–54. https://doi.org/10.2337/dci19-0014. Epub 2019 Apr 18. PMID: 31000505; PMCID: PMC7011201.

11. Salvia MG, Quatromoni PA. Behavioral approaches to nutrition and eating patterns for managing type 2 diabetes: a review. Am J Med Open. 2023;9:100034.

12. Jenkins DJ, Wolever TM, Taylor RH, Barker H, Fielden H, Baldwin JM, et al. Glycemic index of foods: a physiological basis for carbohydrate exchange. Am J Clin Nutr. 1981;34(3):362–6. https://doi.org/10.1093/ajcn/34.3.362. PMID: 6259925.

13. Liu S, Willett WC, Stampfer MJ, Hu FB, Franz M, Sampson L, et al. A prospective study of dietary glycemic load, carbohydrate intake, and risk of coronary heart disease in US women. Am J Clin Nutr. 2000;71(6):1455–61. https://doi.org/10.1093/ajcn/71.6.1455. PMID: 10837285.

14. Kulkarni K, Castle GA, Gregory R, Holmes A, Leontos C, Powers M, et al. Nutrition practice guidelines for type 1 diabetes mellitus positively affect dietitian practices and patient outcomes. J Am Diet Assoc. 1998;98(1):62–70.

15. Franz MJ, Monk A, Barry B, McCLAIN KA, Weaver T, Cooper N, et al. Effectiveness of medical nutrition therapy provided by dietitians in the management of non–insulin-dependent diabetes mellitus: a randomized, controlled clinical trial. J Am Diet Assoc. 1995;95(9):1009–17.

16. Chobanian AV, Bakris GL, Black HR, et al. The seventh report of the joint National Committee on prevention, detection, evaluation, and treatment of high blood pressure: the JNC 7 report. JAMA. 2003;289(19):2560–71. https://doi.org/10.1001/jama.289.19.2560.

17. Kearney PM, Blackwell L, Collins R, Keech A, Simes J, Peto R, et al. Efficacy of cholesterol-lowering therapy in 18,686 people with diabetes in 14 randomised trials of statins: a meta-analysis. Lancet (London, England). 2008;371(9607):117–25.

18. Academy of Nutrition and Dietetics. Disorders of lipid metabolism [Internet], 2010. Evidence Analysis Library. Available from http://andevidencelibrary.com/topic.cfm?cat=3582&auth=1. Accessed 20 Mar 2024.

19. Siervo M, Lara J, Chowdhury S, Ashor A, Oggioni C, Mathers JC. Effects of the Dietary Approach to Stop Hypertension (DASH) diet on cardiovascular risk factors: a systematic review and meta-analysis. Br J Nutr. 2015;113(1):1–15. https://doi.org/10.1017/S0007114514003341.

20. Escott-Stump S. Nutrition and Diagnosis-Related Care. 5th ed. Hagerstown, MD: Lippincott Williams & Wilkins; 2002.

21. Reynolds A, Mann J. Update on nutrition in diabetes management. Med Clin North Am. 2022;106(5):865–79. https://doi.org/10.1016/j.mcna.2022.03.003. Epub 2022 Aug 26. PMID: 36154705.

22. Jing T, Zhang S, Bai M, Chen Z, Gao S, Li S, Zhang J. Effect of dietary approaches on glycemic control in patients with type 2 diabetes: a systematic review with network meta-analysis of randomized trials. Nutrients. 2023;15(14):3156. https://doi.org/10.3390/nu15143156. PMID: 37513574; PMCID: PMC10384204.

23. U.S. Department of Agriculture. Learn how to eat healthy with MyPlate. Available at: https://www.choosemyplate.gov, accessed on 15 Mar 2024.

24. Diabetes Care and Education, Ready, Set Start Counting! Carbohydrate Counting – a Tool to Help Manage Your Blood Glucose. Diabetes Care and Education, a dietetic practice group of the Academy of Nutrition and Dietetics 2016.

25. Warshaw HS, Kulkarni K. Complete Guide to Carb Counting, 3rd ed.

26. Choose Your Foods: Food Lists for Diabetes; 2014 Academy of Nutrition and Dietetics, American Diabetes Association.

27. American Diabetes Association Professional Practice Committee. 5. Facilitating positive health behaviors and Well-being to improve health outcomes: standards of Care in Diabetes—2024. Diabetes Care. 2024;47(Supplement_1):S77–S110. https://doi.org/10.2337/dc24-S005.

28. Franz MJ, MacLeod J, Evert A, et al. Academy of nutrition and dietetics nutrition practice guideline for type 1 and type 2 diabetes in adults: systematic review of evidence for medical nutrition therapy effectiveness and recommendations for integration into the nutrition care process. J Acad Nutr Diet. 2017;117:1659–79.

29. American Diabetes Association Professional Practice Committee. 15. Management of diabetes in pregnancy: standards of Care in Diabetes-2024. Diabetes Care. 2024;47(Suppl 1):S282–94. https://doi.org/10.2337/dc24-S015. PMID: 38078583; PMCID: PMC10725801.

30. Weight Gain During Pregnancy: Reexamining the Guidelines, Institute of Medicine (US) and National Research Council (US) Committee to Reexamine IOM Pregnancy Weight Guidelines. (Ed), National Academies Press (US); 2009.

31. Dietary reference intakes: the essential guide to nutrient requirements. The National Academies Press; 2006.

32. Churuangsuk C, Hall J, Reynolds A, et al. Diets for weight management in adults with type 2 diabetes: an umbrella review of published meta-analyses and systematic review of trials of diets for diabetes remission. Diabetologia. 2022;65:14–36. https://doi.org/10.1007/s00125-021-05577-2.

33. Johnston BC, Kanters S, Bandayrel K, et al. Comparison of weight loss among named diet programs in overweight and obese adults: a meta-analysis. JAMA. 2014;312:923–33.

34. Del Corral P, Chandler-Laney PC, Casazza K, Gower BA, Hunter GR. Effect of dietary adherence with or without exercise on weight loss: a mechanistic approach to a global problem. J Clin Endocrinol Metab. 2009;94(5):1602–7. https://doi.org/10.1210/jc.2008-1057. Epub 2009 Mar 3. PMID: 19258409; PMCID: PMC2684471.

35. Garvey WT, Mechanick JI, Brett EM, Garber AJ, Hurley DL, Jastreboff AM, et al. Reviewers of the AACE/ACE obesity clinical practice guidelines. American Association of Clinical Endocrinologists and American college of endocrinology comprehensive clinical practice guidelines for medical care of patients with obesity. Endocr Pract. 2016;22(Suppl 3):1–203. https://doi.org/10.4158/EP161365.GL. Epub 2016 May 24. PMID: 27219496.

36. Klahr S, Levey AS, Beck GJ, Caggiula AW, Hunsicker L, Kusek JW, Striker G. The effects of dietary protein restriction and blood-pressure control on the progression of chronic renal disease. Modification of Diet in Renal Disease Study Group. N Engl J Med. 1994;330(13):877–84. https://doi.org/10.1056/NEJM199403313301301. PMID: 8114857.

37. de Boer IH, Khunti K, Sadusky T, Tuttle KR, Neumiller JJ, Rhee CM, et al. Diabetes management in chronic kidney disease: a consensus report by the American Diabetes Association (ADA) and kidney disease: improving global outcomes (KDIGO). Diabetes Care. 2022;45(12):3075–90. https://doi.org/10.2337/dci22-0027. PMID: 36189689; PMCID: PMC9870667.

38. Murray DP, Young L, Waller J, Wright S, Colombo R, Baer S, et al. Is dietary protein intake predictive of 1-year mortality in dialysis patients? Am J Med Sci. 2018;356(3):234–43. https://doi.org/10.1016/j.amjms.2018.06.010. Epub 2018 Jun 19. PMID: 30286818.

Navigating Nutritional Challenges and Applying Implementation Science and Practice in Kidney Diseases and Transplantation

4

Ekamol Tantisattamo ⓘ and Kamyar Kalantar-Zadeh ⓘ

Learning Objectives

After completing this chapter, you will be able to

1. Understand the pathophysiology of diet-related kidney function and dysfunction, especially from high dietary protein and sodium intakes and higher animal

E. Tantisattamo (✉)
American Heart Association Comprehensive Hypertension Center at the University of California Irvine Medical Center, Division of Nephrology, Hypertension and Kidney Transplantation, Department of Medicine, University of California Irvine School of Medicine, Orange, CA, USA

Nephrology Section, Department of Medicine, Tibor Rubin Veterans Affairs Medical Center, Veterans Affairs Long Beach Healthcare System, Long Beach, CA, USA

Multi-Organ Transplant Center, Section of Nephrology, Department of Internal Medicine, Corewell Health William Beaumont University Hospital, Oakland University William Beaumont School of Medicine, Royal Oak, MI, USA

Pacific Northwest University of Health Sciences, Yakima, WA, USA

Excellent Center for Organ Transplantation, Faculty of Medicine Ramathibodi Hospital, Mahidol University, Bangkok, Thailand
e-mail: etantisa@hs.uci.edu

K. Kalantar-Zadeh
American Heart Association Comprehensive Hypertension Center at the University of California Irvine Medical Center, Division of Nephrology, Hypertension and Kidney Transplantation, Department of Medicine, University of California Irvine School of Medicine, Orange, CA, USA

Nephrology Section, Department of Medicine, Tibor Rubin Veterans Affairs Medical Center, Veterans Affairs Long Beach Healthcare System, Long Beach, CA, USA

Lundquist Biomedical Research Institute at Harbor-UCLA Medical Center, Torrance, CA, USA

protein than plant protein in patients with kidney diseases and after renal transplantation

2. Identify barriers and facilitators of implementing low dietary protein and sodium intake through plant-dominant protein types in clinical practice in patients with kidney diseases and transplantation
3. Apply implementation science and practice to facilitate low dietary protein and sodium intake in clinical practice in patients with kidney diseases and transplantation at the levels of the individual, a community, and health policy
4. Apply frameworks and models to promote changes in dietary protein and sodium intakes in patients with kidney diseases and transplantation

Introduction

Generally, chronic kidney disease (CKD) is an irreversible disease state, and no curative intervention is known to reverse or regain kidney function except through kidney transplantation. Recent pharmacologic interventions have shown promising clinical outcomes in slowing the progression of kidney diseases. Yet limitations remain, especially in patients with advanced CKD, who are generally not included in clinical studies and therefore are not eligible to receive pharmacologic interventions. Nonpharmacologic interventions such as lifestyle modifications have been complementary with pharmacologic interventions. Among those, the diet shows evidence of slowing CKD progression and delaying dialysis initiation and has long been of interest to patients and providers. However, implementing a diet to improve kidney health through a so-called kidney-healthy diet (KHD) faces several challenges from six domains of influence as contextual determinants of barriers and facilitators, including biological factors, behavioral factors, the physical or built environment, the sociocultural environment, the policy or political environment, and the healthcare system.

In this chapter, we will briefly review evidence of diet that patients with kidney diseases and kidney transplantation should adhere to, specifically protein and sodium. We will analyze the root cause and propose current and future implementation strategies to improve dietary access and adherence that are based on theories, frameworks, and models. Dietary potassium, phosphorus, and calcium intakes as well as calorie intake as part of dietary energy for weight management, obesity prevention, and post-transplant diabetes intervention are integral parts of nutrition management, but these topics are beyond the scope of this chapter.

Diet as Part of Medical Therapy in Kidney Diseases and Transplantation

Mortality

Although conditions or diseases that lead to dysmetabolic syndromes such as diabetes, hypertension, and hyperlipidemia are risk factors for mortality in patients with CKD, the syndrome becomes protective for mortality in patients with end-stage kidney disease (ESKD) as the so-called reverse epidemiology [1]. A recent systematic review and meta-analysis including 29 studies reporting the nutritional status and mortality rate of 11,063 patients with ESKD requiring dialysis revealed that patients with malnutrition status had a 49% significantly greater risk of mortality compared to patients with healthy nutritional status (HR 1.49, 95% CI: 1.36, 1.64, $p < 0.0001$) [2, 3]. However, after successful kidney transplantation, a reversal of the reverse epidemiology may ensue. A retrospective cohort study including 230 deceased donor kidney transplant recipients with a stable baseline kidney allograft function at 1-year after transplant demonstrated that patients with metabolic syndrome defined by modified Adult Treatment Panel III criteria had significantly higher mortality than did patients without metabolic syndrome after at least 18 months of follow-up from baseline [4].

Kidney Function

The mechanisms of diet and changes in kidney function have been studied. Kidney function is believed to be dynamic and can be adjusted to the need to excrete water, electrolytes, and nitrogenous waste products. Potential mechanisms have been extensively studied in how high dietary protein intake leads to renal hemodynamic and structural changes [5].

For renal hemodynamic changes, high dietary protein intake stimulates glucagon secretion from the pancreas [6, 7]. Glucagon increases renal blood flow and the glomerular filtration rate (GFR) [8]. A high-protein-rich meal or a meal with a high animal vs. plant proportion of dietary protein also causes renal artery vasodilatation [9, 10] and glomerular hyperfiltration, which is defined by an increased GFR from the hyperemia of glomerular capillaries and an increase in intraglomerular pressure [11, 12]. Therefore, renal perfusion and glomerular filtration are related to excretory demand, and no healthy value of GFR is known [13].

Renal structural change is a consequence of renal hemodynamic change. High dietary protein intake leads to intrarenal pressure and flow, and this can contribute to age-related glomerulosclerosis [14, 15]. Although glomerulosclerosis can be seen in nonkidney disease and nonhypertensive patients, 95% of patients ≤40 years old were found to have <10% glomerulosclerosis from kidney tissue obtained from autopsy [14].

Box 4.1: Dietary Protein Intake and Kidney Function

Renal hemodynamic change resulting from high dietary protein intake leads to glomerular hyperfiltration and increased intraglomerular pressure. Subsequently, renal structural change from the renal hemodynamic change ultimately causes secondary focal segmental glomerulosclerosis.

The more obvious example of renal hemodynamic and structural changes is in living kidney donors. After living-donor unilateral nephrectomy, renal arteriolar vasodilation occurs. This leads to increased glomerular capillary flow and pressure on the remaining kidney and subsequently an increased GFR. However, these adaptive or compensatory hyperfunctioning glomeruli of the remaining kidney ultimately cause a decline in kidney function [16]. This pathophysiology of sustained adaptive renal hemodynamic alteration injures the hyperfunctioning nephron and supports the deterioration of kidney diseases from other causes [13] (Fig. 4.1).

Because high dietary protein intake can increase the risk of glomerular damage, low dietary protein intake should mitigate the risk by restoring glomerular hemodynamics so that it becomes close to healthy. In addition to preserved renal hemodynamic change, proteinuria and glomerular structural changes are mitigated by low dietary protein intake [17]. Current clinical practice commonly emphasizes low dietary protein intakes to reduce the workload on the nephrons.

Similarly, dietary sodium intake contributes to poor kidney and patient outcomes in patients with kidney diseases and transplantation (PKTs). High dietary sodium intake causes salt and water retention. These lead to hypertension and volume overload and subsequently left ventricular hypertrophy [18]. Hypertension also leads to kidney damage. These types of major end-organ damage ultimately increase mortality. High dietary sodium intake also decreases the effects of renin-angiotensin-aldosterone system blockages (Fig. 4.2).

According to the 2020 updated Kidney Disease Outcomes Quality Initiative (KDOQI) Clinical Practice Guideline for Nutrition in CKD, adults with stage 3–5 nondiabetic CKD are recommended to have a low dietary protein intake, that of

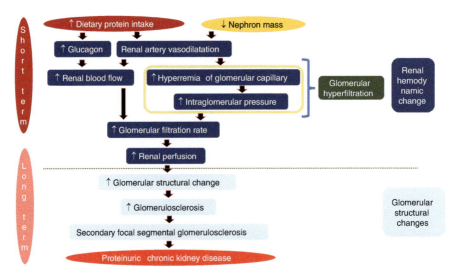

Fig. 4.1 Pathophysiology of renal hemodynamic change from high dietary protein intake or decreased nephron mass, leading to long-term glomerular structural changes

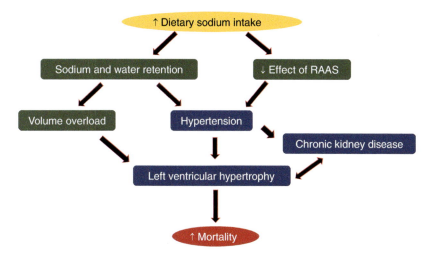

Fig. 4.2 Pathophysiology of major organ damage (blue boxes) from high dietary sodium intake, contributing to the risk of mortality

0.55–0.60 g/kg body weight/day, or a very low dietary protein intake, that of 0.28–0.43 g/kg body weight/day, with additional keto acid/amino acid analogs to reach a daily protein intake of 0.55–0.60 g/kg body weight/day. Adults with stage 3–5 diabetic CKD may be advised to follow a dietary protein intake of 0.6–0.8 g/kg body weight/day to maintain a stable nutritional status and optimize glycemic control. Patients with ESKD with stable metabolic nondiabetes are recommended to consume a dietary protein intake of 1–1.2 g/kg body weight/day to maintain a stable nutritional status, whereas those with diabetes are advised to have a dietary protein intake of 1–1.2 g/kg body weight/day to maintain a stable nutritional status. However, if the patients are at risk for hyper- and/or hypoglycemia, higher levels of dietary protein intake may be considered to maintain glycemic control [19]. No consensus is available to guide the amount of dietary protein and sodium intake in kidney transplant recipients and living kidney donors.

The benefits of low dietary protein intake in kidney transplant recipients to prolong kidney allograft function are uncertain [20]. However, post-transplant timing and the net state of immunosuppression, such as during acute rejection therapy, may guide clinicians in dietary protein management. To slow the progression of kidney allograft dysfunction and to avoid negative nitrogen balance and skeletal muscle mass loss, the proposed amount of dietary protein intake of 1–1.3 g/kg/day during an immediate post-transplant period or when a high protein catabolic rate exists is reasonable. The amount of protein intake may be decreased to 0.8–1 g/kg/day in patients with stable kidney allograft function. However, once kidney allograft function declines and reaches chronic allograft rejection or an estimated GFR < 25 ml/min/1.73 m^2, the dietary protein intake should be decreased to 0.55–0.60 g/kg/day, whereas patients with failed kidney allograft and requiring transition to dialysis should consider increasing their dietary protein intake up to 1–1.2 g/kg/day [21].

In addition to quantity, quality of diet is important for kidney allograft outcomes. Research has provided consistent evidence of the benefits of low dietary protein intake, especially plant-based diets such as the Dietary Approach to Stop Hypertension (DASH) diet, the plant-dominant low-protein diet (PLADO), and the Mediterranean diet, which are associated with a slow decline in kidney allograft function [22–27].

For living kidney donors, no strong evidence supports a recommended amount of dietary protein intake. One cross-sectional study revealed a sigmoid relationship between overnight urinary urea nitrogen and eGFR U-ureaN, with the trend to flatness in the lowest 20% (<5.19 mg/h) and the highest 20% (>10.12 mg/h) of the overnight urinary urea nitrogen. Because the overnight urinary urea nitrogen of 5.19 mg/h approximately corresponds to the recommended daily allowance of protein intake of 0.8 g/kg of ideal weight/day, a dietary protein intake of 0.8–1 g/kg/day should be reasonable for living kidney donors [28].

A plant-based diet should be advised for living kidney donors. One large longitudinal cohort study including 11,952 patients with eGFR $\geq$ 60 mL/min/1.73^2 demonstrated a potential renoprotective association between a plant-based diet and kidney function. Participants consuming more red and processed meat had a greater risk of developing CKD than did those consuming less meat; in contrast, participants with a higher intake of nuts, legumes, and low-fat dairy products had a lower risk of developing CKD than did those consuming fewer plant-based, low-fat dairy products [29].

Similar to dietary protein intake, no consensus exists on the appropriate amount of dietary sodium intake for living kidney donors. One large retrospective cohort study included 3106 participants with and 4871 participants without hypertension, and those participants were categorized into four quartiles on the basis of their amount of daily dietary sodium intake quantified by a 24-h dietary recall Food Frequency Questionnaire (FFQ). Hypertensive participants in quartile 3 (daily sodium intake between 2.93 and 4.03 g/day) had a lower risk of developing CKD than did the participants in quartile 1 (daily sodium intake of <2.08 g/day) and quartile 4 (sodium intake of >4.03 g/day). However, the incidence of CKD was not different among nonhypertensive participants [30].

Challenges in Implementing Dietary Interventions

Barriers and Facilitators for Implementing Dietary Interventions

Although evidence shows that low dietary protein and sodium intake slows the decline in kidney function and possibly improves survival, the proportion of PKTs who adhere to the KHD is low [31, 32]. Several factors contribute to dietary adherence to low protein intake and higher plant vs. animal protein intake. These factors involve the interplay between six complex domains of influence as contextual determinants of barriers and facilitators, including biological factors, behavioral factors, the physical or built environment, the sociocultural environment, the policy or

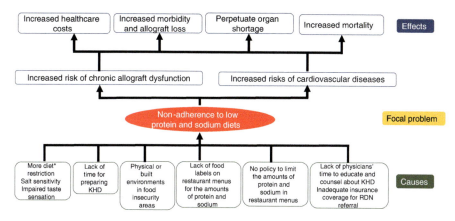

Fig. 4.3 Problem tree analyzing main determinants contributing to the nonadherence to low dietary protein and sodium intake in patients with kidney diseases and kidney transplantation

political environment, and the healthcare system. Therefore, systematically thinking about those contextual determinants of both barriers and facilitators should assist in improving adherence to the KHD (Fig. 4.3).

> **Box 4.2: Domains of Influence for Implementing Dietary Intervention**
> Six contextual determinants as barriers to and facilitators of adhering to low dietary protein and sodium intake include biological factors, behavioral factors, the physical or built environment, the sociocultural environment, the policy or political environment, and the healthcare system. Therefore, systematically thinking about those contextual determinants of both barriers and facilitators should assist in improving adherence to the kidney-healthy diet.

In the biological domain, the recommended daily dietary protein intake is lower in PKTs than in non-kidney-disease patients. In addition, salt sensitivity is common in PKTs [33–36], and this population may need to restrict sodium more than patients without kidney diseases. Taste sensation from the uremic milieu can potentially contribute to salt insensitivity or a loss of salty taste [37] and increase the chance for high dietary sodium consumption. Therefore, PKTs face more challenges in dietary protein and sodium restriction than do patients without kidney diseases. For the behavioral domain, patients with CKD generally have other concomitant comorbidities and are busy with doctor visits. ESKD patients need to spend a significant amount of time on dialysis. Kidney transplant recipients have frequent post-transplant visits, especially during the first year after the transplant. These may contribute to the lack of time that PKTs have to prepare for the KHD.

Regarding the physical or built environment, some proportions of PKTs may reside in areas with food insecurity, such as many big cities with a lot of fast-food restaurants or small towns at a long distance from sources of healthy food. Because the time that PKTs have can be limited by seeking medical attention or performing dialysis, KHD sources that are inconvenient and too far from PKTs may be among of the barriers to dietary adherence. Regarding the sociocultural environment, the most common food type for Americans is the Western diet, with high protein and sodium [38]. Processed or frozen food is also easier to obtain than fresh food. Regarding the policy or political environment, the United States lacks policies on limiting the amount of protein and sodium contained in each menu item in restaurants. Lastly, in the healthcare system domain, although evidence has demonstrated the benefits of low dietary protein and sodium intake in PKTs, no infrastructure facilitates the implementation of these diets in a routine general practice. For example, nephrologists and transplant nephrologists have limited time to provide dietary education and counseling while seeing PKTs during each clinic visit. Even though some practices have or collaborate with dedicated registered dietitian-nutritionists (RDNs), not enough RDNs are available to see all PKTs. In addition, in the United States, RDN referrals may not be covered by some types of insurance. These limit access to dietary education and counseling for PKTs.

Problem-Solving

Theory of Change
If low dietary protein and sodium intake are successfully implemented, a non-KHD should be minimized. This suggestion is made under the assumption that high dietary protein and sodium intake leads to poor clinical outcomes in PKTs and

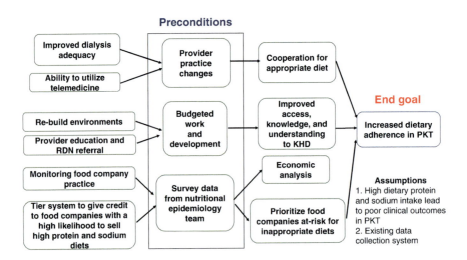

Fig. 4.4 Theory of change for decreasing antibiotic overuse in solid organ transplant recipients *PKTs* patients with kidney diseases and transplantation

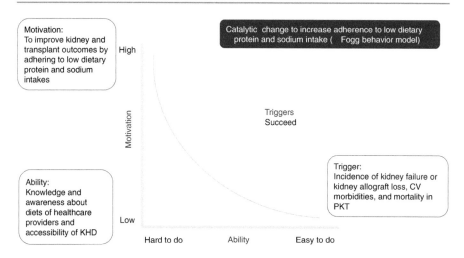

Fig. 4.5 Catalytic change to decrease antibiotic overuse as the target behavior by using the Fogg behavior model
CV cardiovascular, *KHD* kidney-healthy diet, *PKTs* patients with kidney diseases and transplantation

under the precondition that providers and research and development for the dietary interventions are maintained by adequate funding (Fig. 4.4).

Catalytic change to increase adherence to low dietary protein and sodium intake by using the Fogg behavior model involves trigger, motivation, and ability (Fig. 4.5).

Objective Tree

To be efficient and scale up strategies for improving dietary protein and sodium adherence in PKTs, interventions for policies and policy environments are mandatory. Several approaches should be complementary to one another. Among the six domains of influence for nondietary adherence, two of the most relevant (healthcare) system-level interventions for the proposed policy intervention are increasing the implementation of dietary education and counseling and increasing insurance coverage for RDN referrals.

Potential interventions for other domains of influence are changing clinical practice to optimize dialysis adequacy, implementing telemedicine to minimize time spent for several and frequent doctor visits, creating built environments to facilitate access to the KHD, widely implementing food label regulations for the amount of protein and sodium on restaurant menus in addition to calorie labels, and initiating policies to restrict the amounts of protein content and sodium content on restaurant menus. The implementation of regulations and policies to provide more detail on food labels for dietary protein and sodium contents as well as restricted protein and sodium contents may be facilitated by giving incentives to food industries, companies, and business owners.

Stakeholder Analysis

Several stakeholders are involved in the nutrition-related health of PKTs at different positions and levels of influence (Fig. 4.6).

Insurance companies appear to have a high influence but are not in a supportive position in implementing the KHD in PKTs (Fig. 4.6). This is an opportunity to prioritize strategies and engage these stakeholders so that they become more supportive (Table 4.1).

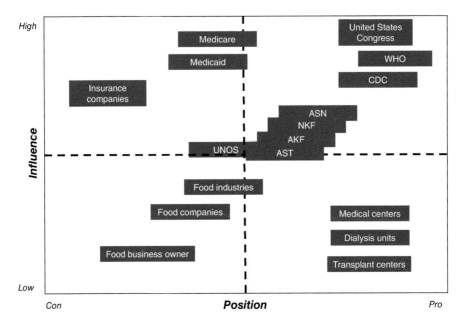

Fig. 4.6 Stakeholder quadrant diagram to analyze the implementation of the kidney-healthy diet in patients with kidney diseases and transplantation

AHA American Heart Association, *AKF* American Kidney Fund, *ASN* American Society of Nephrology, *AST* American Society of Transplantation, *CDC* Centers for Disease Control and Prevention, *CMS* Centers for Medicare and Medicaid Services, *IDSA* Infectious Diseases Society of America, *NKF* National Kidney Foundation, *UNOS* United Network for Organ Sharing, *WHO* World Health Organization

Table 4.1 Stakeholder mapping to analyze the implementation of the kidney-healthy diet in patients with kidney diseases and transplantation

Stakeholder	Goals, motivation, interests	Power and influence (high or low)	Impact on proposed approach (pro vs. con)	Role in proposed approach
US Congress	Keep healthcare costs low and within budget Maintain constituents' approval	High	Pro	Provide funds for new, innovative diagnostic test
CDC	Prevent unhealthy diet consumption Improve the health of patients with kidney diseases or transplantation Enhance kidney healthy diet consumption	High	Pro	Expand system for reporting of unhealthy and kidney heathy diet consumption Provide guidance on how to prepare kidney healthy diet
CMS	Prevent nutrition-related health problems Improve health surveillance	High	Pro	Advocate for amendment and funds from US Congress Include national nutritional therapies or counseling centers
UNOS	Improve the transplant outcomes of recipients	High	Con	Modify criteria to determine transplant outcomes on the basis of patients' medical conditions Assist AST, ASTS, IDSA, or other relevant professional societies—e.g., ASTS, AHA, ASN—to advocate before US Congress
Food industries	Increase revenue from selling food	Low	Con	Provide an adequate food supply

AHA American Heart Association, *ASN* American Society of Nephrology, *AST* American Society of Transplantation, *ASTS* American Society of Transplant Surgeons, *CDC* Centers for Disease Control and Prevention, *CMS* Centers for Medicare and Medicaid Services, *IDSA* Infectious Diseases Society of America, *UNOS* United Network for Organ Sharing

Implementation of Research and Practices to Improve Low Dietary Protein and Sodium Intake

Implementation Science Framework

As mentioned above, the healthcare system domain, specifically dietary education and counseling, is a contextual determinant, potentially an important barrier to adherence to low dietary protein and sodium intake. Although evidence supports the benefits of low dietary protein and sodium intake on the clinical outcomes of PKTs, including slowing the decline in kidney function and decreasing cardiovascular risk factors, morbidity, and mortality, physicians face challenges in providing dietary education and counseling for their patients. To explore the contextual determinants as barriers to dietary education and counseling by physicians, the Consolidated Framework for Implementation Research (CFIR) is utilized [39, 40] (Table 4.2).

The most important barrier is physicians' availability to deliver dietary education and counseling. This barrier is in the inner setting domain among the five CFIR domains and work infrastructure of the CFIR constructs. This barrier has been determined as the top priority because it is crucial in clinical practice and potentially changeable.

Table 4.2 Mapping, rating, and prioritizing contextual determinants with five domains of the Consolidated Framework for Implementation Research

Determinant	CFIR domain	CFIR construct	Importance (0, +, ++)	Changeability (0, +, ++)	Priority?
Available time to deliver dietary education and counseling by physicians	Inner setting	Work infrastructure	++	++	1
Complex PKTs	Characteristics of individuals	Innovative recipients and innovative deliverers	++	+	2
Economic conditions to support implementation	Outer setting	Local conditions	+	++	3
QI processes	Implementation process	Reflecting and evaluating	+	+	4
Unaffordable dietitian fees	Intervention characteristics	Innovation costs	+	0	5

CFIR the Consolidated Framework for Implementation Research (CFIR), *PKT* patients with kidney diseases and transplantation, *QI* quality improvement

The 73 discrete strategies from the Expert Recommendations for Implementing Change (ERIC) [41] fall into nine categories of implementation strategies. The seven categories of implementation strategies that support the implementation of the intervention to overcome the barrier hampering physicians' availability to deliver dietary education and counseling are as follows: adapting and tailoring to context, changing infrastructure, developing stakeholder interrelationships, engaging consumers, training and educating stakeholders, using financial strategies, and supporting clinicians [42]. Because physician availability is the main barrier, supporting clinicians should be one of the most relevant categories of implementation strategies, and task shifting is one of the implementation strategies within this category.

Task shifting involves the rational redistribution of specific tasks, where appropriate, among health workforce teams from highly qualified health workers to health workers with shorter training and fewer qualifications to allow the more efficient utilization of the available human resources for health. [43]. It has been shown to support physicians in response to the changing health service demand [44] and allows physicians to provide more-complex care and expand the healthcare capacity in primary care settings [45, 46]. However, the proposed implementation strategy in this context is to shift the task to experts rather than to nonexperts; therefore, the proposed implementation strategy does not perfectly meet the definition of task shifting. According to the ERIC, three of the 73 defined implementation strategies that may partially, but not completely, fit the proposed strategy in this study are creating a new clinical team, identifying and preparing champions, and revising professional roles [41]. Therefore, for the context of this discussion, the proposed implementation strategy will be termed *task redistributing*, which is defined as a reassignment of a specific task from nonexperts to experts who specialize in that task (Table 4.3).

Therefore, redesigning roles among professionals by redistributing responsibility for dietary education and counseling from physicians to RDNs is one strategy that should mitigate the barrier through possible mechanisms of better support to physicians by RDNs and an increase in incentives for RDNs.

According to the Proctor model, the implementation strategy specification for task redistributing includes seven dimensions: actor, action, action targets, temporality, dose, implementation outcomes affected, and justification [47]. RDN is an actor, and PKTs are action targets. Educating providers (physicians) on the RDN referral process, collaboration between the providers and RDNs for the practice goal, and providing financial support for PKTs with low socioeconomic status or limited healthcare access are actions. For temporality, the task redistributing will initiate dietary education and counseling by RDNs and continue throughout the follow-up period. The dose or frequency of patient follow-up by RDNs can be

Table 4.3 Implementation strategy specification for task redistributing

Discrete strategy (ERIC)	Actor	Action	Action target	Temporality	Dose	Justification
What is the individual strategy called?	Who enacts the strategy?	What steps or processes need to be enacted?	At whom or what is the strategy directed?	When was the strategy delivered over the course of implementation?	For how long should the strategy be implemented?	Why was this strategy chosen?
Task redistributing	Registered dietitian-nutritionists (RDNs)	Educating providers for a RDN referral process Collaboration among the actors (RDNs) and providers (referrers) for the goal and practice Providing financial support for PKTs (action targets) with no insurance	PKTs (action targets)	Early to middle phases of the study	Throughout and after the study	This strategy helps support clinicians, is vital, and potentially leads to changeability

ERIC Expert Recommendations for Implementing Change, *PKTs* patients with kidney diseases and transplantation, *RDN* registered dietitian-nutritionist

varied but generally becomes less frequent overtime. The implementation outcomes affected by the implementation strategy or task redistributing are the acceptability of physicians, RDNs, and PKTs on task redistributing; the adoption of task redistributing by physicians, RDNs, and institute practices; the perceived appropriateness of task redistributing according to physicians, RDNs, PKTs, and institute practices; the perceived feasibility of task redistributing according to physicians, RDNs, and institute practices; the fidelity of physicians and RDNs in implementing task redistributing; the implementation cost spent for physicians, RDNs, and institute practices (e.g., the cost of RDN referrals); the reach of task redistributing in institute practices; and the sustainability of task redistributing as analyzed by administrators and institute practices [48, 49].

The justification for selecting task redistributing as the implementation strategy is that task redistributing helps support clinicians by reducing time spent with PKTs, by prioritizing work on more-complex PKTs, and by providing PKTs with the opportunity to follow up with RDNs, who have expertise in diet and nutrition.

To define and evaluate the outcomes of the implementation strategy (task redistributing), the Reach, Effectiveness, Adoption, Implementation, and Maintenance (RE-AIM) framework is used [50]. The implementation outcomes will be measured along with clinical outcomes designed in this context, which are kidney function, the incidence of cardiovascular diseases, morbidity, kidney allograft loss, kidney transplant access, and the mortality of PKTs. The Implementation Research Logic Model (IRLM), which incorporates the CFIR, the Proctor model, and the RE-AIM framework, is utilized to plan and synthesize this implementation research (Fig. 4.7) [51].

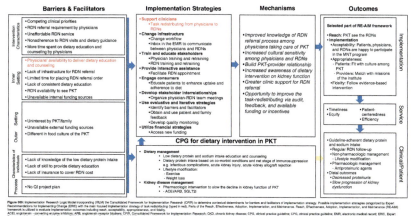

Fig. 4.7 Implementation Research Logic Model for task-redistributing implementation in patients with kidney diseases and transplantation

Although the above implementation frameworks and models can guide providers in implementing changes in dietary intervention, implementation research should be performed to inform changes in future practice. To expedite clinical science translation into practice, one unique study design that can help expedite implementation research and practice to narrow the "know–do" gap is the clinical trial with a hybrid effectiveness–implementation framework [52].

Frameworks

The PRECEDE/PROCEED Framework

The PRECEDE/PROCEED framework includes several steps to follow to analyze situations and design health programs or interventions [53]. The name of this framework is an acronym that is defined in Table 4.4.

Although it includes eight phases, the first four phases (PRECEDE) are the main focuses (Fig. 4.8), and the last four phases (PROCEED) involve implementation and

Table 4.4 Definition of the PRECEDE/PROCEED framework

Abbreviation	Definition	Abbreviation	Definition
P	predisposing	P	policy
R	reinforcing	R	regulatory
E	enabling	O	organizational
C	causes in	C	constructs in
E	educational	E	educational
D	diagnosis	E	environmental
E	evaluation	D	development

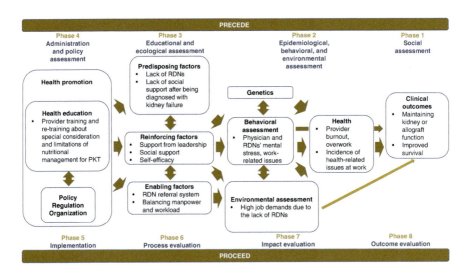

Fig. 4.8 PRECEDE/PROCEED: public health program planning framework to implement low dietary protein and sodium intake in patients with kidney diseases and transplantation
PKTs patients with kidney diseases and transplantation, *RDN* registered dietitian-nutritionist

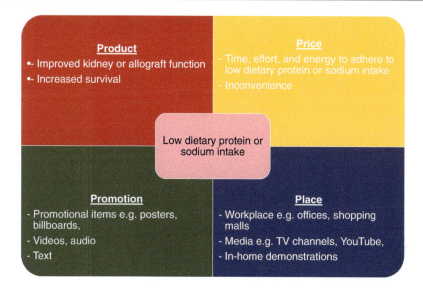

Fig. 4.9 Social marketing framework comprising the four Ps

evaluation. This framework has been proposed to be applied to health behavioral changes through public health program planning for PKTs [54].

Social Marketing Framework

This framework synthesizes social behavior, which benefits the target audience, and communicates a message that the audience can follow. It comprises the four Ps of marketing: product, price, promotion, and place (Fig. 4.9). Product entails the benefits that PKTs will receive after adhering to low dietary protein and sodium intake. Price includes the costs that PKTs will pay to adopt the low dietary protein and sodium intake. Promotion is information about the benefits of low dietary protein and sodium intake to be communicated to PKTs. Place is when and where the promotional information is placed or distributed [53].

Future Directions

Although nutritional recommendations and guidelines that aim to improve clinical outcomes in PKTs can guide public health providers in determining dietary modifications for PKTs, individualized dietary intake is critical to not only optimize clinical outcomes but also improve dietary adherence. The current era of digital technology and artificial intelligence should be able to integrate the complexity of individual medical and environmental factors to individualize dietary modification and achieve an appropriate diet for each individual [55]. Moreover, clinical and translational science research related to diet and nutrition should connect new knowledge and practice from bench to bedside. However, to facilitate and apply the knowledge or clinical practice guidelines in real-world clinical settings, implementation research, especially implementation-effectiveness studies, can allow researchers to answer scientific questions and assess the potentially successful implementation of the study results at the same time and can allow them to ultimately improve equity in research and practice.

Conclusions

Given the multisystemic complexity of implementing strategies to help PKTs adopt the KHD, several interventions should address in parallel the potential contributing factors from the individual domain of influence through the societal level. Integrating health system thinking; the theory of change; stakeholders; and strengths, weaknesses, opportunities, and threats (SWOT) analyses can assist in implementing the KHD at the community and societal (policy) levels. Because successful dietary modification is based heavily on changes in health behavior, integrating health behavioral change models, frameworks, and theories should guide public health providers to navigate and implement dietary modification, especially low dietary protein and sodium intake in PKTs, in a sustainable way.

Further Practice

1. Which of the following is a potentially associated consequence of high dietary protein intake in patients with kidney diseases and transplantation?

   (a) Increased mortality
   (b) Worsened kidney function
   (c) Both

2. What is the main mechanism of worsening kidney function related to high dietary protein intake in patients with kidney diseases and transplantation?

   (a) Glomerular hyperfiltration
   (b) Direct kidney injury from amino acids
   (c) Uremic milieu in the kidneys
   (d) All of the above

3. Which of the following is a contributing factor for high dietary sodium intake–related mortality in patients with kidney diseases and transplantation?

   (a) Hypertension
   (b) Left ventricular hypertrophy
   (c) Chronic kidney disease
   (d) All of the above

4. What is a possible cause of nondietary adherence for patients with kidney diseases and transplantation?

(a) A loss of taste
(b) A lack of time to research and adopt the kidney-healthy diet
(c) A lack of provider time to provide dietary education and counseling
(d) The built environment and food insecurity
(e) All of the above

5. Which of the following is an approach to improve nondietary protein and sodium adherence for patients with kidney diseases and transplantation?

(a) Improve practice to achieve adequate dialysis
(b) Improve the environment that facilitates food security
(c) Implement policies that limit the amount of dietary protein and sodium
(d) Enhance opportunities for patients to receive dietary education and counseling
(e) All of the above

6. Which of the following includes or classifies different implementation strategies for implementation research and practice that can be applied to dietary intervention for patients with kidney diseases and transplantation?

(a) The Expert Recommendations for Implementing Change (ERIC)
(b) The Consolidated Framework for Implementation Research (CFIR)
(c) The Reach, Effectiveness, Adoption, Implementation, and Maintenance (RE-AIM) framework
(d) The Implementation Research Logic Model (IRLM)

7. Which of the following is a helpful framework to determine barriers to or facilitators for implementing dietary intervention for patients with kidney diseases and transplantation?

(a) The Expert Recommendations for Implementing Change (ERIC)
(b) The Consolidated Framework for Implementation Research (CFIR)
(c) The Reach, Effectiveness, Adoption, Implementation, and Maintenance (RE-AIM) framework
(d) The Implementation Research Logic Model (IRLM)

8. Which of the following is a framework for defining and evaluating the outcomes of an implementation strategy (e.g., task redistributing) for dietary intervention for patients with kidney diseases and transplantation?

(a) The Expert Recommendations for Implementing Change (ERIC)
(b) The Consolidated Framework for Implementation Research (CFIR)
(c) The Reach, Effectiveness, Adoption, Implementation, and Maintenance (RE-AIM) framework
(d) The Implementation Research Logic Model (IRLM)

9. Which of the following is a comprehensive framework that incorporates other frameworks to plan and synthesize this implementation research and practice for dietary intervention for patients with kidney diseases and transplantation?

   (a) The Expert Recommendations for Implementing Change (ERIC)
   (b) The Consolidated Framework for Implementation Research (CFIR)
   (c) The Reach, Effectiveness, Adoption, Implementation, and Maintenance (RE-AIM) framework
   (d) The Implementation Research Logic Model (IRLM)

10. What are the benefits of applying theories, frameworks, or models related to health behavioral changes to implement task redistributing as an implementation strategy to improve adherence to low dietary protein and sodium intake for patients with kidney diseases and transplantation?

    (a) The ability to identify the reasons for implementation success
    (b) The ability to identify the reasons for implementation failure
    (c) The ability to evaluate and identify the pitfalls of behavioral interventions
    (d) The ability to plan behavioral interventions
    (e) All of the above

11. The socioecological (ecological) model is one of the oldest models for health behavioral change and can apply to low dietary protein and sodium intake in patients with kidney diseases and transplantation on the basis of the level of the intervention. Which of the following levels is/are included in the model?

    (a) The individual level
    (b) The relationship level
    (c) The community level
    (d) The societal level
    (e) All of the above

12. Educational and ecological assessment is one of the phases of the PRECEDE/ PROCEED framework that may be applied to improve low dietary protein and sodium intake adherence in patients with kidney diseases and transplantation, and it includes three factors. Which of the following contains those three factors?

    (a) Predisposing factors, reinforcing factors, and aggravating factors
    (b) Reinforcing factors, facilitating factors, and aggravating factors
    (c) Reinforcing factors, enabling factors, and blocking factors
    (d) Predisposing factors, reinforcing factors, and enabling factors
    (e) Facilitating factors, enabling factors, and blocking factors

Answer Key

1. (c)
2. (d)
3. (d)
4. (e)
5. (e)
6. (a)
7. (b)
8. (c)
9. (d)
10. (e)
11. (e)
12. (d)

Acknowledgments The authors thank our living kidney donors and our kidney and kidney transplant patients for motivating us to research and expand our knowledge in the field of transplantation and hypertension.

References

1. Kalantar-Zadeh K, Block G, Humphreys MH, Kopple JD. Reverse epidemiology of cardiovascular risk factors in maintenance dialysis patients. Kidney Int. 2003;63(3):793–808.
2. Rashid I, Sahu G, Tiwari P, Willis C, Asche CV, Bagga TK, et al. Malnutrition as a potential predictor of mortality in chronic kidney disease patients on dialysis: a systematic review and meta-analysis. Clin Nutr. 2024;43(7):1760–9.
3. Naderi N, Kleine CE, Park C, Hsiung JT, Soohoo M, Tantisattamo E, et al. Obesity paradox in advanced kidney disease: from bedside to the bench. Prog Cardiovasc Dis. 2018;61(2):168–81.
4. Porrini E, Delgado P, Bigo C, Alvarez A, Cobo M, Checa MD, et al. Impact of metabolic syndrome on graft function and survival after cadaveric renal transplantation. Am J Kidney Dis. 2006;48(1):134–42.
5. Tantisattamo E, Dafoe DC, Reddy UG, Ichii H, Rhee CM, Streja E, et al. Current management of patients with acquired solitary kidney. Kidney Int Rep. 2019;4(9):1205–18.
6. Rocha DM, Faloona GR, Unger RH. Glucagon-stimulating activity of 20 amino acids in dogs. J Clin Invest. 1972;51(9):2346–51.
7. Aoki TT, Brennan MF, Muller WA, Soeldner JS, Alpert JS, Saltz SB, et al. Amino acid levels across normal forearm muscle and splanchnic bed after a protein meal. Am J Clin Nutr. 1976;29(4):340–50.
8. Johannesen J, Lie M, Kiil F. Effect of glycine and glucagon on glomerular filtration and renal metabolic rates. Am J Phys. 1977;233(1):F61–6.
9. Hiatt EP, Hiatt RB. The effect of food on the glomerular filtration rate and renal blood flow in the harbor seal (Phoca Vitulina L.). J Cell Comp Physiol. 1942;19(2):221–7.
10. Pitts RF. The effects of infusing glycin and of varying the dietary protein intake on renal hemodynamics in the dog. Am J Physiol Legacy Content. 1944;142(3):355–65.
11. Kalantar-Zadeh K, Fouque D. Nutritional management of chronic kidney disease. N Engl J Med. 2017;377(18):1765–76.

12. Naber T, Purohit S. Chronic kidney disease: role of diet for a reduction in the severity of the disease. Nutrients. 2021;13(9).
13. Brenner BM, Meyer TW, Hostetter TH. Dietary protein intake and the progressive nature of kidney disease: the role of hemodynamically mediated glomerular injury in the pathogenesis of progressive glomerular sclerosis in aging, renal ablation, and intrinsic renal disease. N Engl J Med. 1982;307(11):652–9.
14. Kaplan C, Pasternack B, Shah H, Gallo G. Age-related incidence of sclerotic glomeruli in human kidneys. Am J Pathol. 1975;80(2):227–34.
15. Kappel B, Olsen S. Cortical interstitial tissue and sclerosed glomeruli in the normal human kidney, related to age and sex. A quantitative study. Virchows Arch A Pathol Anat Histol. 1980;387(3):271–7.
16. Tantisattamo E, Kalantar-Zadeh K. Paradigm shift in lifestyle modification for solitary kidney after donor nephrectomy. Curr Opin Nephrol Hypertens. 2023;32(1):67–75.
17. Dworkin LD, Hostetter TH, Rennke HG, Brenner BM. Hemodynamic basis for glomerular injury in rats with desoxycorticosterone-salt hypertension. J Clin Invest. 1984;73(5):1448–61.
18. Borrelli S, Provenzano M, Gagliardi I, Michael A, Liberti ME, De Nicola L, et al. Sodium intake and chronic kidney disease. Int J Mol Sci. 2020;21(13).
19. Ikizler TA, Burrowes JD, Byham-Gray LD, Campbell KL, Carrero JJ, Chan W, et al. KDOQI clinical practice guideline for nutrition in CKD: 2020 update. Am J Kidney Dis. 2020;76(3 Suppl 1):S1–S107.
20. Tantisattamo E, Kalantar-Zadeh K, Molnar MZ. Nutritional and dietary interventions to prolong renal allograft survival after kidney transplantation. Curr Opin Nephrol Hypertens. 2022;31(1):6–17.
21. Tantisattamo E, Kalantar-Zadeh K. Dietary protein intake and plant-dominant diets to mitigate risk of allograft dysfunction progression in kidney transplant recipients. Curr Opin Nephrol Hypertens. 2024;33(1):43–52.
22. Oste MCJ, Gomes-Neto AW, Corpeleijn E, Gans ROB, de Borst MH, van den Berg E, et al. Dietary Approach to Stop Hypertension (DASH) diet and risk of renal function decline and all-cause mortality in renal transplant recipients. Am J Transplant. 2018;18(10):2523–33.
23. Nafar M, Noori N, Jalali-Farahani S, Hosseinpanah F, Poorrezagholi F, Ahmadpoor P, et al. Mediterranean diets are associated with a lower incidence of metabolic syndrome one year following renal transplantation. Kidney Int. 2009;76(11):1199–206.
24. Oste MC, Corpeleijn E, Navis GJ, Keyzer CA, Soedamah-Muthu SS, van den Berg E, et al. Mediterranean style diet is associated with low risk of new-onset diabetes after renal transplantation. BMJ Open Diabetes Res Care. 2017;5(1):e000283.
25. Gomes-Neto AW, Oste MCJ, Sotomayor CG, van den Berg E, Geleijnse JM, Berger SP, et al. Mediterranean style diet and kidney function loss in kidney transplant recipients. Clin J Am Soc Nephrol. 2020;15(2):238–46.
26. Said MY, Rodriguez-Nino A, Post A, Schutten JC, Kieneker LM, Gomes-Neto AW, et al. Meat intake and risk of mortality and graft failure in kidney transplant recipients. Am J Clin Nutr. 2021;114(4):1505–17.
27. Yeung SMH, Gomes-Neto AW, Oste MCJ, van den Berg E, Kootstra-Ros JE, Sanders JSF, et al. Net endogenous acid excretion and kidney allograft outcomes. Clin J Am Soc Nephrol. 2021;16(9):1398–406.
28. Cirillo M, Zingone F, Lombardi C, Cavallo P, Zanchetti A, Bilancio G. Population-based dose-response curve of glomerular filtration rate to dietary protein intake. Nephrol Dial Transplant. 2015;30(7):1156–62.
29. Haring B, Selvin E, Liang M, Coresh J, Grams ME, Petruski-Ivleva N, et al. Dietary protein sources and risk for incident chronic kidney disease: results from the atherosclerosis risk in communities (ARIC) study. J Ren Nutr. 2017;27(4):233–42.

30. Yoon CY, Noh J, Lee J, Kee YK, Seo C, Lee M, et al. High and low sodium intakes are associated with incident chronic kidney disease in patients with normal renal function and hypertension. Kidney Int. 2018;93(4):921–31.
31. Ichimaru N, Nakazawa S, Yamanaka K, Kakuta Y, Abe T, Kaimori JY, et al. Adherence to dietary recommendations in maintenance phase kidney transplant patients. Transplant Proc. 2016;48(3):890–2.
32. Falbo E, Porchetti G, Conte C, Tarsitano MG. Adherence to Mediterranean diet in individuals on renal replacement therapy. Int J Environ Res Public Health. 2023;20(5).
33. Koomans HA, Roos JC, Boer P, Geyskes GG, Mees EJ. Salt sensitivity of blood pressure in chronic renal failure. Evidence for renal control of body fluid distribution in man. Hypertension. 1982;4(2):190–7.
34. Bovee DM, Cuevas CA, Zietse R, Danser AHJ, Mirabito Colafella KM, Hoorn EJ. Salt-sensitive hypertension in chronic kidney disease: distal tubular mechanisms. Am J Physiol Renal Physiol. 2020;319(5):F729–F45.
35. Koomans HA, Ligtenberg G. Mechanisms and consequences of arterial hypertension after renal transplantation. Transplantation. 2001;72(6 Suppl):S9–12.
36. Hoorn EJ, Walsh SB, McCormick JA, Furstenberg A, Yang CL, Roeschel T, et al. The calcineurin inhibitor tacrolimus activates the renal sodium chloride cotransporter to cause hypertension. Nat Med. 2011;17(10):1304–9.
37. Ciechanover M, Peresecenschi G, Aviram A, Steiner JE. Malrecognition of taste in uremia. Nephron. 1980;26(1):20–2.
38. Carrera-Bastos P, Fontes-Villalba M, O'Keefe JH, Lindeberg S, Cordain L. The Western diet and lifestyle and diseases of civilization. Res Rep Clin Cardiol. 2011;2:15–35. https://doi.org/10.2147/RRCC.S16919.
39. Damschroder LJ, Aron DC, Keith RE, Kirsh SR, Alexander JA, Lowery JC. Fostering implementation of health services research findings into practice: a consolidated framework for advancing implementation science. Implement Sci. 2009;4:50.
40. Consolidated Framework for Implementation Research. Accessed 28 June 2024. https://cfir-guide.org/.
41. Powell BJ, Waltz TJ, Chinman MJ, Damschroder LJ, Smith JL, Matthieu MM, et al. A refined compilation of implementation strategies: results from the Expert Recommendations For Implementing Change (ERIC) project. Implement Sci. 2015;10:21.
42. Waltz TJ, Powell BJ, Matthieu MM, Damschroder LJ, Chinman MJ, Smith JL, et al. Use of concept mapping to characterize relationships among implementation strategies and assess their feasibility and importance: results from the Expert Recommendations For Implementing Change (ERIC) study. Implement Sci. 2015;10:109.
43. World Health Organization, PEPFAR & UNAIDS. Task shifting: rational redistribution of tasks among health workforce teams: global recommendations and guidelines. 2007. Accessed 28 June 2024. https://iris.who.int/handle/10665/43821.
44. Leong SL, Teoh SL, Fun WH, Lee SWH. Task shifting in primary care to tackle healthcare worker shortages: an umbrella review. Eur J Gen Pract. 2021;27(1):198–210.
45. Callaghan M, Ford N, Schneider H. A systematic review of task-shifting for HIV treatment and care in Africa. Hum Resour Health. 2010;8:8.
46. Okpechi IG, Chukwuonye II, Ekrikpo U, Noubiap JJ, Raji YR, Adeshina Y, et al. Task shifting roles, interventions and outcomes for kidney and cardiovascular health service delivery among African populations: a scoping review. BMC Health Serv Res. 2023;23(1):446.
47. Proctor EK, Powell BJ, McMillen JC. Implementation strategies: recommendations for specifying and reporting. Implement Sci. 2013;8:139.
48. Proctor E, Silmere H, Raghavan R, Hovmand P, Aarons G, Bunger A, et al. Outcomes for implementation research: conceptual distinctions, measurement challenges, and research agenda. Admin Pol Ment Health. 2011;38(2):65–76.

49. Peters DH, Adam T, Alonge O, Agyepong IA, Tran N. Republished research: implementation research: what it is and how to do it: implementation research is a growing but not well understood field of health research that can contribute to more effective public health and clinical policies and programmes. This article provides a broad definition of implementation research and outlines key principles for how to do it. Br J Sports Med. 2014;48(8):731–6.
50. Glasgow RE, Vogt TM, Boles SM. Evaluating the public health impact of health promotion interventions: the RE-AIM framework. Am J Public Health. 1999;89(9):1322–7.
51. Smith JD, Li DH, Rafferty MR. The implementation research logic model: a method for planning, executing, reporting, and synthesizing implementation projects. Implement Sci. 2020;15(1):84.
52. Tantisattamo E. Implementation science: a tool to narrow know-do gap and widen equity in kidney diseases and transplantation. Kidney Int. 2024;105(6):1322–3.
53. Glanz K, Rimer B, Viswanath K. Health behavior: theory, research, and practice. San Francisco: John Wiley & Sons, Inc; 2015.
54. Tantisattamo E, Kalantar-Zadeh K. PRECEDE/PROCEED framework for public health program planning in preparation for current and future unprecedented events for patients with kidney failure and living with a kidney transplant. Kidney Int. 2023;104(1):202–3.
55. Ercolano L. One size doesn't fit all: an AI approach to creating healthy personalized diets. Accessed 19 July 2024. https://hub.jhu.edu/2022/11/17/artificial-intelligence-healthy-personalized-diets/.

Antioxidant Food for Sarcopenia

5

Divya Vanoh ⓘ

Learning Objectives
After completing this chapter, you will be able to

1. Understand the meaning of sarcopenia
2. Become familiar with the diagnostic method for sarcopenia
3. Identify dietary patterns rich in antioxidants beneficial for sarcopenia
4. Understand the concept of the antioxidant defence mechanism against sarcopenia
5. Identify the antioxidant flavonoids that have protective effects against sarcopenia

Introduction

The term *sarcopenia* originates from the Greek words *sarcos*, meaning 'flesh', and *penia*, meaning 'poverty or loss', which together means a loss of muscle mass and strength. Clinically, sarcopenia is defined as a syndrome characterized by a progressive and generalized loss of skeletal muscle mass and strength that occurs due to ageing [1]. It is correlated with physical disability, poor quality of life and death [2]. Based on ICD-10-CM code (M62.84), sarcopenia is considered a disease entity [3]. In 2000, the World Health Organization identified sarcopenia as a major threat to functional independence and one of the predictors of comorbidities with advancing age. Sarcopenia is associated with various negative consequences, such as frailty, disabilities, a loss of autonomy and increased mortality.

D. Vanoh (✉)
Dietetics Programme, School of Health Sciences, Universiti Sains Malaysia,
Kubang Kerian, Kelantan, Malaysia
e-mail: divyavanoh@usm.my

A. K. Mitra, D. Vanoh (eds.), *Essentials of Clinical and Public Health Nutrition*,
Nutrition and Health, https://doi.org/10.1007/978-3-031-95373-6_5

A decline in skeletal muscle mass interferes with glucose utilization and insulin sensitivity, increases the risk of type 2 diabetes and has negative impacts on cardiorespiratory fitness [4]. According to a meta-analysis of 263 studies conducted by the European Working Group on Sarcopenia in Older People (EWGSOP), the prevalence of sarcopenia varied widely, from 8% to 36% among people <60 and from 10% to 27% among people ≥60 [5]. Another meta-analysis of the studies from Asia, Europe and the United States demonstrated that the pooled prevalence of sarcopenia is 11%. Differences in the prevalence of sarcopenia were due to the different definitions used for diagnosis [6].

The age-associated loss of skeletal muscle quantity and function are critical determinants of independent physical functioning in later life. A 3-year follow-up study of older adults aged 70–85 years (mean ± standard deviation (SD), 75.5 ± 4.3 years) from the Greater Boston area showed that declining muscle mass, strength, power, and physical performance are independent contributors of the fear of falling, and declining muscle mass and physical performance significantly contribute to poor quality of life [7]. A community-based study conducted among 632 older adults in Ho Chin Minh City, Vietnam, found that sarcopenia was due to advancing age, low education, a lack of employment, poor socioeconomic status and frailty. Prefrailty and frailty increase the risk of sarcopenia by 4.8-fold and 21.16-fold, respectively [8]. Various definitions have been established for the diagnosis of sarcopenia, as are shown in Table 5.1.

Sarcopenia is also known as muscle-wasting syndrome, which is often confused with other conditions, such as cachexia, muscle disuse atrophy and frailty. Sarcopenia and cachexia are different: Sarcopenia is a decline in skeletal muscle function due to a reduction in functional motor units, lower anabolic hormone levels and protein synthesis, whereas cachexia is a consequence of systemic inflammatory impairments such as cancer, organ failure, respiratory illness and critical illness, which may lead to anorexia and a prolonged hypermetabolic state. Cachexia is often associated with drastic weight loss and a lower fat mass, which may contribute to sarcopenia. However, sarcopenia patients may not be cachectic [9]. Patients with diseases have a higher prevalence of sarcopenia compared to the general population. Sarcopenia was found in 18% of diabetics, 66% of patients with unresectable oesophageal cancer, 41% of those in an intensive care unit, 37% of colorectal patients, 40.3% of patients with endovascular aortic aneurysm repair, 52% of patients with lung cancer and 43% of patients with renal cell carcinoma [10].

Muscle mass decline is associated with multiple pathways, namely insulin resistance (secondary to increased body fat and inactivity), inflammation, lower testosterone and growth hormone production. Skeletal muscle dysfunction in ageing is caused by mitochondrial dysfunction due to a decline in the adenosine triphosphate level and excessive reactive oxygen species (ROS), which leads to abnormalities in cellular functioning [9].

Table 5.1 Definitions for the diagnosis of sarcopenia

Diagnostic test	Assessment criteria	Cutoff point
EWGSOP2 (2019)	Criterion 1: low muscle strength Criterion 2: low muscle quantity or quality Criterion 3: low physical performance Only criterion 1 is present: probable sarcopenia is indicated The presence of criteria 1 and 2: sarcopenia is indicated All three criteria are present: severe sarcopenia is indicated	Muscle strength: Grip strength < 27 kg (men); < 16 kg (women) Chair stand: > 15 s for five rises
		Muscle quantity: ASM < 20 kg (men); < 15 kg (women) ASMI: ASM/height^2: < 7.0 kg/m^2, < 5.5 kg/m^2
		Muscle performance: 1. Gait speed $\leq$ 0.8 m/s 2. SPPB $\leq$ 8-point score 3. TUG: $\geq$ 20 s 4. 4-metre walk: noncompletion or $\geq$ 6 min for completion
EWGSOP (2010)	Presarcopenia: only having low muscle mass Sarcopenia: low muscle mass with either low muscle strength or low muscle performance Severe sarcopenia: low muscle mass, low muscle strength and low muscle performance	Muscle mass: SMI < 7.0 kg/m^2 Muscle strength: hand grip strength < 30 kg Muscle performance: gait speed $\leq$ 0.8 m/s
AWGS (2014)	Low muscle mass with either low hand grip strength or low gait speed	Muscle mass: SMI < 8.87 kg/m^2 (men); SMI < 6.42 kg/m^2 (women) (SMI is calculated by total skeletal muscle mass (kg)/square of height(m^2) × 100)
		Muscle strength: hand grip – men < 22.4 kg; women < 14.3 kg
		Physical performance: gait speed – men < 1.27 m/s; women < 1.19 m/s; SPPB score < 9
AWGS (2019)	Possible sarcopenia: low muscle strength with or without low physical performance Sarcopenia: low muscle mass with either low muscle strength or low muscle performance Severe sarcopenia: low muscle mass, low muscle strength and low muscle performance	Muscle mass: ASMI: ASM/height^2 Dual-energy X-ray absorptiometry (men < 7.0 kg/m^2; women < 5.4 kg/m^2) or bioelectrical impedance analysis (men < 7.0 kg/m^2; women < 5.7 kg/m^2)
		Muscle strength Hand grip strength: men < 28 kg; women: < 18 kg
		Muscle performance: 6-metre walk < 1.0 m/s Or 5-time chair stand test $\geq$ 12 s Or short physical performance battery $\leq$ 9

(continued)

Table 5.1 (continued)

Diagnostic test	Assessment criteria	Cutoff point
FNIH (2014)	Sarcopenia is indicated by low muscle mass and low muscle strength	Muscle mass: SMI: men: < 0.789; women: < 0.512 Muscle strength: men < 26 kg; women: < 16 kg
IWGS (2011)	Low muscle mass and muscle function indicates sarcopenia	DXA (ALM/height^2): men: < 7.23 kg/m^2; women: < 5.67 kg/m^2 4-metre gait speed: < 1.0 m/s or standing up from a chair

ASM Appendicular Skeletal Muscle Mass, *ASMI* Appendicular Skeletal Muscle Mass Index, *ALM* appendicular lean muscle mass, *AWGS* Asian Working Group for Sarcopenia, *DXA* dual-energy X-ray absorptiometry, *EWGSOP* European Working Group on Sarcopenia in Older People, *IWGS* International Working Group on Sarcopenia, *SDOC* Sarcopenia Definition and Outcomes Consortium, *SMI* skeletal muscle index, *SPPB* short physical performance battery

Diagnosis of Sarcopenia

Sarcopenia has been given an ICD-10-CM code, namely M62.84, without any specific diagnostic criteria. Sarcopenia diagnoses have been challenging due to the lack of consensus in the definition of sarcopenia [11]. In 1989, sarcopenia was defined as a loss of muscle mass and muscle function. Subsequently, multiple definitions have been proposed. In 2010, the European Working Group on Sarcopenia in Older People (EWGSOP) established specific criteria for diagnosing sarcopenia by combining low muscle strength, low muscle mass and low physical performance. The definition of sarcopenia using EWGSOP is the presence of reduced muscle mass with either low muscle strength or low muscle performance. EWGSOP cutoff points were revised in 2018 as EWGSOP2. In the revised EWGSOP2 criteria, sarcopenia is defined as having low muscle mass and low muscle strength with normal muscle performance [12, 13].

In Asia, the Asian Working Group for Sarcopenia (AWGS) was established in 2014, which included similar components to those in EWGSOP [14]. In 2020, AWGS was updated as AWGS 2019 with an improved diagnostic algorithm. In AWGS 2019, early screening for sarcopenia by using calf circumference or the SARC-F questionnaire was recommended [15]. In AWGS 2019, sarcopenia is defined as having low muscle mass with either low muscle strength or low muscle performance. In addition to that, sarcopenia is also defined by using some other criteria, such as those from the Foundation for the National Institutes of Health (FNIH) and the International Working Group on Sarcopenia, which include similar components, namely the appendicular skeletal muscle mass and muscle function [16, 17]. Table 5.2 summarizes the criteria for the stages of sarcopenia, such as probable sarcopenia, possible sarcopenia, sarcopenia, and severe sarcopenia.

Table 5.2 Simplified stages of sarcopenia based on EWGSOP2 and AWGS2019

Sarcopenia status	Muscle mass	Muscle strength	Muscle performance
Probable sarcopenia (EWGSOP2)	Reduced	Normal	Normal
Possible sarcopenia (AWGS 2019)	Normal	Reduced	Normal
		Normal	Reduced
Sarcopenia (AWGS 2019)	Reduced	Reduced	Normal
		Normal	Reduced
Sarcopenia (EWGSOP2 2019)	Reduced	Reduced	Normal
Severe sarcopenia	Reduced	Reduced	Reduced

Risk Factors of Sarcopenia

Box 5.1: Assessment Methods for Sarcopenia Parameters

Muscle strength: hand grip strength

Muscle mass: the skeletal muscle index (total skeletal muscle mass (kg)/ square of height $(m^2) \times 100$) and the appendicular skeletal muscle mass index

Muscle performance: gait speed, a short physical performance battery, the timed up and go test and the chair stand test

However, multiple factors accelerate the rate of muscle loss, such as diseases, inflammatory pathway activation, mitochondrial abnormalities, the loss of neuromuscular junctions, lower satellite cell numbers, hormonal changes and poor nutritional status.

To date, no drug has been made available to treat sarcopenia. Nutrition is recognized as one of the important components for the prevention of sarcopenia. Nutritional problems leading to sarcopenia are a lack of calorie and protein intake, a low serum vitamin D level, and an insufficient intake of antioxidants and carotenoids [18]. Moreover, sarcopenia is caused by increased oxidative stress due to excessive levels of pro-oxidant mitochondrial radicals and a reduction in antioxidant enzymes in muscle cells – which stimulates the accumulation of reactive oxygen species, leading to sarcopenia [19]. Oxidative stress markers are higher in older adults with sarcopenia [20, 21]. Food rich in antioxidants may scavenge the effects of free radicals, thus reducing the damage to skeletal muscle (Baharirad et al. 2022). Nazri et al. (2021) [22] reported that vegetable and fruit intake lowered the risk of sarcopenia due to the presence of dietary antioxidants, especially vitamin C, carotenoids and vitamin E. Vitamin C is found in high concentrations in vegetables such as Brussels sprouts, peppers and broccoli, whereas carrots, apricots, lettuce, sweet potatoes, butternut squash and spinach are high in carotene. Mushrooms, avocados, almonds, sunflower seeds, asparagus and whole grains are high in excellent sources of vitamin E. Antioxidant vitamins have important roles in the synthesis of viscoelastic collagen, which is involved in maintaining the structural properties of skeletal muscle cells, connective tissue and tendons. Meanwhile, dietary antioxidants such as alpha-carotene, beta-carotene, beta-cryptoxanthin, lutein, lycopene and zea-xanthin are able to destroy free radicals, thus interfering with lipid peroxidation and reducing the redox-sensitive transcription factors involved in the production of pro-inflammatory cytokines.

Another systematic review of cross-sectional studies revealed that the consumption of fruits, adherence to the Mediterranean dietaray pattern and the consumption of diet rich in antioxidants may improve muscle mass and muscle strength among older adults thus, lowering the risk of sarcopenia [23]. The Mediterranean diet is rich in antioxidant nutrients such as vitamins, minerals and omega-3 fatty acids from fish, vegetables, legumes, nuts, grains and olive oil and is low in red meat and poultry. Studies conducted in Italy, Spain and Finland have demonstrated significant improvement in muscle mass, muscle strength and physical performance among those practising the Mediterranean diet [24–27]. Fruits and vegetables are rich in antioxidant vitamins and phytochemicals, and bioactive compounds in whole grains, such as polyphenols, beta-sitosterol, alkylresorcinols and beta-glucan, may promote muscle anabolism. Moreover, the Mediterranean diet emphasizes consuming fish, which has omega-3 fatty acid, selenium, vitamin D and other polar lipids with anti-inflammatory effects [28]. One of the most important components of the Mediterranean diet is extra virgin olive oil (EVOO), which has various antioxidants compounds such as phenyl ethyl alcohol (hydroxytyrosol and tyrosol), cinnamic acid (caffeic acid and p-coumaric acid), benzoic acid (vanillic acid), flavones (api-genin and luteolin) and secorroids (oleuropein and ligtroside derivatives). Improvements in muscle tissue morphology and function have been observed with the regular consumption of EVOO. EVOO can increase the expression of IGF-1, which can reduce inflammation, lower the production of reactive oxygen species and prevent alterations to mitochondrial biogenesis [29].

Silveira et al. (2020) [30] conducted a 12-week three-armed randomized con-trolled trial involving severely obese adults. In this study, participants were ran-domly assigned to one of the following three groups: (1) 52 ml/day of extra virgin olive oil; (2) a traditional Brazilian diet (DieTBra); or (3) DieTBra + olive oil (52 ml/day). The group provided with DieTBra and EVOO had lower total body fat and a reduction in body weight. However, the group provided with DieTBra alone showed significant improvement in hand grip strength and walking speed. DieTBra is a well-balanced meal with sufficient antioxidant-rich fruits and vegetables as well as minimal ultra-processed food. Lunch and dinner consist of rice, beans, a small portion of lean meat and raw or cooked vegetables. Bread and dairy products are consumed in small quantities in this meal. Another type of diet which has high anti-oxidant properties is the Nordic diet. The Nordic diet originated from the Nordic countries. This diet emphasizes a high intake of fruits (especially berries), vegeta-bles (e.g., roots, legumes, cabbage and peas, but not potatoes), Nordic cereals (e.g., rye, oats and barley), Nordic fish (salmon, mackerel and herring) and low-fat and fat-free milk and uses canola oil rich in omega-3 fatty acid. Similar to the Mediterranean diet, the Nordic fish diet emphasizes a low intake of red meat, pro-cessed meat and alcohol [31, 32].

A study by Mahmoodi et al. (2024) [33] investigated the association between oxidative balance score (OBS) and sarcopenia. OBS is a specific formula calculated by the intake of nondietary antioxidants, physical activity, nondietary pro-oxidant components (represented by obesity and smoking), dietary antioxidant components (vitamin E, vitamin C, alpha-carotene, beta-carotene, beta-cryptoxanthin, lutein, lycopene, vitamin B9, zinc, selenium and fibre) and a high intake of dietary pro-oxidant components (saturated fatty acid, polyunsaturated fatty acid and iron). In that study, each OBS component was given a score ranging from 0 to 2, as shown in Table 5.3. The lowest score was 0, indicating high exposure to pro-oxidants, whereas the highest score, that of 34, represented more exposure to antioxidants.

Table 5.3 Oxidative balance score components

OBS components	Score 0	Score 1	Score 2
Nondietary antioxidant components			
Physical activity (MET-min/day)	Low (first tertile)	Medium (second tertile)	High (last tertile)
Nondietary pro-oxidant components			
Obesity	BMI ≥ 30 kg/m^2 AND WC ≥ 0.88 m in women	BMI ≥ 30 kg/m^2 OR WC ≥ 0.88 m in women	BMI < 30 kg/m^2 AND WC < 0.88 m in women
Smoking	Current smoker	Former smoker	Never smoked
Dietary antioxidant components			
	Low (first tertile)	Medium (second tertile)	High (last tertile)
Vitamin E (mg)	0	1	2
Vitamin C (mg)	0	1	2
Alpha-carotene (microgram)	0	1	2
Beta-carotene (microgram)	0	1	2
Beta-cryptoxanthin	0	1	2
Lutein (microgram)	0	1	2
Lycopene (microgram)	0	1	2
Vitamin B9 (microgram)	0	1	2
Zinc (microgram)	0	1	2
Selenium (microgram)	0	1	2
Fibre (gram)	0	1	2
Dietary pro-oxidant components			
SFA (g)	2	1	0
PUFA (g)	2	1	0
Iron (mg)	2	1	0

OBS oxidative balance score, *MET* metabolic equivalent of task, *BMI* body mass index, *WC* waist circumference, *SFA* saturated fatty acid, *PUFA* polyunsaturated fatty acid

OBS scoring is not significantly associated with sarcopenia, due to several limitations. One of them is the multifactorial causes of sarcopenia, namely inflammation, poor nutritional status, a sedentary lifestyle and endocrine changes. OBS scoring requires modification because it assumes similar weights for the intake of oxidants and the intake of pro-oxidants, although some antioxidants have different action potentials, such as alpha-tocopherol, which has a higher redox potential than vitamin C [34]. Another limitation of using OBS is the difficulties in assessing the intake of certain antioxidant nutrients, such as lycopene, lutein and zeaxanthin [33].

The excessive intake of saturated fatty acid increases oxidative stress by activating NF-κB, leading to excessive levels of cytokines, such as tumour necrosis alpha and interleukin 6, and causing insulin resistance [35].

Antioxidant Defence Mechanism for Sarcopenia

A healthy muscle features a balance between the production and breakdown of protein and amino acids. However, in older adults, ageing-related low-grade inflammation and oxidative stress affect this equilibrium due to the enhanced degradation of myofibrillar and mitochondrial proteins [36]. Oxidative stress is the major culprit for sarcopenia in that it activates the redox-sensitive transcription factor nuclear factor kappa B (NF-kB). NF-kB further enhances the secretion of inflammatory cytokines such as interleukin-1, the tumour necrosis factor and interleukin-6, which leads to muscle atrophy and to extensive mitochondrial and nuclear DNA damage [37, 38]. In addition, during the catabolic process, a specific E3 ubiquitin-ligating enzyme that targets protein degradation will be produced. Specifically, two muscle-specific E3 ubiquitin ligases which will be overexpressed during muscle atrophy are atrogin-1/MAFbx and MuRF1 [39]. Oxidative stress occurs due to inequalities in the amount of reactive oxygen species and the endogenous antioxidant. Examples of reactive oxygen species are superoxide anion, hydrogen peroxide, hydroxyl radical, nitric oxide and peroxynitrite. Possible contributing factors to oxidative stress are inflammation, a poor antioxidant defence system, mitochondrial dysfunction, excessive reactive oxygen species, comorbidities, a sedentary lifestyle, heavy metals, drug abuse, alcohol consumption, smoking and exposure to environmental pollutants [40, 41].

In skeletal muscle, reactive oxygen species (ROS) are produced primarily in mitochondrial, nicotinamide adenine dinucleotide phosphate (NADPH) oxidases (NOX), xanthine oxidase and uncoupled nitric oxide synthase (NOS) isoforms [42]. The presence of ROS inhibits anabolic pathways for protein synthesis in skeletal muscle mediated by phosphatidylinositol 3-kinase (P13K)/protein kinase B (Akt)/mammalian target of rapamycin (mTOR) pathways. Components that activate these pathways are insulin, insulin-like growth factors 1(IGF-1), exercise and testosterone. With exposure to oxidative stress, c-Jun-N-terminal kinase (JNK), IkB kinase (IKK) and p38 mitogen-activated protein kinase (p38-MAPK) pathways will be stimulated – which interferes with insulin receptor functioning, promoting insulin resistance in skeletal muscle [43].

Box 5.2: Factors Contributing to Oxidative Stress
1. Inflammation
2. Mitochondrial dysfunction
3. Comorbidities
4. A sedentary lifestyle
5. Alcohol, smoking and other drugs
6. Heavy metals and air pollutants

Antioxidants are required to scavenge free radicals, and they are present in various forms, such as enzymes (superoxide dismutase, catalase, glutathione peroxidase, glutathione reductase), vitamins (vitamin C, vitamin E, vitamin A), elements or minerals (selenium, zinc) and phenolic antioxidants (resveratrol, phenolic acid, flavonoids, selenium, acetylcysteine). Antioxidants can transform free radicals into stable molecules, such as water and molecular oxygen [43].

A cross-sectional study in Japan demonstrated that the Japanese dietary pattern, consisting of a high intake of fish, soybean products, potatoes, most vegetables, mushrooms, seaweed and fruits and a low intake of rice was significantly associated with usual gait speed [44]. The combination of these foods may contribute to nutrient adequacy, which may be lowering the risk of sarcopenia. Rice intake is not harmful, but if it is consumed excessively, the intake of other beneficial food for sarcopenia will be limited. A systematic review of a randomized controlled trial by Besora-Moreno et al. (2022) [23] reported mixed findings on the effectiveness of antioxidant foods and supplements in improving sarcopenic parameters. One of the randomized controlled trials revealed positive findings. The intervention was a three-armed randomized controlled trial conducted for 24 weeks. Group 1 underwent resistance training exposure twice a week; group 2 underwent resistance training twice a week with a healthy diet consisting of whole-grain cereals, fruits, vegetables and berries ($\geq$600 g/day); nuts and seeds, rape seed oil, olive oil and fish and seafood ($\geq$500 g/day); lean meat, low-fat dairy products ($\leq$0.5 L/day); and soft drinks/juice (best to avoid or consume < 1.5 dL juice/day); and the control group was not exposed to any intervention. Findings from this intervention reported that after 24 weeks, groups given the resistance training and a healthy diet showed improved leg lean mass compared to the control group [45].

Fruits and vegetables have been found to be beneficial against sarcopenia due to their containing abundant antioxidant nutrients such as carotenoid and vitamin C. Ageing limits the efficiency of endogenous antioxidant function for protecting cells against damage from reactive oxygen species. Thus, exogenous antioxidant supply is essential for preserving skeletal muscle mass [46]. A study including older Japanese women found a decline in physical performance among women with lower plasma vitamin C concentration [47].

Antioxidant Flavonoid and Sarcopenia

Flavonoids are antioxidant-rich phenolic compounds found abundantly in edible plants. Examples of flavonoids are flavones, flavanols, flavan-3-ols, chalcones, flavanones and isoflavonoids. Flavonoids have antisarcopenic effects [48]. Examples of foods for each subgroup of flavonoids are shown in Table 5.4. Apigenin can reduce mitochondrial superoxide anion, which contributes to oxidative stress; stimulates the activities of antioxidant enzymes such as superoxide dismutase and glutathione peroxidase; and inhibits lipid peroxidation via a reduction in malondialdehyde content [49]. Isobavachalcone is able to increase myogenesis and lower protein degradation [50].

Table 5.4 Subgroups of flavonoids

Subgroup		Examples of food
Flavones	Apigenin	Parsley, celery, oranges, chamomile, broccoli,
	Luteolin	Celery, parsley, broccoli
	5,7-Dimethoxyflavone	Kaempferia parviflora
	Baicalin	Tea, chocolate
	Sinensetin	Citrus fruit peels, celery, parsley, red pepper, mint, gingko biloba
Flavanols	Quercetin, dihydromyricetin, Icartin	Medicinal herbs, vegetables, grapes, berries
Flavan-3-ols (flavanols)	Catechin, epicatechin, epicatechin gallate, epigallocatechin, epigallocatechin gallate	Green tea, apples, carobs, berries, avocados, cocoa
Isoflavonoids	Genistein, daidzein, glabridin	Liquorice, soy, tea, chocolate
Flavanones	Hesperetin, naringenin	Citrus fruits such as lemons, oranges
Chalcones	Isobavachalcone, panduratin A	Citrus fruits, apples, tomatoes, shallots, bean sprouts, potatoes, liquorice

Curcumin and Sarcopenia

Curcumin, which is a polyphenol derived from the rhizome *Curcuma longa L.*, belongs to the Zingiberaceae (ginger) family. It is commonly known as turmeric. *C. longa* has rich therapeutic properties and has been used extensively in traditional Chinese and Ayurvedic medications. Curcumin is a yellow flavonoid with lipophilic characteristics and whose chemical structure is $C_{21}H_{20}O_6$ [51]. Curcumin is an excellent antioxidant thanks to its ability to increase the activity of antioxidant enzyme and decrease the levels of malondialdehyde (MDA). A study involving dexamethasone induced sarcopenia in Institute of Cancer Research (ICR) mice exposed to curcumin water extract for 7 days demonstrated that myostatin, MuRF-1 and atrogin-1 expression declined, which suppressed muscle loss and boosted the levels of antioxidant enzymes [52]. Atrogin-1 and MURF-1 are able to promote protein degradation. The presence of reactive oxygen species activates the regulator of the antioxidant defence system, namely nuclear factor erythroid-2-related-factor-2 (Nrf2). Nrf2 enhances the gene expression of antioxidant enzymes by binding to antioxidant response elements [53, 54]. Animal study findings have reported that turmeric extract was fed to senescence-accelerated mouse prone 8 (SAMP8) mice and showed decreased muscle atrophy–related mRNA expression, especially in the glucocorticoid receptor-FoxO signalling pathway [55].

Green Tea and Sarcopenia

Green tea is rich in catechins, which are categorized into four groups: epigalloca-thechin-3-gallate (EGCG), epicathechin, epigallocathechin and epicathechin gallate. A study by Meador et al. (2015) [56] revealed that 20-month-old Sprague Dawley rats fed with 200 mg/kg/body weight (BW) of an EGCG diet showed improved gastrocnemius muscle mass and muscle atrophy mediators such as 19S, MuRF1, MAFbx and myostatin, which were inhibited more than they were in aged controls. A clinical trial involving older men supplemented with epicathechin (1 mg/kg/BW) for 8 weeks showed improved performance on the timed up and go test and improved appendicular skeletal muscle mass [57]. Catechin is able to inhibit the expression of ubiquitin ligase in muscle atrophy–related genes, slow the breakdown of skeletal muscle mass and reduce the apoptotic pathways related to muscle atrophy [58]. The consumption of catechin from green tea with protein and resistance exercise further promotes muscle protein synthesis [59].

Resveratrol and Sarcopenia

Resveratrol (3,4,5-trihydroxystilb), a polyphenol present in the skin of red grapes, berries, dark chocolate, red grape juice, red wine, raw peanuts and cocoa powder, has positive effects on skeletal muscle by inhibiting protein degradation [60]. Resveratrol mimics the effect of caloric restriction by promoting MPK/Sirt1 signalling, which lowers inflammation, promotes longevity, improves mitochondrial biogenesis and lowers oxidative stress [61]. Resveratrol promotes the functions of antioxidant enzymes, such as superoxide dismutase and catalase, which inhibit reactive oxygen species [62]. A study on aged male Fischer 344 × Brown Norway rats found that treatment with resveratrol, calorie restriction or a combination of calorie restriction and resveratrol can improve mitochondrial functioning and reduce apoptotic signalling pathways in glycolytic muscle and protects against muscle loss [63]. Another study showed improved muscle strength and muscle performance in aged mice treated with resveratrol and exercise training when compared to mice treated with resveratrol or exercise alone [64].

Some of the clinical trials using dietary antioxidants on humans are presented in Table 5.5.

Table 5.5 Antioxidant effect on sarcopenia in randomized controlled trials

Author (year)	Study design/ sample size	Intervention strategy	Study parameters	Findings
Nasimi et al. (2020) [65]	Randomized double-blind, controlled trial on 33 participants aged 65 years and above with sarcopenia in each treatment and control group	Duration: 12-weeks. Control group: 300 g of plain yogurt with lunch and/or dinner (0 g vitamin C, vitamin D and β-Hydroxy-β-Methylbutyrate (HMB)) administered daily. Treatment group: 300 g of yogurt fortified with HMB, vitamin D and vitamin C (3 g HMB, 1000 IU vitamin D, and 500 mg vitamin C) administered daily	Primary: lean mass, appendicular lean mass (ALM), skeletal muscle index, body weight, height, BMI, waist circumference, hip circumference, Mini-Nutritional Assessment (MNA), diet, physical activity. Secondary: hand grip strength; gait speed; metabolic, inflammatory and oxidative stress biomarkers	Total lean mass (0.56 vs. 0.30 kg) and ALM (0.20 vs. 0.03 kg) increased in the intervention group. Significant fat mass decreased in the control group. Significant increase in vitamin D and IGF-1 in the intervention group. Decreased level of malondialdehyde level in the intervention group (−0.49 μM/l) compared to the control group (−0.21 μM/l)

(continued)

Table 5.5 (continued)

Author (year)	Study design/ sample size	Intervention strategy	Study parameters	Findings
Bountry-Regard et al. (2020) [66]	Double-blind, randomized controlled trial involving older adults with limited mobility	Duration: 12 weeks Subjects were given 1 out of 3 beverages with 7 capsules + electrical muscle stimulation (EMS) 1. Control: beverage with 20 g of carbohydrate (maltodextrin glucose syrup 21 DE) + placebo capsules with dextrin and medium chain triglyceride ($n = 12$) 2. Beverage with 20 g of whey protein isolate (95% whey) + placebo capsules ($n = 15$) 3. Beverage with 20 g of whey protein + hard capsule containing rutin (500 mg per day) + fish oil–derived omega-3 fatty acid/curcumin in soft capsules (1.5 g/day of fish oil with 18% EPA and 7% DHA and 500 mg/day curcumin with 95% curcuminoids) ($n = 10$)	Muscle thickness, MNA, isometric knee extensions, gait speed, blood parameters, body composition	Knee extension strength improved in the group receiving protein + capsule with omega-3 fatty acid, rutin, curcumin

McDermott et al. (2020) [67]	Double-blind randomized controlled trial involving older adults with lower-extremity peripheral artery disease (PAD)	Duration: 6 months 1. Intervention: 15 g of cocoa + 75 mg of epicatechin daily 2. Control: matching placebo powder, where 3 packets drank daily with either water or milk	Primary: 6-minute walking distance (assessed at 2.5 hours and 24 hours after beverage was consumed) Secondary: 6-month change in brachial artery flow–mediated dilation, change in maximal and pain-free treadmill walking distance (measured 48 hours after beverage intervention), 6-minute walk test, brachial artery flow–mediated dilation, calf muscle perfusion, epicatechin metabolites, 5-(3,4-dihydroxyphenyl)-γ-valerolactone metabolites, calf muscle biopsy	The intervention group showed statistically significant improvement in walking speed at the 2.5-hour time point but not the 24-hour time point The intervention group had improved calf muscle perfusion and calf muscle cytochrome c oxidase (COX) enzyme activity, improved capillary density and increased central nuclei compared to placebo
Alway et al. (2021) [68]	Double-blind randomized controlled trial on healthy older adults	Duration: 12 weeks Intervention: 500 mg resveratrol/day in capsule form + exercise Control: 500 mg/day of corn starch placebo in capsule form + exercise Exercise: 3 sets of 10–12 repetitions of bilateral leg presses, knee extensions, pull down, chest presses and shoulder presses, three consecutive days each week for 12 weeks	Maximal oxygen uptake, blood chemistry, mitochondrial metabolism, muscle myosin composition and morphology, satellite cell and myonuclei, DNA oxidative damage	Intervention group had improved mitochondrial density, knee extensor muscle peak torque, average peak torque and power, mean muscle fibre area, total myonuclei from the vastus lateralis

(continued)

Table 5.5 (continued)

Author (year)	Study design/ sample size	Intervention strategy	Study parameters	Findings
Tokuda and Mori (2021) [59]	Open-label, pilot, randomized controlled trial on older adults with sarcopenia	Duration: 24 weeks 1. Resistance exercise group ($n = 18$) 2. Resistance exercise with essential amino acid ($n = 18$) 3. Resistance exercise with essential amino acid and tea catechin ($n = 18$) Essential amino acid consists of 1200 mg leucine, 330 mg valine and 320 mg isoleucine Tea catechin consists of 540 mg of powder that amounts to 19 kcal Exercise included 20-minute warmup exercise and 40 minutes of resistance exercises using resistance elastic band and body weight resistance exercise	Primary outcome: skeletal muscle mass Secondary outcomes: grip strength, knee extension strength, gait speed, health-related quality of life	Skeletal muscle mass improved in the resistance exercise group with essential amino acid and tea catechin supplementation

Further Practice

1. Sarcopenia is defined as

    A. Low muscle mass
    B. Low muscle mass and muscle strength
    C. Low muscle strength
    D. Low muscle performance and low muscle strength
    E. Low muscle performance

2. Muscle mass can be assessed by using

    A. Measuring tape
    B. A hand grip dynamometer
    C. A stadiometer
    D. Dual-energy X-ray absorptiometry
    E. A short physical performance battery

3. The following are all muscle performance assessment methods for sarcopenia except for

    A. Gait speed
    B. Bioelectrical impedance analysis
    C. Usual walking
    D. Time up and go
    E. Balance tests

4. Choose from among the following the nutrient that is considered dietary pro-oxidant.

    A. Iron
    B. Monounsaturated fatty acid
    C. Vitamin C
    D. Potassium
    E. Vitamin E

5. Which of the following is categorized as a flavanol?

    A. Naringenin
    B. Quercetin
    C. Apigenin
    D. Daidzein
    E. Sinensetin

6. Which of the following factors does *not* promote the production of reactive oxygen species?

    A. Comorbidities
    B. Air pollutants
    C. Physical inactivity

D. Soy-rich food

E. Inflammation

7. Which of the following is *not* an antioxidant vitamin or mineral?

A. Vitamin A

B. Vitamin C

C. Zinc

D. Calcium

E. Vitamin E

8. What is the major component present in green tea that is beneficial against sarcopenia?

A. Epigallocathechin-3-gallate

B. Luteolin

C. Apigenin

D. Naringenin

E. Quercetin

9. Among the following, which is not rich in resveratrol?

A. Grapes

B. Peanuts

C. Red wine

D. Green tea

E. Cocoa powder

10. The following are the components in the Nordic diet except for

A. Salmon

B. Rye

C. Extra virgin olive oil

D. Canola oil

E. Low-fat milk

11. Extra virgin olive oil is rich in antioxidants such as phenyl ethyl alcohol (hydroxytyrosol and tyrosol) and cinnamic acid (caffeic acid and p-coumaric acid).

True/false

12. The following foods are rich in vitamin E except for

A. Mushrooms

B. Avocados

C. Almonds

D. Sunflower seeds

E. Rice

13. The skeletal muscle index is calculated by dividing an individual's total skeletal muscle mass by the square of their height.

   True/false

14. According to FNIH (2014), sarcopenia is indicated by low muscle performance and low muscle mass.

   True/false

15. Muscle strength can be assessed by using a gait speed test.

   True/false

Answer Keys

1. B
2. D
3. B
4. A
5. B
6. D
7. D
8. A
9. D
10. C
11. False
12. True
13. E
14. True
15. False

References

1. Santilli V, Bernetti A, Mangone M, Paoloni M. Clinical definition of sarcopenia. Clin Cases Miner Bone Metab. 2014;11(3):177–80.
2. Roubenoff R. Origins and clinical relevance of sarcopenia. Can J Appl Physiol. 2001;26(1):78–89. https://doi.org/10.1139/h01-006.
3. Gustafsson T, Ulfhake B. Sarcopenia: what is the origin of this aging-induced disorder? Front Genet. 2021;12:688526. https://doi.org/10.3389/fgene.2021.688526.
4. Barazzoni R, Cederholm T, Zanetti M, Cappellari GG. Defining and diagnosing sarcopenia: is the glass now half full? Metabolism. 2023;143:155558.
5. Petermann-Rocha F, Balntzi V, Gray SR, Lara J, Ho FK, Pell JP, Celis-Morales C. Global prevalence of sarcopenia and severe sarcopenia: a systematic review and meta-analysis. J Cachexia Sarcopenia Muscle. 2022;13(1):86–99.
6. Carvalho do Nascimento PR, Bilodeau M, Poitras S. How do we define and measure sarcopenia? A meta-analysis of observational studies. Age Ageing. 2021;50(6):1906–13.

7. Trombetti A, Reid KF, Hars M, Herrmann FR, Pasha E, Phillips EM, Fielding RA. Age-associated declines in muscle mass, strength, power, and physical performance: impact on fear of falling and quality of life. Osteoporos Int. 2016;27:463–71.

8. Pham LAT, Nguyen BT, Huynh DT, Nguyen BMLT, Tran PAN, Van Vo T, et al. Community-based prevalence and associated factors of sarcopenia in the Vietnamese elderly. Sci Rep. 2024;14(1):17.

9. Wiedmer P, Jung T, Castro JP, Pomatto LC, Sun PY, Davies KJ, Grune T. Sarcopenia–Molecular mechanisms and open questions. Ageing Res Rev. 2021;65:101200.

10. Yuan S, Larsson SC. Epidemiology of sarcopenia: prevalence, risk factors, and consequences. Metabolism. 2023;144:155533.

11. Evans WJ, Guralnik J, Cawthon P, Appleby J, Landi F, Clarke L, Vellas B, Ferrucci L, Roubenoff R. Sarcopenia: no consensus, no diagnostic criteria, and no approved indication – how did we get here? GeroScience. 2024;46(1):183–90.

12. Liu X, Hou L, Zhao W, Xia X, Hao Q, Yue J, Dong B. Comparison of sarcopenia diagnostic criteria using AWGS 2019 with the other five criteria in western China. Asian J Gerontol Geriatr. 2020;15(2):103. Hong Kong Academy of Medicine.

13. Voulgaridou G, Tyrovolas S, Detopoulou P, Tsoumana D, Drakaki M, Apostolou T, et al. Diagnostic criteria and measurement techniques of sarcopenia: a critical evaluation of the up-to-date evidence. Nutrients. 2024;16(3):436.

14. Chen LK, Liu LK, Woo J, Assantachai P, Auyeung TW, Bahyah KS, et al. Sarcopenia in Asia: consensus report of the Asian Working Group for Sarcopenia. J Am Med Dir Assoc. 2014;15(2):95–101.

15. Chen LK, Woo J, Assantachai P, Auyeung TW, Chou MY, Iijima K, et al. Asian Working Group for Sarcopenia: 2019 consensus update on sarcopenia diagnosis and treatment. J Am Med Dir Assoc. 2020;21(3):300–7.

16. Fielding RA, Vellas B, Evans WJ, Bhasin S, Morley JE, Newman AB, et al. Sarcopenia: an undiagnosed condition in older adults. Current consensus definition: prevalence, etiology, and consequences. International working group on sarcopenia. J Am Med Dir Assoc. 2011;12(4):249–56.

17. Studenski SA, Peters KW, Alley DE, Cawthon PM, McLean RR, Harris TB, et al. The FNIH sarcopenia project: rationale, study description, conference recommendations, and final estimates. J Gerontol A Biol Sci Med Sci. 2014;69(5):547–58.

18. Yakout SM, Alkahtani SA, Al-Disi D, Aljaloud KS, Khattak MNK, Alokail MS, et al. Coexistence of pre-sarcopenia and metabolic syndrome in Arab men. Calcif Tissue Int. 2019;104:130–6.

19. Kadoguchi T, Shimada K, Miyazaki T, Kitamura K, Kunimoto M, Aikawa T, et al. Promotion of oxidative stress is associated with mitochondrial dysfunction and muscle atrophy in aging mice. Geriatr Gerontol Int. 2020;20(1):78–84.

20. Küçükdiler AHE, Varli MURAT, Yavuz Ö, Yalçin A, Öztorun HS, Devrim ERDİNÇ, Aras SEVGİ. Evaluation of oxidative stress parameters and antioxidant status in plasma and erythrocytes of elderly diabetic patients with sarcopenia. J Nutr Health Aging. 2019;23(3):239–45.

21. Bernabeu-Wittel M, Gómez-Díaz R, González-Molina Á, Vidal-Serrano S, Díez-Manglano J, Salgado F, et al. Oxidative stress, telomere shortening, and apoptosis associated to sarcopenia and frailty in patients with multimorbidity. J Clin Med. 2020;9(8):2669.

22. Nazri NSM, Vanoh D, Soo KL. Natural food for sarcopenia: a narrative review. Malays J Med Sci. 2022;29(4):28.

23. Besora-Moreno M, Llauradó E, Valls RM, Tarro L, Pedret A, Solà R. Antioxidant-rich foods, antioxidant supplements, and sarcopenia in old-young adults≥ 55 years old: a systematic review and meta-analysis of observational studies and randomized controlled trials. Clin Nutr. 2022;41(10):2308–24.

24. Milaneschi Y, Bandinelli S, Corsi AM, Lauretani F, Paolisso G, Dominguez LJ, et al. Mediterranean diet and mobility decline in older persons. Exp Gerontol. 2011;46(4):303–8.

25. Shahar DR, Houston DK, Hue TF, Lee JS, Sahyoun NR, Tylavsky FA, et al. Adherence to Mediterranean diet and decline in walking speed over 8 years in community-dwelling older adults. J Am Geriatr Soc. 2012;60(10):1881–8.
26. Granic A, Jagger C, Davies K, Adamson A, Kirkwood T, Hill TR, et al. Effect of dietary patterns on muscle strength and physical performance in the very old: findings from the Newcastle 85+ study. PLoS One. 2016;11(3):e0149699.
27. León-Muñoz LM, Guallar-Castillón P, López-García E, Rodríguez-Artalejo F. Mediterranean diet and risk of frailty in community-dwelling older adults. J Am Med Dir Assoc. 2014;15(12):899–903.
28. Papadopoulou SK, Detopoulou P, Voulgaridou G, Tsoumana D, Spanoudaki M, Sadikou F, et al. Mediterranean diet and sarcopenia features in apparently healthy adults over 65 years: a systematic review. Nutrients. 2023;15(5):1104.
29. Salucci S, Bartoletti-Stella A, Bavelloni A, Aramini B, Blalock WL, Fabbri F, Vannini I, Sambri V, Stella F, Faenza I. Extra virgin olive oil (EVOO), a Mediterranean diet component, in the management of muscle mass and function preservation. Nutrients. 2022;14(17):3567.
30. Aparecida Silveira E, Danésio de Souza J, dos Santos Rodrigues AP, Lima RM, de Souza Cardoso CK, de Oliveira C. Effects of extra virgin olive oil (EVOO) and the traditional Brazilian diet on sarcopenia in severe obesity: a randomized clinical trial. Nutrients. 2020;12(5):1498.
31. Jang EH, Han YJ, Jang SE, Lee S. Association between diet quality and sarcopenia in older adults: systematic review of prospective cohort studies. Life. 2021;11(8):811.
32. Van Elswyk ME, Teo L, Lau CS, Shanahan CJ. Dietary patterns and the risk of sarcopenia: a systematic review and meta-analysis. Curr Dev Nutr. 2022;6(5):nzac001.
33. Mahmoodi M, Shateri Z, Nazari SA, Nouri M, Nasimi N, Sohrabi Z, Dabbaghmanesh MH. Association between oxidative balance score and sarcopenia in older adults. Sci Rep. 2024;14(1):5362.
34. Hernández-Ruiz Á, García-Villanova B, Guerra-Hernández E, Amiano P, Ruiz-Canela M, Molina-Montes E. A review of a priori defined oxidative balance scores relative to their components and impact on health outcomes. Nutrients. 2019;11(4):774.
35. Mazza E, Ferro Y, Maurotti S, Micale F, Boragina G, Russo R, et al. Association of dietary patterns with sarcopenia in adults aged 50 years and older. Eur J Nutr. 2024;63(5):1651–62.
36. Bagheri A, Soltani S, Hashemi R, Heshmat R, Motlagh AD, Esmaillzadeh A. Inflammatory potential of the diet and risk of sarcopenia and its components. Nutr J. 2020;19:1–8.
37. Bagheri A, Hashemi R, Heshmat R, Motlagh AD, Esmaillzadeh A. Patterns of nutrient intake in relation to sarcopenia and its components. Front Nutr. 2021;8:645072.
38. Cerullo F, Gambassi G, Cesari M. Rationale for antioxidant supplementation in sarcopenia. J Aging Res. 2012;2012:1.
39. Meng SJ, Yu LJ. Oxidative stress, molecular inflammation and sarcopenia. Int J Mol Sci. 2010;11(4):1509–26.
40. Liguori I, Russo G, Curcio F, Bulli G, Aran L, Della-Morte D, et al. Oxidative stress, aging, and diseases. Clin Interv Aging. 2018;13:757–72.
41. Phaniendra A, Jestadi DB, Periyasamy L. Free radicals: properties, sources, targets, and their implication in various diseases. Indian J Clin Biochem. 2015;30:11–26.
42. Agrawal S, Chakole S, Shetty N, Prasad R, Lohakare T, Wanjari M. Exploring the role of oxidative stress in skeletal muscle atrophy: mechanisms and implications. Cureus. 2023;15(7)
43. Gonzalez A, Simon F, Achiardi O, Vilos C, Cabrera D, Cabello-Verrugio C. The critical role of oxidative stress in sarcopenic obesity. Oxidative Med Cell Longev. 2021;2021
44. Yokoyama Y, Kitamura A, Seino S, Kim H, Obuchi S, Kawai H, et al. Association of nutrient-derived dietary patterns with sarcopenia and its components in community-dwelling older Japanese: a cross-sectional study. Nutr J. 2021;20:1–10.
45. Strandberg E, Edholm P, Ponsot E, Wåhlin-Larsson B, Hellmén E, Nilsson A, et al. Influence of combined resistance training and healthy diet on muscle mass in healthy elderly women: a randomized controlled trial. J Appl Physiol. 2015;119(8):918–25.

46. Koyanagi A, Veronese N, Solmi M, Oh H, Shin JI, Jacob L, et al. Fruit and vegetable consumption and sarcopenia among older adults in low-and middle-income countries. Nutrients. 2020;12(3):706.

47. Saito K, Yokoyama T, Yoshida H, Kim H, Shimada H, Yoshida Y, et al. A significant relationship between plasma vitamin C concentration and physical performance among Japanese elderly women. J Gerontol A Biol Sci Med Sci. 2012;67(3):295–301.

48. Jung UJ. Sarcopenic obesity: involvement of oxidative stress and beneficial role of antioxidant flavonoids. Antioxidants. 2023;12(5):1063.

49. Wang D, Yang Y, Zou X, Zhang J, Zheng Z, Wang Z. Antioxidant apigenin relieves age-related muscle atrophy by inhibiting oxidative stress and hyperactive mitophagy and apoptosis in skeletal muscle of mice. J Gerontol A. 2020;75(11):2081–8.

50. Kim J, Lee JY, Kim CY. A comprehensive review of pathological mechanisms and natural dietary ingredients for the management and prevention of sarcopenia. Nutrients. 2023;15(11):2625.

51. Vargas-Mendoza N, Madrigal-Santillán E, Álvarez-González I, Madrigal-Bujaidar E, Anguiano-Robledo L, Aguilar-Faisal JL, et al. Phytochemicals in skeletal muscle health: effects of curcumin (from Curcuma longa Linn) and sulforaphane (from Brassicaceae) on muscle function, recovery and therapy of muscle atrophy. Plan Theory. 2022;11(19):2517.

52. Kim S, Kim K, Park J, Jun W. Curcuma longa L. Water extract improves dexamethasone-induced sarcopenia by modulating the muscle-related gene and oxidative stress in mice. Antioxidants. 2021;10(7):1000.

53. Saud Gany SL, Chin KY, Tan JK, Aminuddin A, Makpol S. Curcumin as a therapeutic agent for sarcopenia. Nutrients. 2023;15(11):2526.

54. Muthusamy VR, Kannan S, Sadhaasivam K, Gounder SS, Davidson CJ, Boeheme C, et al. Acute exercise stress activates Nrf2/ARE signaling and promotes antioxidant mechanisms in the myocardium. Free Radic Biol Med. 2012;52(2):366–76.

55. Lyu W, Kousaka M, Jia H, Kato H. Effects of turmeric extract on age-related skeletal muscle atrophy in senescence-accelerated mice. Life. 2023;13(4):941.

56. Meador BM, Mirza KA, Tian M, Skelding MB, Reaves LA, Edens NK, et al. The green tea polyphenol epigallocatechin-3-gallate (EGCg) attenuates skeletal muscle atrophy in a rat model of sarcopenia. J Frailty Aging. 2015;4(4):209–15.

57. Liu HW, Chang SJ. Effects of green tea–derived natural products on resistance exercise training in sarcopenia: a retrospective narrative mini-review. J Food Drug Anal. 2023;31(3):381.

58. Wang H, Lai YJ, Chan YL, Li TL, Wu CJ. Epigallocatechin-3-gallate effectively attenuates skeletal muscle atrophy caused by cancer cachexia. Cancer Lett. 2011;305(1):40–9.

59. Tokuda Y, Mori H. Essential amino acid and tea catechin supplementation after resistance exercise improves skeletal muscle mass in older adults with sarcopenia: an open-label, pilot, randomized controlled trial. J Am Nutr Assoc. 2023;42(3):255–62.

60. Chachay VS, Kirkpatrick CM, Hickman IJ, Ferguson M, Prins JB, Martin JH. Resveratrol–pills to replace a healthy diet? Br J Clin Pharmacol. 2011;72(1):27–38.

61. Liao ZY, Chen JL, Xiao MH, Sun Y, Zhao YX, Pu D, et al. The effect of exercise, resveratrol or their combination on sarcopenia in aged rats via regulation of AMPK/Sirt1 pathway. Exp Gerontol. 2017;98:177–83.

62. Zhou DD, Luo M, Huang SY, Saimaiti A, Shang A, Gan RY, Li HB. Effects and mechanisms of resveratrol on aging and age-related diseases. Oxidative Med Cell Longev. 2021;2021(1):9932218.

63. Joseph AM, Malamo AG, Silvestre J, Wawrzyniak N, Carey-Love S, Nguyen LMD, et al. Short-term caloric restriction, resveratrol, or combined treatment regimens initiated in late-life alter mitochondrial protein expression profiles in a fiber-type specific manner in aged animals. Exp Gerontol. 2013;48(9):858–68.

64. Kan NW, Ho CS, Chiu YS, Huang WC, Chen PY, Tung YT, Huang CC. Effects of resveratrol supplementation and exercise training on exercise performance in middle-aged mice. Molecules. 2016;21(5):661.

65. Nasimi N, Sohrabi Z, Dabbaghmanesh MH, Eskandari MH, Bedeltavana A, Famouri M, Talezadeh P. A novel fortified dairy product and sarcopenia measures in sarcopenic older adults: a double-blind randomized controlled trial. J Am Med Dir Assoc. 2021;22(4):809–15.
66. Boutry-Regard C, Vinyes-Parés G, Breuillé D, Moritani T. Supplementation with whey protein, omega-3 fatty acids and polyphenols combined with electrical muscle stimulation increases muscle strength in elderly adults with limited mobility: a randomized controlled trial. Nutrients. 2020;12(6):1866.
67. McDermott MM, Criqui MH, Domanchuk K, Ferrucci L, Guralnik JM, Kibbe MR, et al. Cocoa to improve walking performance in older people with peripheral artery disease: the COCOA-PAD pilot randomized clinical trial. Circ Res. 2020;126(5):589–99.
68. Alway SE, McCrory JL, Kearcher K, Vickers A, Frear B, Gilleland DL, Bonner DE, Thomas JM, Donley DA, Lively MW, Mohamed JS. Resveratrol enhances exercise-induced cellular and functional adaptations of skeletal muscle in older men and women. J Gerontol A Biol Sci Med Sci. 2017;72(12):1595–606.

Nourishing Oral Health for a Radiant Smile

6

Jylana L. Sheats and Melissa D. Porter

Learning Objectives

After completing this chapter, you will be able to

- Understand the global burden of oral health and why it is a national priority for the United States
- Explore the relationship between oral and systemic health, including disparities and determinants
- Learn about essential nutrients for strong teeth and gums and how to source them from food and dietary supplements
- Discover the impact of sugar-sweetened and acidic foods and beverages on oral health
- Identify best practices for healthy meals and snacks, including insights into mindful eating
- Examine the significance of integrated oral health care and the value of engagement across sectors, stakeholders, and communities

J. L. Sheats (✉)
Tulane University Celia Scott Weatherhead School of Public Health & Tropical Medicine, New Orleans, LA, USA
e-mail: jsheats@tulane.edu

M. D. Porter
Meharry Medical College, Department of Pediatric Dentistry, Nashville, TN, USA
e-mail: melissa.porter@mmc.edu

Introduction

Optimal oral health is essential for overall health and well-being [1]. Yet like its definition, oral health is multifaceted. According to the World Health Organization [2], *oral health* is defined as "the state of the mouth, teeth, and orofacial structures that enables individuals to perform essential functions such as eating, breathing, and speaking, and encompasses psychosocial dimensions such as self-confidence, well-being and the ability to socialize and work without pain, discomfort, and embarrassment." The definition, as presented, represents three core facets that may independently or collectively affect one's health: [3, 4] (1) *disease and condition status* (i.e., severity, progression), *physiological function* (i.e., the performance of key behaviors, such as speaking, smiling, chewing, and swallowing), and *psychosocial function* (i.e., the mental health implications associated with one's ability to perform physiological functions and comfortably engage in social or professional settings).

The most common preventable oral diseases and conditions are dental caries (i.e., tooth decay, also known as cavities), severe periodontal (gum) disease, edentulism (i.e., tooth loss), and lip and oral cavity cancers [5, 6]. When left untreated, they may result in hypersensitivity, pain, infection, morbidities, and mortality [7, 8]. Increased sugar consumption, along with tobacco use, alcohol use, oral trauma or injury, and poor oral hygiene (e.g., not regularly brushing, flossing, or receiving regular oral healthcare from an oral health professional), are the primary factors increasing their prevalence [2]. This chapter explores the intersection of oral health, nutrition, and overall health and well-being, focusing on ensuring that optimal oral health outcomes can be achieved for all.

The Global Burden of Oral Health

Globally, 3.5 billion people, from infants to older adults, are affected by oral diseases and conditions [4]. According to the World Health Organization's Oral Health Status Report: Towards Universal Health Coverage for Oral Health by 2030, "the combined estimated number of cases of oral diseases globally is about 1 billion higher than cases of all five primary non-communicable diseases (mental disorders, cardiovascular diseases, diabetes mellitus, chronic respiratory diseases, and cancers)" [4]. Dental caries is the most common noncommunicable disease in the world and "develops when bacteria in the mouth metabolize sugars to produce acid that demineralizes the hard tissues of the teeth (enamel and dentin)," which covers and gives shape to the crowns of teeth [9, 10]. The incidence of oral diseases and conditions is lower in industrialized countries [4], such as the United States, where 73% of cities have fluoridated water systems to strengthen teeth and prevent tooth decay [11]. Despite these and other protective public health measures in the United States to reduce dental caries, it remains a significant public health issue impacting individuals from childhood into adulthood [12].

Oral health population surveillance data show that in the United States, "the prevalence of total dental caries (untreated and treated) in primary or permanent teeth among youth aged 2–19 years was 43.1%. Prevalence increased with age, going from 17.7% among youth aged 2–5 to 45.2% among those aged 6–11 to 53.5% among those aged 12–19" [13]. Tooth decay remains high among adults, where 90% of those aged 20 years and older have experienced at least one cavity [6]. The prevalence of complete tooth loss among older adults increased with age from 8.9% among those aged 65 to 69 years to 10.6% among those aged 70 to 74 years to 17.8% among those aged 75 years and older. Race and ethnicity are also factors given the greater percentage of non-Hispanic Black adults (25.4%) who have experienced complete tooth loss relative to Hispanic (15.3%) and non-Hispanic White adults [14].

Oral Health: A National Priority Connected to Dietary Patterns

The prevalence of oral health conditions and diseases increases as individuals age [15]. Given the magnitude and impact of poor oral health and the implications for systemic health, a national call to action for oral health conditions can be found in Healthy People 2030, the nation's roadmap for improving health and well-being, preventing morbidity and mortality, and improving quality of life among all people [16]. The objectives are organized by category—life course (i.e., children and adolescents, adults, and older adults), healthcare access and quality, healthy policy, nutrition and healthy eating, preventive care, and public health infrastructure. The life course and nutrition and healthy eating oral health objectives include the following:

- Reduce the proportion of children and adolescents with active and untreated tooth decay.
- Reduce the proportion of children and adolescents with lifetime tooth decay.
- Reduce the proportion of adults with active and untreated tooth decay.
- Reduce the proportion of adults aged 45 years and over who have lost all their teeth.
- Reduce the proportion of older adults with active and untreated tooth decay.
- Reduce the proportion of older adults with untreated root surface decay.
- Reduce the proportion of adults aged 45 years and over with moderate and severe periodontitis.
- Reduce the consumption of added sugars by people aged 2 years and over.

Data on the country's progress in achieving the objectives are reported to be at "baseline," "improving," or "met or exceeded." Some strides have been made, but to date, "little or no detectable change" has been detected in the consumption of added sugars among children aged 2 years and older or the proportion of children and adolescents with lifetime tooth decay. Further, the proportion of adults aged 45 years and older who have lost all their teeth is reportedly "getting worse" [16]. Nutrition and dietary patterns, which are the combination of foods and beverages that make up an individual's overall nutritional intake over time [17], play vital roles in advancing the country's progress in meeting the Healthy People 2030 oral health objectives.

Oral Health Determinants and Disparities

Although largely preventable, dental caries is a combination of genetic, physiological, environmental, behavioral, and social determinants [12, 18]. Examples of genetic determinants include tooth and enamel structure and development, saliva production, and regulation, biofilm (plaque) production, and tooth mineralization [19]. Genetic determinants of oral health are inherently physiological; other physiological determinants, such as saliva composition, immune responses, and microbial interactions, also significantly shape oral health and disease susceptibility [12]. Key behavioral determinants of dental caries include inadequate fluoride intake, poor oral hygiene practices, and the frequent consumption of added sugars (e.g., glucose, fructose, sucrose, and maltose) [12]. Below are examples of strategies that could be implemented to prevent dental caries and other oral conditions and diseases [20]:

- Brushing one's teeth twice per day
- Using an interdental cleaner (e.g., floss)
- Rinsing one's mouth with water or a mouth rinse that contains fluoride, after eating
- Visiting a dentist for professional cleanings and regular checkups
- Using dental sealants (a recommendation for all school-age children)
- Drinking tap water (most public water has fluoride in it)
- Consuming foods that will not get stuck on or between teeth
- Checking with a dentist about fluoride treatments, antiseptic and disinfecting treatments, and/or combined treatments to prevent or treat tooth decay

Fillings, root canal therapy, crowns and bridges, and dental implants are procedures used to save, repair, or replace teeth impacted by an oral health condition or disease. Common treatments for gum disease are scaling, root planting, periodontal surgery, antibiotic therapy, and ongoing disease management. An oral health professional should guide an individual in the appropriate preventive measures or treatment.

Although behaviors are essential in preventing and addressing oral health conditions and diseases, factors beyond the individual also play important roles. Thus, social determinants—the nonmedical factors associated with health outcomes that drive oral health inequities—must also be recognized [18]. Factors such as socioeconomic status, the cost of and access to oral healthcare, food insecurity, and cultural beliefs and practices (e.g., gender norms and fatalistic beliefs) affect oral health outcomes and disparities [14, 16, 21, 22]. For example, Black and Hispanic adults were twice as likely to cite cost as a barrier to dental care relative to White adults [23]. Individuals without dental insurance and those with at least one oral health symptom have reported experiencing significantly more food insecurity than those with dental insurance or oral health symptoms, respectively [24]. Further, children living in low-income households are two times more likely to have untreated dental caries relative to children from high-income households [6].

Understanding these and other broader behavioral, societal, and contextual factors impacting oral health outcomes will not only help address oral health disparities but also illuminate systemic health implications that underscore the significance of oral health from a holistic perspective.

Systemic Health Implications of Oral Health

In the landmark 2000 report Oral Health in America: A Report of the Surgeon General, former US surgeon general Dr. David Satcher stated that the "mouth is the window to all the diseases of the body" [25]. In other words, oral health is intricately connected to systemic health, where poor oral health plays a role in developing and exacerbating systemic health issues. For example, the oral cavity and pathogens related to periodontal diseases can influence the development of systemic diseases. The inflammation initiated by periodontal disease has the potential to cause systemic inflammation, thereby playing a role in the development of noncommunicable diseases [23] such as Alzheimer's disease, diabetes and insulin resistance, cardiovascular diseases, chronic obstructive pulmonary disease (COPD), respiratory tract infections and bacterial pneumonia, oral/colorectal carcinoma, and gastrointestinal diseases [23, 26].

Dietary patterns significantly influence the composition and balance of the oral microbiome. The oral microbiome is an essential component of oral health that refers to "a community of bacteria, viruses, and fungi that reside in the mouth," where the composition of bacteria varies depending on the specific location within the oral cavity (e.g., inner cheeks, tongue, saliva, teeth, or periodontal pocket) [27]. Diet represents just one of several factors that influence the oral microbiome, a connection that researchers have associated with the potential development of systemic illnesses [28]. Engaging in good oral hygiene practices, regular dental care, and a nutrient-dense diet helps maintain a healthy oral microbiome. Understanding the oral microbiome and the interconnectedness of oral health and overall health is fundamental to implementing personalized dietary recommendations that can optimize oral health outcomes and contribute to holistic health and well-being.

Essential Nutrients for Strong Teeth and Gums

A holistic approach to oral health that considers dietary factors alongside oral health practices is critical given that a clear bidirectional, symbiotic relationship exists between diet, oral health, and nutrition in maintaining oral health homeostasis within the oral cavity—ensuring equilibrium in the gums, teeth, saliva, and oral microbiota [27, 29]. Nutrients are substances that the body uses to function and grow and are essential in maintaining oral and systemic health [28, 30]. They prevent previously noted oral diseases and conditions and systemic conditions [7, 23]. There are two types of nutrients: macronutrients and micronutrients. Macronutrients include nutrients that humans consume large quantities of—namely proteins, carbohydrates, and fats—and are essential energy sources for humans [28]. Micronutrients are consumed in small quantities and comprise essential vitamins and minerals. Deficiencies in macro- and micronutrients can impact growth, development, and bodily functions [31]. The sections below provide insight into the macro- and micronutrients vital for oral health and sources from which to obtain them.

Macronutrients and the Oral Cavity

Understanding the role and importance of macronutrients is fundamental to maintaining health and well-being. Each of the three classes of macronutrients—carbohydrates, proteins, and fats—is vital for overall human health and development [28]. Briefly, carbohydrates are categorized into two types: simple and complex. Simple carbohydrates include "added sugars," such as refined sugar and sugary beverages, which lack minerals and vitamins and contribute to poor oral health [17, 28]. In contrast, complex carbohydrates are naturally occurring and contain minerals, vitamins, and fiber (e.g., fruits, vegetables, and whole grains). Sugars and refined carbohydrates can contribute to developing dental caries and other conditions and diseases [28].

In contrast, "proteins are vital structural and functional components within every cell of the body and are essential for growth and repair and maintenance of health" [32]. They also play a role in oral health in that proteins are "building blocks" for bones and periodontia, which are composed of hard and soft tissues that hold teeth in place—supporting oral functions such as biting and chewing. In addition to slowing wound healing and reducing salivary flow, protein deficiencies can impact teeth strength, thereby compromising dentition integrity [32, 33] and increasing the risk of gingivitis, periodontal disease, and tooth loss.

Lipids are significant energy sources present in all physiological functions of the body [34]. They occur as fats, oils, phospholipids, steroids, and carotenoids [35]. "Healthy fats" (i.e., monounsaturated and polyunsaturated fats) are found primarily in oils, nuts, and seeds and are known to reduce inflammation. Evidence suggests that omega-3 fatty acids, a polyunsaturated fat found in fish, seeds, and nuts [36], may aid in reducing periodontitis due to their anti-inflammatory effects [35]. Because all fats are not created equal, the Dietary Guidelines for Americans recommends limiting the intake of saturated fats (found primarily in meats, dairy products, and processed foods) and replacing them with unsaturated fats to support cardiovascular health and lower cholesterol levels [17].

Macronutrients are critical for oral health, and micronutrients, such as minerals and vitamins, are essential for supporting oral health functions. The section below will underscore the crucial nature of nutrition and dietary patterns in maintaining optimal oral health.

Micronutrients and the Oral Cavity

Minerals work in conjunction with vitamins to reinforce and fortify teeth. Although not an exhaustive list, minerals, calcium, fluoride, magnesium, phosphorus, and vitamins A, C, and D are essential in maintaining optimal health and well-being when combined with regular dental hygiene and care [37, 38].

Minerals

Calcium Calcium is the body's most abundant and essential mineral. Over 99% is stored within the bones and teeth, making it vital in maintaining their strength and integrity [38]. It is also a primary component of dental enamel, the outer and strongest layer of the tooth that protects teeth against acids that cause tooth decay [39]. In addition to its role in bone and enamel health, calcium supports normal bodily movement by keeping tissue rigid, strong, and flexible, aiding in blood vessel contraction and dilation, muscle function, blood clotting, nerve transmission, and hormone secretion [40, 41], all of which impact oral health (e.g., chewing, swallowing, sensations in the teeth and mouth, and muscle function).

Fluoride "Fluoride is the ionic form of the element fluorine, and it inhibits or reverses the initiation and progression of dental caries (tooth decay) and stimulates new bone formation" [38]. This mineral has been added to tap water in most cities across the United States per the recommendation of the US Public Health Service, with established guidelines from the Environmental Protection Agency (EPA) [38]. Fluoride is also available in oral health products such as toothpaste and mouth rinses, medications (not the active ingredient), and dietary supplements.

Magnesium Magnesium is an essential and abundant mineral in the body, found predominantly in the bones (60%) and soft tissues (40%)—with less than 1% in the blood [42]. It serves several functions in the body, such as muscle and nerve function, blood glucose control, bone development and health, regulating the inflammatory response (systemically and locally), maintaining the functioning of the immune system, and transporting calcium and potassium [28, 34]. Magnesium contributes to the development of tooth enamel, "has an impact on the quality and anatomy of dental hard tissues," [10] and helps prevent tooth decay [39].

Phosphorus Phosphorus is key in developing bones, teeth, cell membranes, and genes (DNA and RNA) [43]. The second-most-abundant mineral in the body (after calcium), phosphorus is stored mainly (85%) in the bones and teeth. Phosphorus and calcium work synergistically to support nutrient absorption and bodily functions [38]. Although not a primary component of saliva, phosphorus in saliva assists in balancing pH in the oral cavity, which supports tooth enamel remineralization, thereby helping maintain tooth mineral integrity and strength [44].

Vitamins

Vitamin A Vitamin A is a fat-soluble vitamin involved in strengthening the immune system to combat disease, supporting cell growth and differentiation, which develops and maintains vital organs (e.g., heart, lungs, eyes); enabling vision in low-light conditions; and maintaining the health of the skin and mucous membranes and that of other bodily functions [38]. The human diet has two vitamin A sources: (1) preformed vitamin A and (2) provitamin A carotenoids. Preformed vitamin A is found in animal-based foods (e.g., dairy, eggs, fish, and organ meats). In contrast, provitamin A is found in plant-based pigments (i.e., beta-carotene, alpha-carotene, and beta-cryptoxanthin) that can be converted into active vitamin A, which has implications for those following a plant-based dietary pattern [38]. Vitamin A is essential for maintaining mucosal membranes that line various parts of the oral cavity (e.g., cheeks, gums, tongue, and other internal surfaces) [38, 45].

Vitamin C Vitamin C, also known as ascorbic acid, is a water-soluble vitamin that is involved in strengthening the immune system to combat disease, protecting cells from damage caused by free radicals, promoting skin health and wound healing, enhancing iron absorption, and it is essential for maintaining healthy skin, bones, blood vessels, neurological functions, gums, and teeth [38, 46]. Because vitamin C is important for synthesizing collagen, it promotes healthy gums and protects against gum diseases and associated inflammation and bleeding. Research suggests that vitamin C, a natural antioxidant, may reduce the risk of oral cancer and slow its progression [47].

Vitamin D Vitamin D, often known as calciferol, is a vital fat-soluble vitamin that the body requires for multiple functions and is crucial for bone health and immune function. Vitamin D is produced mainly in the skin when exposed to sunlight but can also come from certain foods or supplements. The body transforms inactive vitamin D into an active form, aiding calcium absorption for bone strength and muscle functioning [38, 48]. Vitamin D is vital for maintaining healthy teeth and gums and reducing the risk of tooth decay and diseases of the gums [48].

Sources of Minerals and Vitamins

Food Sources

Table 6.1 provides examples of the micronutrient food and beverage sources highlighted in this chapter. For more information on these and other micronutrients, access the US National Institutes of Health Office of Dietary Supplements Dietary Supplement Fact Sheets [38]. Fact sheets are available for health professionals and consumers and can provide more in-depth information on each mineral or vitamin source, recommended intakes, deficiencies, and impacts on health. These fact sheets are available via the following weblink: https://ods.od.nih.gov/factsheets/list-all/.

Table 6.1 Micronutrient food sources to support optimal oral health [45, 48–51]

Mineral	Food sources	Sample consequences of oral health-related deficiencies
Calcium	Vegetables (e.g., bok choy, broccoli, kale, kidney beans, lima beans, soybeans, spinach)	Hypomineralization
	Fruits (e.g., apples (Golden Delicious with skin))	Delayed eruption of the tooth
	Grains (e.g., breakfast cereal (fortified))	Periodontitis
	Dairy and fortified soy alternatives (e.g., milk (nonfat), soymilk, mozzarella cheese (partly skim), sour cream (reduced fat))	Increased bleeding of the gums
	Protein-rich foods (e.g., almonds, chia seeds, pine nuts, pink salmon, sardines, tofu)	Tooth looseness and premature tooth loss
	Beverages (e.g., grapefruit juice (100% fortified), orange juice (100% fortified))	Inadequate jawbone density and strength to anchor tooth structure
Fluoride	Vegetables (e.g., asparagus, carrots, potatoes)	Tooth decay Weakened enamel
	Fruits (e.g., apples, avocados, bananas, tomatoes)	
	Grains (e.g., bread (white or whole wheat), oatmeal, macaroni (plain), rice, tortilla)	
	Dairy and fortified soy alternatives (e.g., cheese (cheddar), milk (fat-free or 1%))	
	Protein-rich foods (e.g., beef, chicken, egg, lamb chop, pork chop, shrimp, tuna (light))	
	Beverages (e.g., black tea (brewed), coffee (brewed), grapefruit juice, water with added fluoride)	
Magnesium	Vegetables (e.g., carrots, lima beans, squash (yellow), tomatoes)	Soft dental enamel, which cannot resist the acids causing tooth decay
	Fruits (e.g., apples, avocados, grapefruit, peaches)	
	Grains (e.g., barley flour or meal, bread (whole grain), corn meal (whole grain, white), oatmeal, pasta (whole wheat), rice (brown))	Increased bleeding
	Dairy and fortified soy alternatives (e.g., milk, soymilk, yogurt (plain, low fat))	
	Protein-rich foods (e.g., almonds, beef patty, chicken (breast), crab, halibut, peanuts, salmon (Atlantic), sunflower seeds)	Tooth looseness and premature tooth loss

(continued)

Table 6.1 (continued)

Mineral	Food sources	Sample consequences of oral health-related deficiencies
Phosphorus	Vegetables (e.g., asparagus, cashews, cauliflower, kidney beans, lentils, nuts, peas (green))	Weakened tooth enamel
	Fruits (e.g., apple, clementine)	
	Grains (e.g., rice (brown), bread (whole wheat), oatmeal, tortilla (corn))	
	Dairy and fortified soy alternatives (e.g., milk (2%), mozzarella cheese (part-skim), yogurt (plain, low fat))	A predisposition to tooth decay
	Protein-rich foods (e.g., chicken breast, eggs, salmon (Atlantic), scallops)	
	Beverage (e.g., green tea (brewed))	Impairment of the proper mineralization of teeth
Vitamin A	Vegetables (e.g., black-eyed peas, broccoli, carrots, spinach, summer squash, sweet potatoes)	Decreased oral epithelial development (oral mucosa, preventing infections, and aiding in the healing process of oral wounds)
	Fruits (e.g., apricots, cantaloupe, mangoes)	Impaired tooth formation
	Grains (e.g., cereal that's ready to eat and fortified with vitamin D)	Enamel hypoplasia (thin enamel layer)
	Dairy and fortified soy alternatives (e.g., milk (skim with added vitamin A and vitamin D), cheese (ricotta), yogurt (plain, low fat))	Periodontitis
	Protein-rich foods (e.g., chicken breast, eggs, herring (Atlantic), pistachio nuts, salmon (sockeye), tuna (light))	Increased risk of tooth decay
		Hypomineralization
		Delayed eruption of the tooth
		Increased bleeding of the gums
		Xerostomia (dry mouth)
Vitamin C	Vegetables (e.g., broccoli, brussels sprouts, cabbage, green peas, peppers (raw red or green), spinach)	Hypomineralization
	Fruits (e.g., grapefruit, orange, strawberries, kiwifruit)	Delayed eruption of the tooth
	Beverage (e.g., grapefruit juice, orange juice, tomato juice)	Periodontitis
		Inflammation of the gums
		Swollen, bleeding gums
		Tooth loosening or loss of teeth

(continued)

Table 6.1 (continued)

Mineral	Food sources	Sample consequences of oral health-related deficiencies
Vitamin D	Vegetables (e.g., broccoli, carrots, lentils, mushrooms (white))	Periodontitis
	Fruits (e.g., apples, bananas)	Onset and progression of certain oral cancers
	Grains (e.g., cereal that's ready to eat and fortified with vitamin D, rice (brown))	Higher risk of tooth defects, caries, and the failure of oral treatment (e.g., orthodontic-related tooth movement)
	Dairy and fortified soy alternatives (e.g., cheese (cheddar), milk (2%) or vitamin D–fortified soy, almond, or oat milk)	Hypomineralization
	Protein-rich foods (e.g., chicken breast, eggs, liver (beef), sardines, trout (rainbow), tuna fish (light), salmon (sockeye))	Delayed eruption of the tooth
		Increased bleeding of the gums
		Xerostomia (dry mouth)
		Inadequate jawbone density and strength to anchor tooth structure

Dietary Supplements

Consuming nutrient-dense foods and beverages containing essential vitamins, minerals, and other beneficial elements while low in added sugars, saturated fat, and sodium [17] is necessary for maintaining good oral health. Poor oral health accompanied by pain and/or infection, for example, may lead to an inadequate intake of vitamins and minerals, resulting in nutritional deficiencies [7]. Food and/or dietary supplements provide essential minerals that form the basic structure of teeth [48]. In the United States, consuming vitamin and mineral dietary supplements is common across all ages [52]. According to a National Center for Health Statistics (NCHS) Data Brief, one-third of children and adolescents have consumed them in the past 30 days compared to over half (58%) of adults. Relative to men, the use of supplements is higher among women (64%). They also report that multivitamin-mineral, vitamin D, and omega-3 fatty acid supplements are the most commonly consumed across all age groups [52]. Monitoring nutrient intakes from dietary supplements and all other sources, such as one's diet, products (e.g., toothpaste and mouth rinses), and other sources, is necessary to ensure that nutritional needs are met and not exceeded.

Food Access and Food Insecurity

Obtaining essential nutrients is more difficult when access to healthy foods is limited or if an individual is food insecure [24]. Although access to food is a fundamental element and indicator of well-being [53], in 2022, 44.2 million people in the United States lived in 17 million food-insecure households—with evidence

Table 6.2 US government programs to address food access and food insecurity

Supplemental Nutrition Assistance Program (SNAP) https://www.fns.usda.gov/snap/supplemental-nutrition-assistance-program	Senior Farmers Market Nutrition Program (SFMNP) https://www.fns.usda.gov/sfmnp/senior-farmers-market-nutrition-program
Special Supplemental Nutrition Program for Women, Infants, and Children (WIC) https://www.fns.usda.gov/wic	Commodity Supplemental Food Program (CSFP) https://www.fns.usda.gov/csfp/commodity-supplemental-food-program
National School Lunch Program (NSLP) https://www.fns.usda.gov/nslp/national-school-lunch-program-nslp	Home-Delivered Nutrition Services https://acl.gov/senior-nutrition/basics-home-delivered-meals
National School Breakfast Program (NSBP) https://www.fns.usda.gov/sbp/school-breakfast-program	Farmers Market and Local Food Promotion Program (FMLFPP) https://www.fns.usda.gov/fmnp/farmers-market-nutrition-program
Summer Food Service Program (SUN Meals) https://www.fns.usda.gov/summer/sunmeals	Healthy Food Financing Initiative (HFFI) https://www.rd.usda.gov/about-rd/initiatives/healthy-food-financing-initiative
Child and Adult Care Food Program (CACFP) https://www.fns.usda.gov/cacfp	

demonstrating disproportionate rates among some racial and ethnic population subgroups relative to others [54]. According to Martin and colleagues [24], dentists and healthcare providers can play a vital role in connecting people to healthier food choices. In addition to sharing local resources, government programs are available to reduce food insecurity and promote food access, such as those listed in Table 6.2.

In addition to federal programs that support food access, connecting dietary and oral health guidance empowers individuals to make informed choices for improved dietary patterns and health outcomes.

Sugar-Sweetened and Acidic Foods and Beverages: Impacts on Oral Health

An interplay between oral health and dietary patterns has already been established. The consumption of sugars is one of the primary drivers of poor oral health, which often leads to dental caries. There are two types of sugars: (1) intrinsic and (2) extrinsic sugars. Intrinsic sugars are naturally occurring (versus being processed) and are found in whole fruits, vegetables, and dairy foods. Extrinsic sugars are "added" sugars [55] and should comprise no more than 10% of an individual's dietary pattern [17]. "Worldwide, data suggest that added sugar intake rises starting from one year of age and is highest among school-age children and adolescents compared to adults" [56].

Moreover, the Dietary Guidelines for Americans states that "added sugars account on average for almost 270 calories—or more than 13 percent of total calories—per day in the US population" [17]. The top two sources and average intakes of added sugar among the US population aged 1 year or older are sugar-sweetened beverages (24%) and desserts and sweet snacks (19%). Within the sugar-sweetened beverages subcategory, carbonated beverages (i.e., soft drinks), fruit drinks, and sports and energy drinks ranked highest, whereas within the subcategory of desserts and sweet snacks, cookies and brownies, ice cream and frozen dairy desserts, and cakes and pies were ranked highly for containing added sugar [17].

Briefly, when an individual consumes a sugary food or a sugar-sweetened beverage, the bacteria in the oral cavity produce acids as byproducts. These acids, in turn, attack the tooth's enamel, which leads to the breakdown, or demineralization, of said tooth. Over time, demineralization can lead to the softening of the tooth and, ultimately, the formation of dental caries (shaped like holes) in the teeth [57]. Additionally, when individuals consume acidic foods or drinks, they directly attack the tooth's mineral layer, weakening and thinning it over time, leading to one of the most commonly reported dental symptoms—sensitivity. The more prolonged and frequent the exposure to foods with added sugar and sugar-sweetened beverages, the greater the risk of tooth decay. Introducing fluoride through oral health products and combined treatments and saliva can reverse the demineralization process via a process referred to as remineralization. During remineralization, fluoride, a mineral, strengthens the tooth enamel and structure, thereby increasing resistance to tooth decay [12]. If left untreated, dental caries can progress to more-extensive oral diseases, conditions, and complications that can affect overall health, including systemic infections, abscesses, and, in severe cases, life-threatening diseases and conditions [4, 7].

The worldwide messaging about reducing or limiting sugar intake has been consistent [9, 17, 56]. Also of note are acidic foods associated with the erosion of tooth enamel, such as citrus foods (lemons, oranges, and grapefruits), vinegar-based foods (pickled vegetables and salad dressings), carbonated drinks (sodas and sparkling waters), and sports drinks [57]. The harmful effects of sugary and acidic foods and drinks on oral health demonstrate why patients must make informed dietary choices, practice proper daily oral hygiene, and receive regular professional oral health care to prevent oral diseases and conditions.

From Meals to Snacks: Best Practices for a Healthy Smile

As people progress through different life stages, their dietary patterns and preferences evolve. These "shifts" are often shaped by myriad influences extending beyond individual beliefs, knowledge, and behaviors. Factors ranging from interpersonal connections (such as family, friends, and social networks) to organizational settings (e.g., schools and workplaces), community aspects (e.g., food access, availability, and quality), and societal elements (e.g., food-related policies and community infrastructure) all play roles in shaping food choices during meals [17, 58].

Defining Meals and Snacks

Although global agreement has been reached on defining a *meal* as "a certain amount of food eaten at a specific time" [59], meals' symbolic meanings and their timing vary across individuals, groups, societies, and cultures [60]. In Western society, the notion that daily food consumption should be structured around three core meals—breakfast (morning), lunch (midday), and dinner (evening)—is embedded in American culture [61, 62]. Although the word *snack* is often defined as the consumption of food and beverages outside of the three core meals (breakfast, lunch, and dinner), neither it nor the related terms *snacking* and *snack foods* has a clear definition [63]. Among US adults, 55% consume three meals and at least one snack [62]. Regarding snack frequency, among US adults, 88% reported consuming one snack daily, and 63% reported consuming two or more snacks daily [62].

Generally, the Dietary Guidelines for Americans recommends consuming various fruits, vegetables, whole grains, protein-rich foods, and dairy or fortified soy alternatives [17]. They advise limiting the intake of saturated fat, high-sodium foods, and added sugars, advice that is important given their documented association with dental caries [17, 64]. Evidence has also shown that snacking is associated with overall diet quality among adult populations [65]. Snacking has the potential to enhance dietary patterns by providing essential vitamins and minerals while supplementing energy and nutrient intake between core meals [63]. However, snack foods are often composed of energy-dense and nutrient-poor foods and beverages high in carbohydrates, sodium, added sugars, and/or fat (e.g., packaged snacks, carbonated beverages, desserts, and candies) [62, 66]. People who consume more significant amounts of sugar-sweetened beverages (daily or multiple times per week) are at increased risk of developing dental caries and erosion and tend to have higher rates of cavities compared to those who consume smaller quantities (less than twice weekly) [67]. Implementing food choice and preparation strategies that align with recommendations from the Dietary Guidelines for Americans [17] will benefit general and oral health by ensuring an adequate consumption of nutrient-dense foods and reducing the risk of poor oral health. Table 6.3 provides examples of practical strategies that foster the consumption of healthy meals and snack foods to lower the risk of tooth decay, gum disease, and enamel erosion, for example.

Table 6.3 Examples of food selection and preparation strategies to promote optimal general and oral health [11, 17, 68–73]

Categories	Examples
Select the rainbow	Select a colorful array of crisp raw fruits and vegetables into snacks for optimal nutrition and disease prevention. For example, dip broccoli, colorful peppers, zucchini strips, or baby carrots into hummus, guacamole, or low-fat yogurt.
Combine food groups	Combine different food groups to create a satisfying snack or meal. For example, pair dairy (e.g., low-fat yogurt) with berries or apples; pair celery with nut or seed butter; or pair whole-grain crackers with turkey and avocado.
Prep in advance	Prepare snacks in advance and incorporate diverse nutrient-rich options to promote healthier dietary choices. Wash and cut fresh vegetables and then divide them into reusable containers for an easy grab-and-go option for snacks or meals.
Wash and go	Fresh fruits such as apples, pears, grapes, and bananas are always quick and simple snack choices because they can be consumed whole and travel well.
Make it convenient	Ensure that nutritious snacks, like fruits and vegetables, are prominently displayed and easily accessible in the fridge or on the counter for a convenient snack option at any time.
Create your own	Create a custom snack mix using unsalted nuts, such as seeds, cereals (unsweetened), dried fruit (e.g., dried raisins or cranberries), and plain popcorn.
Enjoy "nature's candy"	Swap sugary snacks like candy and desserts for fresh fruits or crunchy vegetables like apples, carrots, or celery. These can help stimulate saliva production, which helps naturally clean teeth by removing food particles and bacteria. Vitamin A in carrots can also repair tooth enamel.
Hydrate for oral health	Drink water or unsweetened herbal teas instead of sugar-sweetened beverages such as carbonated beverages or fruit juices (that are not 100% juice). Drinking water washes away food particles and bacteria, keeps the mouth hydrated, and reduces the risk of tooth decay. Not all bottled water contains fluoride. Check the label or contact the brand's manufacturer for fluoride content. If you are concerned about a child's lack of fluoride consumption, talk to their dentist and/or pediatrician. Green tea, known for its antioxidant properties and potent antibacterial effects, has been shown to inhibit the growth of periodontal-associated bacteria, thereby reducing the risks of halitosis (i.e., bad breath), tooth decay, gingivitis, and periodontitis.
Say cheese!	Selecting low-fat dairy products high in calcium and phosphorus can help strengthen tooth enamel, prevent tooth decay, and neutralize acids.
Acid defense for tooth enamel	Limit the intake of acidic foods and beverages by rinsing the mouth with water (tap, bottled, or alkaline electrolyzed), which restores the oral pH to a neutral level. Using a straw will also minimize contact time between acidic beverages (e.g., carbonated beverages) and teeth.
Nutty nourishment	Choose nuts and seeds instead of chips or crackers. Nuts and seeds contain antioxidants that prevent or treat oral diseases and conditions such as periodontal disease, tooth decay, and oral cancer. They are also rich in vitamins C and E and healthy fats.

Timing Matters: Meals, Brushing, and Interdental Cleaning

Understanding the optimal timing for meals, brushing, and interdental cleaning (e.g., with dental floss, a dental floss pick, powered water, or air flossers) promotes regular, healthy oral hygiene practices and preserves the long-term integrity of teeth and gums. Studies have shown that the timing of meals can have significant implications for overall health, including oral health [74, 75]. For example, nocturnal eating (i.e., eating during the night) was shown to be a predictor of tooth loss among adults aged 30 to 60 years, [75] and another study among adults found nocturnal eating to be a predictor of not only missing teeth but also periodontal disease and active decay [76]. Among a sample of youth aged 12 to 14, an association was found between tooth erosion and the consumption of acidic beverages at bedtime, for example [77].

Like eating, the timing of when one brushes one's teeth is also important. The American Dental Association recommends brushing for 2 minutes twice daily with fluoride toothpaste to remove food and plaque and lower the risk of dental caries [78]. Evidence has shown that brushing immediately after a meal may result in pain from tooth abrasion or erosion due to high levels of acidity in saliva from food. Waiting at least 30 minutes to brush allows acids in the mouth to allow the pH in saliva to return to its premeal state and strengthen (or reharden) tooth enamel before brushing is recommended. Although people are advised to rinse their mouth with water after meals [70], guidelines in the United States and other countries generally recommend to "spit and avoid rinsing/excessive rinsing with water" after brushing with fluoride toothpaste [79]. An alternative to rinsing with water may be the use of oral rinses that contain fluoride because evidence has shown that they have a protective effect against caries among children with limited exposure to fluoride and that their use should be targeted toward individuals at high risk of caries. Interdental cleaning is also important as part of an oral care routine. Interdental cleaning removes debris and plaque from between the teeth [80]. In a systematic review and meta-analysis, Silva and colleagues examined whether flossing before or after dental brushing was more effective in reducing plaque and found no significant effect on reducing plaque for either condition [81].

More research is generally needed on the timing of meals, dental brushing, and flossing. Additional research in these areas may help uncover potential correlations, guide best practices by dental health professionals, and contribute to advancing preventive dental care strategies.

Mindful Eating During Meals

Mindfulness is another factor to consider in the relationship between nutrition and oral health. *Mindfulness* is defined as "the awareness that arises out of intentionally attending in an open and discerning way to whatever is arising in the present moment" [82]. Applying this concept of eating behavior has proven difficult due to the lack of a clear definition of *mindful eating* [83]. In assessing multiple definitions [84–86], a common thread is the emphasis on being fully present and aware during the eating experience and "shifting one's attention to the food and mind–body connection" [87]—paying more attention to the sensory qualities of food (e.g., taste and texture) and the overall experience. The literature has documented key principles and practices of mindful eating [85, 88]. Examples include the following:

- *Eat slowly.* Slowing down the eating pace allows internal cues for hunger, fullness, and satiation to register in the brain (i.e., estimated to take about 20 minutes) versus external cues, such as the amount of food on the plate.
- *Serve smaller portion sizes.* Serving and consuming smaller portions and using smaller dishware (e.g., 9 inches/23 centimeters in diameter) may increase satiation.
- *Reduce distractions while eating.* Distractions by external stimuli (e.g., television or device screens) may reduce "the ability to assess internal sensory cues such as taste perception and satiation" [85].
- *Savor and chew food thoroughly.* Engaging the senses to note colors, aromas, taste, and texture influences food choice, consumption, and the overall experience during a meal.

Experimental research examining the sensory aspects of food and energy consumption is variable, where some studies have found significant reductions in the consumption of energy-dense food, whereas others have not [89]. More research is needed on the connection between mindful eating and oral health. In doing so, researchers will better identify strategies that promote eating behaviors and dietary patterns that may reduce oral diseases and conditions.

Oral Health–Nutrition Relationship: Working Across Sectors for Optimal Oral Health Behaviors and Outcomes

Establishing good oral hygiene practices starting from childhood will aid in maintaining healthy teeth and gums and preventing oral health diseases and conditions. School-based oral health programs aim to prevent dental caries, which has implications for overall health and academic success [90, 91]. Given the progressive nature of tooth decay, school-based programs offer a variety of services, such as educating and promoting oral health, conducting dental screenings and making referrals, applying dental sealants, administering fluoride mouth rinses or tablets, applying fluoride varnish, managing cases, helping establish a dental care routine, and providing necessary restorative treatments [92]. This is particularly important for children from underserved and vulnerable communities and/or those who have limited or no access to oral healthcare. Such programs should align with the student-centered Whole School, Whole Community, Whole Child (WSSC) model by the Centers for Disease Control and Prevention (CDC), a model that represents a more holistic approach to health by integrating traditional health and wellness (including a component focused on nutrition environment and services) with community engagement and a goal to promote overall health and well-being and academic success [91].

As noted earlier, the incidence of dental caries increases with age, and a higher proportion of older adults experience tooth loss. Taking a more holistic perspective will require consideration of traditional and nontraditional stakeholders to promote oral health well-being and address inequities. A more holistic approach endorsed by the Institute of Medicine is integrating oral health with primary care providers [93]. Coordination between oral health professionals and primary care providers will be necessary given the systemic nature and implications of oral health. This approach may improve accessibility to dental care, facilitate more-efficient health management (especially for those with oral health symptoms), and increase awareness about the relationship between oral health and overall health and well-being.

While an emerging area of research [94], the "provision of nutrition care to optimize oral health is within the scope of practice of different health professions, including registered dietitians and oral health professionals. In addition, healthy eating has been identified as a priority area by the World Health Organization when initiating and strengthening oral health programs." The Academy of Nutrition and Dietetics "supports the integration of oral health with nutrition services, education, and research. Collaboration between registered dietitian nutritionists (RDNs); dietetic technicians, registered (DTRs); and oral healthcare professionals is recommended for oral health promotion and disease prevention and intervention" [95]. However, a review paper by Lieffers and colleagues indicated that nutrition care is delivered to patients by oral health professionals at least some of the time (94). Nutrition and dietetic professionals utilize the nutrition care process (NCP), a systematic approach for individualized care. NCP consists of four key steps [96]: (1) nutrition assessment and reassessment, (2) nutrition diagnosis, (3) nutrition intervention, and (4) nutrition monitoring and evaluation. The integration of nutrition care with oral healthcare may be a viable strategy to address obstacles identified by oral health professionals when intervening, such as time constraints. Dietitians can dedicate more time to nutrition care and address patient motivation issues by using motivational interviewing techniques. Their specialized education and training would fill gaps in knowledge and confidence that oral health professionals may feel about delivering nutrition care and advisement [94]. All groups could benefit from such an integrative oral healthcare model. For example, children and adults with developmental disabilities often have complex healthcare needs and impairments (e.g., physical and cognitive) [97, 98]. Tooth decay, periodontal gum disease, oral malformations, delayed tooth eruption, and malocclusion (i.e., tooth position when the jaw is closed and has implications for chewing) are examples of oral health diseases and conditions often experienced by this population [97]. Thus, in addition to an oral healthcare professional and/or a medical doctor, having the patient's caregiver and a registered dietitian on the care team—at a minimum—could be ideal (depending on the patients' needs and diagnosis).

In closing, a clear relationship exists between nutrition and oral health—with a range of implications for overall health and well-being. In alignment with the Bronfenbrenner socioecological model [99], health-related behaviors, including oral health-related behaviors, influence and are influenced by multiple factors across different levels of an intricate and ever-evolving socioecological system [100]. Individual, interpersonal, organizational, community, and societal/policy factors need to be considered when addressing oral healthcare and disparities. Diversifying stakeholder type and expanding across the above-mentioned levels may help improve oral health literacy, change oral health-related behaviors, enable inter- and cross-sector collaboration for oral health services, drive the design of innovative care models (e.g., mobile dental clinics in underserved areas), and facilitate support for more-comprehensive and more-effective strategies in promoting oral health equity.

Further Practice

1. Which one of the following is a micronutrient?

   (a) Carbohydrates
   (b) Proteins
   (c) Vitamins
   (d) Fiber

2. Which one of the following nutrients is most important for dental health?

   (a) Calcium
   (b) Sodium
   (c) Iron
   (d) Fat

3. Poor oral hygiene can contribute to the development of certain systemic health conditions such as cardiovascular disease and diabetes.

   True/false

4. Which of the following is considered a macronutrient?

   (a) Iron
   (b) Vitamin C
   (c) Protein
   (d) Zinc

5. Brushing your teeth immediately after consuming acidic foods or beverages can help prevent tooth erosion.

   True/false

6. What role does phosphorus play in maintaining overall oral health?

    (a) It helps with saliva production.
    (b) It supports the remineralization of tooth enamel.
    (c) It aids in the absorption of calcium.
    (d) All of the above.

7. Demineralization of enamel is primarily caused by the interactions of sugars and bacteria.

    True/false

8. Which one of the following is a recommended brushing timing practice for good oral health?

    (a) Brushing once a day before bedtime
    (b) Brushing immediately after every meal
    (c) Brushing for 30 seconds in the morning
    (d) Brushing twice a day for 2 minutes each time

9. Which of the following is an example of a micronutrient?

    (a) Proteins
    (b) Carbohydrates
    (c) Vitamin D
    (d) Omega-3 fatty acids

10. Which statement accurately distinguishes between intrinsic and extrinsic sugars regarding their impact on oral health?

    (a) Intrinsic sugars are naturally present in foods and are less likely to contribute to tooth decay than extrinsic sugars.
    (b) Extrinsic sugars are found naturally in fruits and vegetables, whereas intrinsic sugars are added to processed foods.
    (c) Extrinsic sugars are less likely to adhere to the tooth surface and promote bacterial growth than intrinsic sugars.
    (d) Intrinsic sugars are more commonly associated with dental caries due to their natural occurrence, whereas extrinsic sugars pose a lower risk.

11. Excessive consumption of acidic foods and beverages can lead to tooth enamel erosion.

    True/false

12. Rinsing your mouth with water after consuming acidic or sugary foods and drinks can

    (a) Neutralize the acids and reduce the risk of tooth decay
    (b) Increase the risk of tooth erosion
    (c) Whiten the teeth
    (d) Have no effect on oral health

13. Mindful eating involves attention to the taste, texture, and eating experience.

    True/false

14. What are some of the tools that can be used for interdental cleaning?

    (a) Dental floss
    (b) Water flossers
    (c) Air flossers
    (d) All of the above

15. Which statement accurately reflects the intricate relationship between consuming nutrient-dense meals and oral health?

    (a) Nutrient-dense meals have a limited impact on oral health outcomes.
    (b) Nutrient-dense meals can positively affect oral health by replenishing essential nutrients vital for periodontal health.
    (c) Nutrient-dense meals focus primarily on enhancing the appearance of teeth rather than their overall health.
    (d) Nutrient-dense meals have no significant role in tissue regeneration within the oral cavity.

Answer Key

1. (c)
2. (a)
3. True
4. (c)
5. False
6. (d)
7. True
8. (d)
9. (c)
10. True
11. (a)
12. True
13. (d)
14. (b)
15. (a)

References

1. Yap AU. Oral health equals total health: a brief review. J Dent Indonesia. 2017;24(2):59–62.
2. World Health Organization (WHO). Oral Health. 2024. Retrieved from https://www.who.int/health-topics/oral-health#tab=tab_1.
3. Glick M, Williams DM, Kleinman DV, Vujicic M, Watt RG, Weyant RJ. A new definition for oral health developed by the FDI World Dental Federation opens the door to a universal definition of oral health. Br Dent J. 2016;221(12):792793.
4. World Health Organization. Global oral health status report: towards universal health coverage for oral health by 2030. Geneva: License: CC BYNCSA 3.0 IGO; 2022.
5. WHO. Oral health: key facts. 2023. Retrieved from https://www.who.int/news-room/fact-sheets/detail/oral-health#:~:text=Overview,tooth%20loss%20and%20oral%20cancers.
6. Centers for Disease Control and Prevention (CDC). Oral health surveillance report: trends in dental caries and sealants, tooth retention, and Edentulism, United States, 1999–2004 to 2011–2016. US Dept of Health and Human Services; 2019.
7. Kane SF. The effects of oral health on systemic health. Gen Dent. 2017;65(6):30–4.
8. Inchingolo AM, Malcangi G, Ferrante L, Del Vecchio G, Viapiano F, Mancini A, et al. Damage from carbonated soft drinks on enamel: a systematic review. Nutrients. 2023;15(7):1785.
9. WHO. Sugars and dental caries. 2017. Retrieved from https://www.who.int/news-room/fact-sheets/detail/sugars-and-dental-caries.
10. Klimuszko E, Orywal K, Sierpinska T, Sidun J, Golebiewska M. Evaluation of calcium and magnesium contents in tooth enamel without any pathological changes: in vitro preliminary study. Odontology. 2018;106:369376.
11. CDC. Community water fluoridation facts. 2024. Retrieved from https://www.cdc.gov/oral-health/data-research/facts-stats/fast-facts-community-water-fluoridation.html.
12. Pitts NB, Zero DT, Marsh PD, et al. Dental caries. Nat Rev Dis Primers. 2017;3:17030.
13. Fleming E, Afful J. Prevalence of total and untreated dental caries among youth: United States, 2015–2016. 2018.
14. Fleming E, Afful J, Griffin SO. Prevalence of tooth loss among older adults: United States, 2015–2018. 2020.
15. Ruiz-Roca JA, Martín Fuentes D, Gómez García FJ, Martínez-Beneyto Y. Oral status of older people in medium to long-stay health and social care setting: a systematic review. BMC Geriatr. 2021;21(1):363.
16. Office of Disease Prevention and Health Promotion (ODPHP). Oral conditions. In: Healthy people 2030. U.S. Department of Health and Human Services; n.d.
17. USDA and the U.S. Department of Health and Human Services. Dietary Guidelines for Americans, 2020–2025, 9th ed. 2020.
18. Tellez M, Zini A, Estupiñan-Day S. Social determinants and oral health: an update. Curr Oral Health Rep. 2014;1:148–52.
19. American Dental Association. Genetics and oral health. 2023. Retrieved from https://www.ada.org/en/resources/adalibrary/oralhealthtopics/geneticsandoralhealth.
20. Mayo Clinic. Cavities and tooth decay. 2024. Retrieved from https://www.mayoclinic.org/diseases-conditions/cavities/symptoms-causes/syc-20352892.
21. Borrell LN, Reynolds JC, Fleming E, Shah PD. Access to dental insurance and oral health inequities in the United States. Community Dent Oral Epidemiol. 2023;51(4):615620.
22. Walker KK, Martínez-Mier EA, Soto-Rojas AE, Jackson RD, Stelzner SM, Galvez LC, et al. Midwestern Latino caregivers' knowledge, attitudes and sense-making of the oral health etiology, prevention and barriers that inhibit their children's oral health: a CBPR approach. BMC Oral Health. 2017;17:1–11.
23. American Dental Association. Dental care utilization among the US population by race and ethnicity. Infographic: Health Policy Institute; 2021a.
24. Martin P, Santoro M, Heaton LJ, Preston R, Tranby EP. Hunger pains: how food insecurity affects oral health. 2023. https://doi.org/10.35565/CQI.2023.2006.

25. U.S. Department of Health and Human Services. Oral health in America: a report of the surgeon general. Rockville, MD: U.S. Department of Health and Human Services, National Institute of Dental and Craniofacial Research, National Institutes of Health; 2000.

26. Bui FQ, Almeida-da Silva CLC, Huynh B, Trinh A, Liu J, Woodward J, et al. Association between periodontal pathogens and systemic disease. Biom J. 2019;42(1):2735.

27. MaritanThompson D. Links between the oral microbiome imbalance and disease. 2024. Retrieved from https://blog.mdpi.com/2024/02/15/oralmicrobiome/.

28. Santonocito S, Giudice A, Polizzi A, Troiano G, Merlo EM, Sclafani R, et al. A cross-talk between diet and the oral microbiome: balance of nutrition on inflammation and immune system's response during periodontitis. Nutrients. 2022;14(12):2426.

29. Pisano M, Giordano F, Sangiovanni G, Capuano N, Acerra A, D'Ambrosio F. The interaction between the Oral microbiome and systemic diseases: a narrative review. Microbiol Res. 2023;14(4):1862–78.

30. Chan AKY, Tsang YC, Jiang CM, Leung KCM, Lo ECM, Chu CH. Diet, nutrition, and oral health in older adults: a review of the literature. Dent J. 2023;11(9):2.

31. Savarino G, Corsello A, Corsello G. Macronutrient balance and micronutrient amounts through growth and development. Ital J Pediatr. 2021;47(1):109.

32. Zohoori FV. Nutrition and diet. The impact of nutrition and diet on oral health. 2020;28:113.

33. Fluitman KS, van den Broek T, Reinders I, Wijnhoven HA, Nieuwdorp M, Visser M, et al. The effect of dietary advice aimed at increasing protein intake on Oral health and Oral microbiota in older adults: a randomized controlled trial. Nutrients. 2023;15(21):4567.

34. Li XY, Wen MZ, Liu H, Shen YC, Su LX, Yang XT. Dietary magnesium intake is protective in patients with periodontitis. Front Nutr. 2022;9:976518.

35. Heo H, Bae JH, Amano A, Park T, Choi YH. Supplemental or dietary intake of omega-3 fatty acids for the treatment of periodontitis: a meta-analysis. J Clin Periodontol. 2022;49(4):362377.

36. Kapoor B, Kapoor D, Gautam S, Singh R, Bhardwaj S. Dietary polyunsaturated fatty acids (PUFAs): uses and potential health benefits. Curr Nutr Rep. 2021;10:232242.

37. Cagetti MG, Wolf TG, Tennert C, Camoni N, Lingström P, Campus G. The role of vitamins in oral health. A systematic review and meta-analysis. Int J Environ Res Public Health. 2020;17(3):938.

38. National Institutes of Health. Dietary supplement fact sheets for health professionals. 2024. Retrieved from https://ods.od.nih.gov/factsheets/list-all/.

39. Chen H, Liu Y. Teeth. In: Advanced ceramics for dentistry. ButterworthHeinemann; 2014. p. 521.

40. Institute of Medicine. Dietary reference intakes for calcium and vitamin D. Washington, DC: The National Academies Press; 2011. https://doi.org/10.17226/13050.

41. Del Valle HB, Yaktine AL, Taylor CL, Ross AC, editors. Dietary reference intakes for calcium and vitamin D. Washington: National Academies Press; 2011.

42. Piuri G, Zocchi M, Della Porta M, Ficara V, Manoni M, Zuccotti GV, et al. Magnesium in obesity, metabolic syndrome, and type 2 diabetes. Nutrients. 2021;13(2):320.

43. Heaney RP. Phosphorus. In: Erdman JW, Macdonald IA, Zeisel SH, editors. Present knowledge in nutrition. 10th ed. Washington, DC: Wiley Blackwell; 2012. p. 447458.

44. Farooq I, Bugshan A. The role of salivary contents and modern technologies in the remineralization of dental enamel: a narrative review. F1000Research. 2020:9.

45. Alotaibi T. Malnutrition and diet role in prevention of oral disease. EC Dent Sci. 2019;18(9):220613.

46. Murererehe J, Uwitonze AM, Nikuze P, Patel J, Razzaque MS. Beneficial effects of vitamin C in maintaining optimal oral health. Front Nutr. 2022;8:805809.

47. Zhou J, Chen C, Chen X, Fei Y, Jiang L, Wang G. Vitamin C promotes apoptosis and cell cycle arrest in oral squamous cell carcinoma. Front Oncol. 2020;10:976.

48. Uwitonze AM, Murererehe J, Ineza MC, Harelimana EI, Nsabimana U, Uwambaye P, et al. Effects of vitamin D status on oral health. J Steroid Biochem Mol Biol. 2018;175:190–4.

49. United States Department of Agriculture (USDA). 2019. Agricultural Research Service. FoodData Central. Retrieved from fdc.nal.usda.gov; and National Institutes of Health. 2023.
50. Botelho J, Machado V, Proença L, Delgado AS, Mendes JJ. Vitamin D deficiency and oral health: a comprehensive review. Nutrients. 2020;12(5):1471.
51. Gossweiler AG, MartinezMier EA. Vitamins and oral health. The Impact of Nutrition and Diet on Oral Health. 2020;28:5967.
52. Mishra S, Stierman B, Gahche JJ, Potischman N. Dietary supplement use among adults: United States, 2017–2018. No: NCHS Data Brief; 2021. p. 399.
53. Maslow AH. A theory of human motivation. Psychol Rev. 1943;50(4):370–96. https://doi.org/10.1037/h0054346.
54. USDA. Economic Research Service. Key statistics and graphics. 2023. Retrieved from https://www.ers.usda.gov/topics/food-nutrition-assistance/food-security-in-the-u-s/key-statistics-graphics.
55. Redruello-Requejo M, Samaniego-Vaesken MDL, Partearroyo T, Rodríguez-Alonso P, Soto-Méndez MJ, Hernández-Ruiz Á, et al. Dietary intake of individual (intrinsic and added) sugars and food sources from Spanish children aged one to< 10 years—results from the EsNuPI study. Nutrients. 2022;14(8):1667.
56. Chatelan A, Gaillard P, Kruseman M, Keller A. Total, added, and free sugar consumption and adherence to guidelines in Switzerland: results from the first national nutrition survey menuCH. Nutrients. 2019;11(5):1117.
57. Kianoush N, Adler CJ, Nguyen KAT, Browne GV, Simonian M, Hunter N. Bacterial profile of dentine caries and the impact of pH on bacterial population diversity. PLoS One. 2014;9(3):e92940.
58. Ziegler AM, Kasprzak CM, Mansouri TH, Gregory AM, Barich RA, Hatzinger LA, et al. An ecological perspective of food choice and eating autonomy among adolescents. Front Psychol. 2021;12:654139.
59. Alkhulaifi F, Darkoh C. Meal timing, meal frequency and metabolic syndrome. Nutrients. 2022;14(9):1719.
60. Fjellström C. Mealtime and meal patterns from a cultural perspective. Scand J Nutr. 2004;48(4):161–4.
61. Paoli A, Tinsley G, Bianco A, Moro T. The influence of meal frequency and timing on health in humans: the role of fasting. Nutrients. 2019;11(4):719.
62. Kant AK. Eating patterns of US adults: meals, snacks, and time of eating. Physiol Behav. 2018;193:270278.
63. Potter M, Vlassopoulos A, Lehmann U. Snacking recommendations worldwide: a scoping review. Adv Nutr. 2018;9(2):86–98.
64. Erickson J, Sadeghirad B, Lytvyn L, Slavin J, Johnston BC. The scientific basis of guideline recommendations on sugar intake: a systematic review. Ann Intern Med. 2017;166(4):257267.
65. Zizza CA, Xu B. Snacking is associated with overall diet quality among adults. J Acad Nutr Diet. 2012;112(2):291296.
66. Hess JM, Jonnalagadda SS, Slavin JL. What is a snack, why do we snack, and how can we choose better snacks? A review of the definitions of snacking, motivations to snack, contributions to dietary intake, and recommendations for improvement. Adv Nutr. 2016;7(3):466475.
67. Valenzuela MJ, Waterhouse B, Aggarwal VR, Bloor K, Doran T. Effect of sugar-sweetened beverages on oral health: a systematic review and meta-analysis. Eur J Pub Health. 2021;31(1):122–9.
68. USDA. Learn how to eat healthy with MyPlate. 2025. Retrieved from https://www.myplate.gov/.
69. Khan AS, Zulfiqar N, Waheed M. Fueling your smile: the importance of nutrition for dental wellness. Asian J Dent Sci. 2023;6(1):308317.

70. Kondo K, Kanenaga R, Tanaka Y, Hotta K, Arakawa S. The neutralizing effect of mouth rinsing with alkaline electrolyzed water on different regions of the oral cavity acidified by acidic beverages. J Oral Sci. 2022;64(1):17–21.
71. Arab H, Maroofian A, Golestani S, Shafaee H, Sohrabi K, Forouzanfar A. Review of the therapeutic effects of Camellia sinensis (green tea) on oral and periodontal health. J Med Plants Res. 2011;5:54655469.
72. Koh SGS, Sim YF, Sim CJ, Hu S, Hong CHL, Duggal MS. Rinsing with water for 1 min after milk formula increases plaque pH. Eur Arch Paediatr Dent. 2021;22:611618.
73. Manna A, Khan T. Antioxidants: their role in oral health a short review. J Dent Panacea. 2024;6(2):7780. https://doi.org/10.18231/j.jdp.2024.017.
74. Smith HA, Betts JA. Nutrient timing and metabolic regulation. J Physiol. 2022;600(6):1299–312.
75. Lundgren JD, Smith BM, Spresser C, Harkins P, Zolton L, Williams K. The relationship of night eating to oral health and obesity in community dental clinic patients. Age (years). 2010;57(15):12.
76. Lundgren JD, Williams KB, Heitmann BL. Nocturnal eating predicts tooth loss among adults: results from the Danish MONICA study. Eat Behav. 2010;11(3):170174.
77. Hamasha AAH, Zawaideh FI, Al-Hadithy RT. Risk indicators associated with dental erosion among Jordanian school children aged 12–14 years of age. Int J Paediatr Dent. 2014;24(1):5668.
78. American Dental Association. Toothbrushes. 2022. Retrieved https://www.ada.org/en/resources/adalibrary/oralhealthtopics/toothbrushes.
79. Pitts N, Duckworth RM, Marsh P, Mutti B, Parnell C, Zero D. Post-brushing rinsing for the control of dental caries: exploration of the available evidence to establish what advice we should give our patients. Br Dent J. 2012;212(7):315–20.
80. American Dental Association. Floss/interdental cleaners. 2021. Retrieved from https://www.ada.org/en/resources/ada-library/oral-health-topics/floss#.
81. Silva C, Albuquerque P, de Assis P, Lopes C, Anníbal H, Lago MCA, Braz R. Does flossing before or after brushing influence the reduction in the plaque index? A systematic review and meta-analysis. Int J Dent Hyg. 2022;20(1):18–25.
82. Shapiro SL. The integration of mindfulness and psychology. J Clin Psychol. 2009;65(6):555–60.
83. Mantzios M. (re) defining mindful eating into mindful eating behaviour to advance scientific enquiry. Nutr Health. 2021;27(4):367371.
84. Framson C, Kristal AR, Schenk JM, Littman AJ, Zeliadt S, Benitez D. Development and validation of the mindful eating questionnaire. J Am Diet Assoc. 2009;109(8):14391444.
85. Monroe JT. Mindful eating: principles and practice. Am J Lifestyle Med. 2015;9(3):217220.
86. Taylor MB, Daiss S, Krietsch K. Associations among self-compassion, mindful eating, eating disorder symptomatology, and body mass index in college students. Transl Issues Psychol Sci. 2015;1(3):229.
87. Cherpak CE. Mindful eating: a review of how the stress digestion mindfulness triad may modulate and improve gastrointestinal and digestive function. Integr Med. 2019;18(4):48.
88. Hanh TN, Cheung L. Savor: mindful eating, mindful life. San Francisco: HarperOne; 2011.
89. Tapper K. Mindful eating: what we know so far. Nutr Bull. 2022;47(2):168–85.
90. American Academy of Pediatrics. Oral health. 2023. Retrieved from https://www.aap.org/en/patient-care/oral-health/.
91. CDC. Whole School, Whole Community, Whole Child (WSSC). 2023. Retrieved from https://www.cdc.gov/healthyschools/wscc/index.htm.
92. CDC. School sealant programs. 2024. Retrieved from https://www.cdc.gov/oral-health/php/school-dental-sealant-programs/.
93. Institute of Medicine. Improving access to oral health care for vulnerable and underserved populations. Washington, DC: The National Academies Press; 2011.

94. Lieffers JR, Vanzan AGT, Rover de Mello J, Cammer A. Nutrition care practices of dieti- tians and oral health professionals for oral health conditions: a scoping review. Nutrients. 2021;13(10):3588.
95. Mallonee LFH, Boyd LD, Stegeman C. Practice paper of the academy of nutrition and dietet- ics abstract: oral health and nutrition. J Acad Nutr Diet. 2014;114(6):958.
96. Academy of Nutrition and Dietetics. Nutrition care process. 2024. Retrieved from https:// www.eatrightpro.org/practice/nutrition-care-process/ncp-overview/nutrition-assessment.
97. National Institute of Dental and Craniofacial Research. Developmental disabili- ties and oral health. 2023. Retrieved from https://www.nidcr.nih.gov/health-info/ developmental-disabilities.
98. Sarvas E, Webb J, Landrigan-Ossar M, Yin L. Oral health Care for Children and Youth with Developmental Disabilities: clinical report. Pediatrics. 2024:e2024067603.
99. Bronfenbrenner U. Toward an experimental ecology of human development. Am Psychol. 1977;32(7):513.
100. Do LG, Song YH, Du M, Spencer AJ, Ha DH. Socioecological determinants of child oral health—a scoping review. Community Dent Oral Epidemiol. 2023;51(5):1024–36.

Rebuilding Swallowing Strength: A Specialized Diet Approach for Post-Stroke Dysphagia Recovery

7

Madiha Ajaz, Misbah Ajaz, and Sanowber Ajaz

Learning Objectives

After completing this chapter, you will be able to

- Understand the impact of dysphagia and its types
- Learn about the various methods and tools used for the assessment
- Learn about the specialized diets for dysphagia
- Apply meal-planning strategies for dysphagia

Introduction

Swallowing is a complex process involving coordinated muscle movements that propel food or liquid to the stomach from the mouth. This activity involves intricate sensorimotor control to ensure the safety of the airway and prevent aspiration, where foreign substances enter the respiratory tract [1–5]. Dysphagia entails patients' experiencing difficulty swallowing due to weakened or improperly coordinated muscles involved in swallowing or when a patient has impairment in the neural pathways that control swallowing [6]. Stroke, a prevalent cerebrovascular

M. Ajaz (✉)
School of Pharmacy and Medical Sciences, Griffith University, Gold Coast, QLD, Australia
e-mail: madiha.ajaz@griffithuni.edu.au

M. Ajaz
College of Human Nutrition and Dietetics – Allied Health Sciences, Ziauddin University, Karachi, Pakistan
e-mail: misbah.ajaz@zu.edu.pk

S. Ajaz
Nutrition and Aging Lab, University of Waterloo, Ontario, Canada
e-mail: s2ajaz@uwaterloo.ca

© The Author(s), under exclusive license to Springer Nature Switzerland AG 2025
A. K. Mitra, D. Vanoh (eds.), *Essentials of Clinical and Public Health Nutrition*, Nutrition and Health, https://doi.org/10.1007/978-3-031-95373-6_7

141

disease, frequently contributes to disruptions in the swallowing process, leading to the onset of post-stroke dysphagia (PSD) [7–9]. The specific neuroanatomical localization of brain lesions, supra- and infratentorial, leads to dysphagia. The prevalence of dysphagia is higher due to brainstem lesions as opposed to hemispheric strokes. However, lesions affecting both the brain regions lead to more-extensive impairments in swallowing function [10]. Motor deficit–induced dysphagia is due mostly to infratentorial lesions, whereas supratentorial stroke leads to afferent sensory dysfunction–induced dysphagia [11]. The estimated global annual incidence for neurogenic dysphagia is between 400,000 and 800,000 individuals [12]. The sensitivity of assessment measures influences the prevalence estimates of dysphagia; the utilization of instruments in assessment identifies a prevalence of 64–78% for dysphagia; and clinical examination indicates a prevalence of 51–55% in the post-acute stroke phase, whereas chronic dysphagia is observed in roughly half of all instances [13, 14]. The use of instruments for dysphagia screening offers superior diagnostic precision and enables a more comprehensive evaluation of swallowing abilities than clinical examination does [15].

Dysphagia incurs a substantial financial and societal burden by straining healthcare facilities, reducing bed space availability and increasing medical costs [16, 17]. A recent study has reported that annual healthcare costs were higher for acute ischemic stroke patients with dysphagia, ranging from $67,100 to $112,400. In comparison, for acute ischemic stroke patients without dysphagia, the costs were lower, ranging from $54,310 to $51,979.80 in the United States [18]. Dysphagia exerts a profound influence not just on an individual's physiological health but also on their psychological health [19]. Alongside the physical implications, including pneumonia, dehydration, sarcopenia, malnutrition, and mortality, dysphagia exerts a considerable toll on both an individual's quality of life and their mental health [20–23]. The mortality rate among stroke patients with dysphagia is concerning, where a considerable proportion succumb to fatal chest infections and malnutrition [24, 25]. Stroke patients experiencing malnutrition and/or dehydration carry a significantly higher risk of subsequent complications, dependence, and mortality [26, 27]. Inadequate nutritional intake undermines the immune system's ability to fight infections, and reduced fluid consumption leads to dehydration, which potentially exacerbates swallowing difficulties and related issues [28]. Nutritional screening helps in evaluating patients' severity of malnutrition, nutritional intake, quality of life, and appropriate post-intervention follow-up monitoring [29, 30]. Henceforth, assessing the nutritional status of all dysphagia patients and optimizing their nutritional status with a modified diet plan is recommended [31–33]. The International Dysphagia Diet Standardization Initiative (IDDSI) will be incorporated into this chapter, along with several recipes. The holistic approach outlined here aims to empower recovery, improve quality of life, and mitigate the challenges associated with dysphagia, thus contributing to a more effective and compassionate post-stroke care paradigm.

Types and Symptoms of Dysphagia

Dysphagia is categorized into two types according to the affected anatomical site: esophageal dysphagia and oropharyngeal dysphagia. Motility dysfunction or anatomical blockage below the upper esophageal sphincter leading to impaired food transit into the stomach characterizes esophageal dysphagia. Mechanical obstruction typically results in difficulty in swallowing solids, while motility dysfunction can cause difficulty in swallowing both solids and liquids. Esophageal spasm, systemic sclerosis, achalasia, and ineffective esophageal motility cause motility-linked dysphagia, whereas stricture, tumor, Schatzki ring, and eosinophilic esophagitis are common causes of anatomical blockage dysphagia [34, 35].

In the context of stroke, oropharyngeal dysphagia is of primary interest because it is a dysfunction within the oral and pharyngeal regions, culminating in impaired swallowing function. Approximately 37% of stroke survivors experience oropharyngeal dysphagia in the acute phase, and this figure increases to 78% in the chronic phase. These individuals encounter challenges in effectively transferring liquid or solid food boluses from the oral cavity to the esophagus. Additionally, an enumeration of discerning symptoms aids in the differentiation of oropharyngeal dysphagia from its esophageal counterpart. These symptomatic indices, comprising manifestations such as excessive drooling, compromised mastication function, reflexive coughing, and instances of choking, offer insights into the underlying neuromuscular dysfunctions within the oropharyngeal milieu [14, 34, 36].

Malnutrition and oropharyngeal dysphagia usually coexist among the elderly population aged 65 and above, and there is a significant association between oropharyngeal dysphagia and sarcopenia [37, 38]. Multiple studies have emphasized the importance of swallowing and nutritional therapy in PSD patients [27, 39–41]. Post-stroke patients with oropharyngeal dysphagia suffer from both compromised swallowing efficacy and compromised swallowing safety. Food residue remaining in the mouth and/or throat reflects the impaired ability to ingest food, leading to inadequate nutrient intake and dehydration. Similarly, laryngeal penetration and tracheobronchial aspiration indicate compromised swallowing safety [42–44]. The combination of suboptimal dietary intake and recurrent airway infections, stemming from aspiration events, can trigger numerous complications, potentially culminating in fatality [45–47]. Table 7.1 provides a concise overview of different types of dysphagia, including their descriptions, causes, and manifestations.

Clinical signs of oropharyngeal dysphagia [48] include a wet voice; coughing; choking; repeatedly clearing the throat; nasal regurgitation; reduced tongue pressure; reduced dietary intake; spending more time to finish a meal; sluggish swallowing; anterior sialorrhea; impaired mastication; impaired tongue and lip movements; spitting food out; consuming fluids with meals; food residue in the oral cavity; sensations of food sticking in the oral cavity or neck region; xerostomia; and food discharge from the oropharynx.

Table 7.1 Types of dysphagia

Type	Description	Cause	Manifestation
Oropharyngeal dysphagia	Oropharyngeal dysphagia refers to difficulty with moving food (solid or liquid) from the mouth to the cervical esophagus.	Neuromuscular disorders or anatomic anomalies of the oropharynx are common culprits. Dysfunction in the upper esophageal sphincter, either due to failure to relax or a lack of coordination with pharyngeal contraction, is a frequent cause.	Symptoms of oropharyngeal dysphagia include difficulty in initiating or transporting food boluses, sensations of food sticking in the oral cavity or neck region, and symptoms of pulmonary aspiration.
Esophageal dysphagia	Esophageal dysphagia refers to difficulty with moving food (solid or liquid) below the upper esophageal sphincter to the stomach.	Motility dysfunction or mechanical obstruction is the common culprit.	A feeling of sluggish movement of food in the chest.

Screening and Assessing the Swallowing Function After Stroke

Initial Screening and Assessment

Dysphagia management begins with screening as the initial step, aiming to identify individuals at risk. Screening helps identify those in need of further assessment for dysphagia and minimizes the occurrence of aspiration [49]. Hence, prompt dysphagia screening within 24 hours of stroke onset is recommended. Patients who do not pass the screening test should receive a further clinical evaluation by a dysphagia expert to examine their swallowing function [50]. Practitioners can utilize instrumental tools, noninstrumental tools, or a combination of both in clinical assessment to explore the determinants of dysphagia onset and evaluate the swallowing effectiveness and safety of aspiration risk, which facilitates determining various oral or feeding strategies [51].

In cases where cognitive or health issues impede dysphagia screening, the screening should be delayed. The complete restriction of oral intake is typically enforced in such cases until patients undergo screening. In some instances where health or cognitive function improvement is not anticipated, patients may undergo screening or assessment that uses alternative methods or pathways [50]. Utilizing screenings and assessments with validated and reliable diagnostic and psychometric qualities is vital [52, 53]. Ensuring feasibility requirements, such as user-friendliness for training clinicians, easy implementation, and noninvasiveness, is crucial before adopting any screening method [54, 55]. Diverse screening and assessment tools are available for dysphagia evaluation, where instrumental tools are widely accepted as the gold standard [51]. Table 7.2 provides a comprehensive list of dysphagia screening and assessment methods.

Comprehensive Clinical Assessment

In-depth clinical assessment may incorporate the results of instrumental/noninstrumental assessments with findings from medical records; evaluations of cognitive impairments; physiological and anatomical examinations of the oral cavity, larynx, and pharynx functioning; dietary intake; and nutritional status evaluations and interventions, such as a trial on texture-modified food, adjustments to posture, and sensory simulations. Table 7.3 provides examples of questionnaires for assessing nutritional status and dietary intake, and Box 7.1 provides an example of an assessment method.

Table 7.2 Dysphagia screening and assessment methods

Screening/assessment type	Examples
Screening	Bedside swallow screening tool [56]
	Volume–Viscosity Swallow Test [57]
	Gugging Swallow Screen [58]
	Dysphagia Trained Nurse Assessment [59]
	2 Volume, 3 texture test [60]
Instrumental assessment	Videofluoroscopic swallowing study (VFSS)
	The flexible endoscopic evaluation of swallowing (FEES) [61]
	Ultrasonography [62, 63]
	High-resolution manometry [64]
Noninstrumental assessment	American Speech–Language–Hearing Association national outcomes measurement system dysphagia scale [65]
	Dysphagia disorders survey [66]
	Dysphagia management staging scale [66]
	Dysphagia severity rating scale [67]
	Eating and drinking ability classification system [68]
	Easy dysphagia symptom questionnaire [69]
	Functional oral intake scale [70]
	International Dysphagia Diet Standardization Initiative functional diet scale [71]
	The Mann assessment of swallowing ability [72]
	The Mann assessment of swallowing ability—cancer [73]
	McGill ingestive skills assessment [74]
	The modified Mann assessment of swallowing ability [75]
	The swallowing portion of the functional assessment measure [76]
	Swallowing proficiency for eating and drinking [77]
	Swallowing status [78]
	Test for masticating and swallowing solids [79]

Table 7.3 Questionnaires for assessing nutritional status and dietary intake

Clinical assessment	Example questionnaires
Nutritional status evaluation	Mini Nutritional Assessment [81]
	10-Item Eating Assessment Tool [82]

Physiological Examination

- Larynge.al aspiration or vocal cord pathology can be reflected by the timbre and tone of a patient's voice.
- A soft palate, mouth, tongue, and lip examination reveals irregularities or dysfunctions in the movement and coordination of muscles involved in speech and swallowing.
- Palpating the movement of the larynx during swallowing helps in identifying abnormalities in laryngeal ascent.
- Observing chewing and bolus propulsion without choking helps to identify oral swallowing issues.
- Sialorrhea and drooling could indicate swallowing impairment [80].

Box 7.1

The water-swallowing test (WST) is a clinical functional assessment test used to evaluate swallowing function and detect the risk of aspiration, where food or liquid enters the airway instead of the digestive tract [83]. The development of the 3 ml modified water-swallowing test (MWST) stemmed from concerns about aspiration risk in stroke patients and elderly individuals when swallowing large amounts of water [84]. Safety is crucial when assessing swallowing function. Using a small amount of water allows for a thorough examination of various variables while minimizing the risk of aspiration. However, when the mouthful of water is too small, it may not trigger the swallowing reflux [85]. Examples are available where 10, 50, 90, 100, and 150 ml of water was used [86, 87]. Swallowing reflux (choking, coughing, and voice change) during swallowing water examination suggests neurogenic dysphagia [88].

Self-Reported Assessments by Patients

Patient-centered dysphagia assessment is performed by utilizing questionnaires to gather information on functional status and its effect on quality of life. Table 7.4 provides examples of questionnaires for assessing patients' reported functional status and quality of life.

Table 7.4 Questionnaires for assessing patients' reported functional status and quality of life

Type of self-reported assessment	Example questionnaires
Functional health	Sydney Swallow Questionnaire [89]
	Functional Oral Intake Scale [70]
Quality of life	MD Anderson Dysphagia Inventory [90]
	European Dysphagia Group Questionnaire [91]
	SWAL-QOL [92]
	Dysphagia Handicap Index [93]
	Deglutition Handicap Index [94]

Specialized Dietary Approaches for Post-Stroke Dysphagia

The significance of optimal nutrition cannot be understated in post-stroke patients experiencing dysphagia, and if appropriate dietary management is not implemented, individuals will be at a higher risk of experiencing malnutrition, where older patients are at an even higher risk. Effective dysphagia management includes essential dietary modifications because they aim to prevent aspiration while ensuring proper nutrition and hydration.

The specific dietary strategies vary depending on the severity and specific characteristics of the dysphagia. Additionally, patient preferences and the overall health of the patient are important factors in determining a dietary approach. Generally, adjusting diets for post-stroke dysphagia involves texture modification, compensatory strategies, and rehabilitation exercises.

1. Texture modification: modifying the thickness and texture of foods and liquids to ensure safer swallowing
2. Compensatory strategies: employing specific techniques like head turn or chin tuck while swallowing to promote safety
3. Rehabilitation exercises: engaging in swallowing exercises designed to improve function and minimize the likelihood of aspiration [95]

Texture-Modified Diets

Modified-texture diets adjust the consistency of food to enhance safe swallowing for individuals with dysphagia. The International Dysphagia Diet Standardization Initiative (IDDSI) has established a global standardization framework to standardize texture-modified foods and liquids, encompassing seven levels that range from thin to extremely thick textures [96]. Table 7.5 provides a comprehensive description of IDDSI levels with examples. Determining the suitable diet for individuals after a stroke involves assessing the severity of their swallowing challenges and findings from a clinical evaluation of their swallowing function or instrumental

Table 7.5 Description of texture-modified foods by IDDIS level

IDDIS level and particle size	IDDSI flow test	Fork drip test	Spoon tilt test	Fork pressure test	Spoon pressure test	Finger test	Chopstick test
Level 0 (Thin liquids)	Have watery flow. *Example: water, tea*	N/A					
Level 1 (Slightly thick)	Comparatively slow flow than thin liquids. *Example: nectars, creamy soup*	N/A					
Level 2 (Mildly thick)	Comparatively slow flow than level 1 liquids. *Example: milk shakes, smoothies*	N/A					
Level 3 (Moderately thick)	Non-sticky, flow slowly, do not retain shape. Can be sucked using straw but can't be eaten using spoon. *Example: smooth yogurt, fruit puree*			No indention marks when pressed		Can't be held between fingers. Slides leaving a thin coat	N/A

Level	Particle size				
Level 4 (Extremely thick-pureed)	N/A	Non-sticky retains shape, most of the puree slides off the cutlery when tilted but does not flow. Liquids that cannot be drunk from a cup but eaten with a spoon	Indention marks stay when pressed	Slides off when held between fingers leaving a thin coat	N/A
		Example: custard, thickened pureed fruits and vegetables			
Level 5 (Minced and moist)	Pediatric: ≤2 mm × ≤8 mm Adult: ≤4 mm × ≤15 mm	N/A	Sticky, most food remains on cutlery when tilted, retain shape when scooped, foods that are soft and moist, which can be mashed easily. Requires minimal chewing. *Example: mashed ripe banana, cooked soft mashed vegetables*		
Level 6 (Soft and bite-size)	Pediatric: 8 mm Adults: 15 mm = 1.5 cm	N/A	Foods that are soft and tender and easily broken down. Requires chewing before it can be swallowed. *Example: ripe banana, cooked soft vegetables*		
Level 7 (Easy to chew)	Pediatric: 8mm (More or less) Adult: 15 mm = 1.5 cm (more or less)	N/A	Breaks/cut and do not retain original shape. Requires gentle chewing without causing fatigue. *Example: soft and tender meat, fish, boiled/steamed vegetables*		

assessment, such as fiberoptic endoscopic evaluation or a videofluoroscopic swallow study. Additionally, diets must be customized to suit individual tastes, preferences, cultural influences, and nutritional requirements. A collaborative team featuring a registered dietitian, a registered nurse, and a speech-language therapist can work together to develop an individualized texture-modified diet plan that meets the specific swallowing abilities and nutritional goals of the individual.

Benefits of Modified Textures and Consistencies

Modifying the textures and consistencies of foods and liquids plays a vital role in managing post-stroke dysphagia, resulting in significant benefits to individuals recovering from stroke-related swallowing challenges. These modifications promote safer swallowing by reducing the risk of aspiration, where food or liquid enters the airway instead of the digestive tract. Texture modification not only reduces the risk of choking but also facilitates enhanced nutritional intake, ensuring that essential nutrients are consumed despite difficulties in swallowing. Table 7.5 provides a description of texture-modified foods according to the IDDSI level. Some of the benefits of modifying textures and consistencies in the diet include reduced aspiration risk, improved swallowing safety, enhanced nutritional intake, and enhanced quality of life.

Reduced aspiration risk: Modified textures, specifically thicker textures and consistencies can help regulate the speed of foods and liquids, thereby reducing the risk of aspiration.

Improved swallowing safety: Modified textures reduce the risk of choking and aspiration, facilitating managing and controlling the bolus during swallowing for individuals with dysphagia.

Enhanced nutritional intake: By adjusting textures, individuals with dysphagia can safely consume a wider variety of foods and liquids, ensuring that they receive adequate nutrients despite swallowing difficulties.

Enhanced quality of life: Texture-modified diets allow individuals to enjoy meals with reduced discomfort, improving their overall eating experience and boosting their confidence in swallowing [97, 98].

Compensatory Strategies

In addition to texture-modified diets, individuals with post-stroke swallowing difficulties may benefit from using compensatory strategies. Compensatory strategies refer to techniques aimed to improve the safety and efficiency of swallowing, reducing the aspiration risk for individuals affected by post-stroke dysphagia. Some common compensatory strategies include chin tuck, head turn, supraglottic swallow, and super-supraglottic swallow.

Chin tuck: During swallowing, the patient is advised to tilt their chin downward toward their chest, a technique that aids in closing the airway and preventing aspiration.

Head turn: During swallowing, the patient is advised to tilt their head sideways, facilitating the flow of food and liquids toward the more functional side of the pharynx.

Supraglottic swallow: During swallowing, the patient is advised to take a breath, hold it briefly, swallow, and then exhale. This technique assists in protecting the airway while swallowing.

Super-supraglottic swallow: In addition to the supraglottic swallow, during swallowing, the patient is advised to bear down (tighten their stomach and chest muscles as if lifting something heavy) while holding their breath, which offers enhanced airway protection [98].

Rehabilitation Exercises

In addition to texture modification in diet and compensatory strategies, swallowing rehabilitation exercises may also benefit patients with post-stroke dysphagia. These exercises are aimed at enhancing the strength and coordination of the swallowing muscles, thereby reducing the likelihood of aspiration and improving overall swallowing ability. Some common exercises used for swallowing rehabilitation include effortful swallow, the Mendelsohn maneuver, tongue-hold swallow, and the Masako maneuver.

Effortful swallow: Swallowing vigorously, the patient tightens muscles at the back of the throat.

The Mendelsohn maneuver: Holding the swallow for few seconds and maintaining larynx elevation helps the patient to strengthen the swallowing muscles.

Tongue-hold swallow: During swallowing, holding the tongue outside the mouth helps the patient to strengthen the tongue muscles.

The Masako maneuver: While swallowing, gently holding the tongue between the teeth helps the patient to strengthen the pharyngeal muscles [95, 99].

Patients may be advised to perform these exercises several times throughout the day, typically under the supervision of a speech-language therapist or another healthcare professional.

Enteral Nutrition

Sometimes, individuals dealing with post-stroke dysphagia cannot fulfill their nutritional needs solely through oral intake despite using texture-modified diets and thickened liquids. In such circumstances, enteral nutrition, delivering nutrients

Table 7.6 Types of feeding tubes used for enteral nutrition

Type of feeding tube	Description
NG tube (nasogastric)	Inserted via the nose into the stomach Typically used as a temporary measure or when short-term feeding is required
Percutaneous endoscopic gastrostomy (PEG)	Inserted via the abdominal wall directly into the stomach Typically used when long-term feeding is required and can be placed for several years
Percutaneous endoscopic jejunostomy (PEJ)	Inserted directly into the small intestine (jejunum) through the abdominal wall Typically used for individuals who are unable to tolerate the PEG feed [100].

through a feeding tube inserted directly into the gastrointestinal tract, may be initiated to meet the patient's required nutrition and hydration. Details on the types of feeding tubes are given in Table 7.6.

While selecting the enteral formula, a registered dietitian relies on factors such as the patient's medical history, nutritional requirements, and tolerance to different formulas. Typically, the standard polymeric formula is administered to individuals with post-stroke dysphagia without any other medical conditions that may require specialized nutrition. The standard polymeric formula contains balanced levels of macro- and micronutrients (carbohydrates, proteins, fats, vitamins, and minerals). However, in some cases, a specialized enteral formula is required for an individual's post-stroke dysphagia:

- High-protein formulas for patients with wounds or depilated muscle mass to support healing and muscle mass maintenance
- Fiber containing formula for patients who need additional fiber to regulate regular bowel movements
- Disease-specific formulas for specific diseases, such as a renal formula for kidney disorders, where little protein as well as sodium, potassium, and other electrolytes are required [101].

Continuously monitoring patients is essential to avoid any potential complications, such as diarrhea, constipation, aspiration, or skin rupture around the feeding tube site. To ensure that the patient is tolerating food well, that their nutritional requirements are being met, and that any necessary adjustments to the plan are being made, regular follow-ups with a registered dietitian and other healthcare professionals are essential.

Dietary Progression and Transition

As the recovery of post-stroke dysphagia progresses, gradually shifting toward less restriction is recommended. This process involves regularly assessing swallowing function, gradually advancing the diet, and providing appropriate education and training.

Regularly assessing swallowing function: assessment through bedside swallowing and evaluation through fluoroscopic swallowing studies or fiberoptic endoscopy

Gradually advancing the diet: transitioning from IDDSI level 2 to puréed and gradually to solid foods according to patient tolerance

Providing appropriate education and training: making sure that patients and their caregivers are well informed, fully understand dietary recommendations, and know how to properly prepare different textured foods [95, 97, 98, 102]

The specific timeline for dietary progression varies depending on the patient's recovery and the severity of their dysphagia. Close collaboration between patients, caregivers, and the healthcare team is essential to ensure a safe and successful transition to a regular diet.

Meal-Planning Strategies

Portion Size and Frequency

Increasing food intake in elderly individuals with dysphagia is difficult. Symptom management involves the frequent elimination of specific foods from their diet [103]. It also involves offering texture-modified foods and fluids, which might not be taken in adequate portions [104]. The nutritional content of food can be modified to support health in managing dysphagia. Individuals with dysphagia often experience fatigue during meals and may benefit from meals rich in nutrients to lower the chance of malnutrition or dehydration. This can be accomplished by incorporating food enhancers like protein powder or butter, which increase the caloric value of food [105]. Likewise, microgels or soft gels can be added to deliver proteins, fats, and fiber to texture-modified food. Offering smaller, more-frequent meals may help people with dysphagia by reducing fatigue issues [106–108].

Box 7.2: Hydration

Dehydration increases the risk of confusion, urinary tract infection, fatigue, fall-related injuries, delayed healing, and constipation, leading to extended inpatient stays or fatality. The literature indicates that around 55% of people with dysphagia bear high healthcare-related expenses and experience diminished quality of life due to dehydration. On average, in hospital settings, dysphagia patients on a thickened liquid diet manage to fulfill merely 23.4% of their daily fluid requirements [109–112]. Behavioral interventions such as the use of specially designed cups, an open choice of drinks, verbal cues, and providing toilet support improve fluid consumption practices [113]. Fluids provided between meals do not reduce fluid consumption after meals. Therefore, offering fluids between meals could help increase overall fluid intake and reduce the risk of dehydration [114].

Meal Timing and Environment

Also, a patient's usual mealtime habits should also be understood and accounted for. Not everyone eats three meals a day at fixed times. Some patients may hesitate to ask for assistance or company during meals. For these patients, having a friend or relative sit with them during meals can make a significant difference, helping them eat an entire meal rather than nothing at all. This is particularly true for elderly patients. Mealtimes are social events, so patients who eat alone are less likely to consume as much food and drink as patients who are surrounded by other patients or family members [115]. Having good company and fostering meaningful social bonds may increase the success of mealtime [116]. Providing verbal instruction or prompts and giving additional time to eat also assist in safe swallowing.

Environmental distractions such as television, loud sounds, or conversations can impact the meal completion of older individuals [117]. The lighting of the dining area is also important because it makes food visible and appealing [118]. Serving meals in a preferred eating space (table/room) can also enhance eating practice [119].

Meal Appearance

Texture-modified food should be presented in an appealing and appetizing manner. Various methods can be employed to achieve the desired food texture for individuals with dysphagia, thereby improving the convenience and pleasure of meals.

Food molds: Food molds typically refer to silicone molds where puréed food is placed to achieve a specific shape [120].
3D-printed foods: 3D food printing involves an additive manufacturing process where food is layered to form various shapes.
Other methods: Methods such as using piping bags, spherification, gelification, and emulsification can enhance the visual attractiveness of texture-modified food [121].

Adaptive Cups, Plates, and Utensils

Cups
Taking in fluid from a standard cup is associated with an increased risk of aspiration compared to taking in fluid using a spoon or a straw [122]. However, a range of specially designed cups can facilitate safer drinking. Cognitively intact patients can comfortably use *Wonder-Flo* cups while being semi-reclined. The rubber button

feature helps maintain controlled drinking because the liquid does not flow until the user sucks. The oval shape of the *dysphagia cup* facilitates the directed flow of liquid into the lips without escaping. To use the dysphagia cup effectively, patients should tuck their chin in toward their chest. Transparent *nosey cups* with angled rims are useful for patients with limited neck movement or an impaired grip because they can drink without tipping. *Two-handled* transparent spout lid cups or spillproof lid cups benefit people with restricted or impaired hand movement by providing a firm grip [123].

Plates

Plates designed with a deep inner ridge prevent food from sliding off a spoon and facilitate scooping. Similarly, a dish with a side wall 1 ¾ inches high enhances the eating experience by making scooping easier. Scooper bowls and scoop dishes with partitions serve the same purpose [123].

Utensils

A variety of utensils are available for individuals with a weak grip and impaired hand movement, offering easy and secure grip options, such as *Sure-Grip* and *lightweight foam* utensils. The bendable feature of *Sure-Grip*, *flexible*, and *weighted* utensils further enhances the eating experience for individuals with limited hand movement. The additional weight of *weighted* utensils' handles stabilizes holding. Coated cutlery is another user-friendly option, where the cutlery edges are coated and provide protection against food-temperature effects [123].

Antislip Products

These products help secure dinnerware surfaces [123].

Posture

For optimal safety and comfort during mealtime and to prevent reflux, individuals are recommended to maintain an upright sitting position while eating. For bedridden patients, elevating the head side of the bed up to 30° is a usual practice. Additionally, instructing patients to adopt a chin-down or chin-tuck position while swallowing can further mitigate the risk of food aspiration. In cases where patients have paralysis on one side of the body, eating while lying on the nonparalyzed side with the head leaning toward the paralyzed side can aid in the transit of food [117]. These strategies aim to optimize safety and comfort for patients with swallowing difficulties.

A sample meal plan for PSD patients is provided in Table 7.7.

Table 7.7 Sample meal plan for patients with post-stroke dysphagia

Meal	Texture/consistency	Foods
Breakfast	Puréed	Oatmeal with puréed fruits, scrambled eggs
Snack	Soft	Yogurt, a mashed banana
Lunch	Soft	Mashed potatoes, puréed vegetables
Snack	Liquid	Thickened apple juice, pudding
Dinner	Puréed	Puréed chicken, mashed sweet potatoes

Dysphagia-Friendly Recipes

Banana Shake Ingredients: Banana 2 medium size; milk 2 cups; strawberry syrup 2 tsp; honey 2 tbsp

Method: Add all ingredients into a blender. Blend well and serve.

Soft Scrambled Eggs Ingredients: Eggs 4; butter 2 tbsp; cheese cube 2; salt to taste

Method: In a pan, melt butter and add eggs. Turn on the heat and mix the butter and eggs using a spatula. Keep mixing for 30 seconds. Take off heat and keep mixing for 10 seconds. Put on heat again for 30 seconds, then take off heat for 10 seconds. Add two cheese cubes and cook for 30 seconds on heat again. Soft, creamy scrambled eggs are ready to serve.

Broccoli Soup Ingredients: Broccoli 1 cup (boiled and blended); all-purpose flour 2 tbsp; butter 1 tbsp; garlic paste ¾ tsp; milk 1 cup; chicken broth 4 cups; chicken ½ cup (boiled and blended); chicken cube 1 cube; soy sauce 1 tbsp; thyme ½ tsp; oregano ½ tsp; salt to taste; black pepper to taste

Method: In a pot, add butter, garlic paste, and all-purpose flour. Turn on the heat and keep mixing for 1–2 minutes. Take off the heat, cool, add milk, and keep mixing to avoid lumps. Add blended chicken, broccoli, chicken broth, chicken cube, soy sauce, salt, pepper, thyme, and oregano. Cook for 5 minutes or until desired consistency has been achieved.

Bite-Size Sandwich Ingredients: Bread 4 slices; chicken ½ cup (boiled blended); yogurt ½ cup; salt to taste; pepper to taste; cheese slice 4 slices

Method: Cut the edges of the bread slices. Mix blended chicken, salt, pepper, and yogurt. Spread a thin layer of chicken spread on bread slices, top it with a slice of cheese, and microwave for 5-8 seconds. Cut into half-inch pieces and serve.

Fish Ingredients: White fish fillets 180 grams (thin, skinless, boneless); garlic chopped 2 tsp; salt as per taste; green chili ½; mint leaves ¼ cup; coriander leaves ¼ cup; lemon juice 2 tbsp; red chili powder to taste

Method: In a blender, add green chili, mint leaves, coriander leaves, and garlic, then blend. Marinade fish with green paste, salt, red chili powder, and lemon juice. Steam cook.

Baked Custard Ingredients: Eggs 3; 2 tbsp sugar; vanilla 1 tsp; 2 milk ½ cups; nutmeg or cinnamon to taste

Method: Preheat oven to 160 °C. Lightly beat together eggs, sugar, and vanilla. Warm the milk gently on the stove, then gradually add it to the egg mixture while stirring constantly. Transfer the mixture to a shallow ovenproof dish, and sprinkle it with nutmeg and/or cinnamon. Place the dish in a water bath, ensuring that the water comes halfway up the sides of the dish. Bake in the oven for 30 minutes, then reduce the heat to 140 °C and continue baking for another 20–30 minutes until set.

Masoor Daal (Red Lentil) Ingredients: Daal ½ Cup; garlic 8 cloves; red chili powder 1 tbsp; turmeric powder 1 tsp; salt to taste

For tempering: chopped onion 1/4 cup; cumin seeds 1 tsp; oil 1/4 cup
Method: Rinse ½ cup of masoor daal under cool running water for approximately 1 minute. Drain the water. Then add the rinsed red lentils to a pressure cooker/pot along with 2 to 3 cups of water. Add garlic cloves, red chili powder, turmeric powder, and salt. Bring this daal mixture to a boil. Cover with a lid and let the daal mixture cook until tender and softened completely. Use another pan for tempering. Add oil, chopped onion, and cumin seeds. Stir and sauté until golden brown. Add this to the cooked daal. Blend the daal until puréed.

Chicken and Vegetable Pasta Ingredients: Chicken boiled 250 g; pasta cooked 1 cup; boiled vegetables (peas, spinach, green onions) 1 cup; chicken stock 1/4 cup; milk 1/4 cup; black pepper 1 tsp; salt to taste

Method: In a blender, add all the ingredients and blend until puréed.

Further Practice

1. What is the cause of post-stroke dysphagia?
    (a) Weakened or improperly coordinated muscles involved in swallowing
    (b) Difficulty in breathing
    (c) Neural pathway impairments that control swallowing
    (d) Both a and c

2. What is the usual practice of oral intake for dysphagia patients when cognitive or health issues affect dysphagia screening?

    (a) They should be given only liquids.
    (b) They should be allowed only thickened fluids.
    (c) They should be completely restricted from oral intake.
    (d) They should be allowed only small sips of water.

3. What is sarcopenia (a dysphagia-related complication)?

    (a) Reduced skin elasticity
    (b) Bone fragility
    (c) A neurological disorder
    (d) Muscle weakness and loss

4. What is the first step of dysphagia management?

    (a) The complete restriction of oral intake
    (b) Screening
    (c) Physiotherapy
    (d) Nutritional therapy

5. Dysphagia is categorized into which of the following two types according to the affected anatomical site?

    (a) Gastrointestinal dysphagia and esophageal dysphagia
    (b) Esophageal dysphagia and oropharyngeal dysphagia
    (c) Stomach dysphagia and mouth dysphagia
    (d) Throat dysphagia and stomach dysphagia

6. A clinical assessment of dysphagia may include which of the following?

    (a) An instrumental assessment and/or noninstrumental assessment
    (b) Medical records and a nutritional assessment
    (c) A physical examination
    (d) All of the above

7. Stricture, tumor, Schatzki ring, and eosinophilic esophagitis are common causes of what?

    (a) Gastrointestinal dysphagia
    (b) Esophageal dysphagia
    (c) Oropharyngeal dysphagia
    (d) All of the above

8. What is the recommendation for when to initiate dysphagia screening?

    (a) Within 6 hours
    (b) Within 24 hours
    (c) Within 36 hours
    (d) Within 48 hours

9. The addition of protein powder and butter to food helps to improve which of the following?

    (a) Caloric value
    (b) Fluid intake
    (c) Fiber intake
    (d) Sweetness

10. What is coated cutlery is useful for?

    (a) Protection against food temperatures
    (b) Protection against sharp cutlery edges
    (c) Protection against food smells
    (d) Both a and b

11. What is the common feeding practice for bedridden patients?

    (a) Elevating the head side of the bed up to 30°
    (b) Elevating the head side of the bed up to 90°
    (c) Elevating the foot side of the bed up to 30°
    (d) Elevating the foot side of the bed up to 90°

12. Which enteral formula should be used for post-stroke dysphagia patients without any medical complications?

    (a) A high-protein formula
    (b) A standard polymeric formula
    (c) A high-fiber formula
    (d) Both a and c

13. Which rehabilitation exercise requires holding the tongue between the teeth and helps the patient to strengthen their pharyngeal muscles?

    (a) The Masako maneuver
    (b) The Mendelsohn maneuver
    (c) Tongue-hold swallow
    (d) Effortful swallow

14. At which level does the IDDSI recommend the initiation of puréed foods?

    (a) Level 3
    (b) Level 4
    (c) Level 5
    (d) Level 6

15. Nectar-thick juices fall under which of the following categories?

    (a) Liquids that quickly flow from a spoon
    (b) Liquids that flow from a spoon slower than thin liquids do
    (c) Liquids that are thicker than thin liquids and that require effort to drink with a spoon
    (d) Liquids that cannot be poured but rather are drunk from a cup

Answer Key

1. (d)
2. (c)
3. (d)
4. (b)
5. (b)
6. (d)
7. (b)
8. (b)
9. (a)
10. (d)
11. (a)
12. (b)
13. (a)
14. (b)
15. (b)

References

1. Gottlieb D, Kipnis M, Sister E, Vardi Y, Brill S. Validation of the 50 ml3 drinking test for evaluation of post-stroke dysphagia. Disabil Rehabil. 1996;18(10):529–32.
2. DePippo KL, Holas MA, Reding MJ. The burke dysphagia screening test: validation of its use in patients with stroke. Arch Phys Med Rehabil. 1994;75(12):1284–6.
3. Wu MC, Chang YC, Wang TG, Lin LC. Evaluating swallowing dysfunction using a 100-ml water swallowing test. Dysphagia. 2004;19(1):43–7.
4. Hinds NP, Wiles CM. Assessment of swallowing and referral to speech and language therapists in acute stroke. QJM. 1998;91(12):829–35.
5. Wilmskoetter J, Daniels SK, Miller AJ. Cortical and subcortical control of swallowing—can we use information from lesion locations to improve diagnosis and treatment for patients with stroke? Am J Speech Lang Pathol. 2020;29(2S):1030–43.
6. Clavé P, Shaker R. Dysphagia: current reality and scope of the problem. Nat Rev Gastroenterol Hepatol. 2015;12(5):259–70.
7. Cohen DL, Roffe C, Beavan J, Blackett B, Fairfield CA, Hamdy S, et al. Post-stroke dysphagia: a review and design considerations for future trials. Int J Stroke. 2016;11(4):399–411.
8. Hamdy S, Aziz Q, Rothwell JC, Crone R, Hughes D, Tallis RC, et al. Explaining oropharyngeal dysphagia after unilateral hemispheric stroke. Lancet. 1997;350(9079):686–92.
9. Teismann IK, Suntrup S, Warnecke T, Steinsträter O, Fischer M, Flöel A, et al. Cortical swallowing processing in early subacute stroke. BMC Neurol. 2011;11:1–13.
10. Horner J, Buoyer FG, Alberts MJ, Helms MJ. Dysphagia following brain-stem stroke: clinical correlates and outcome. Arch Neurol. 1991;48(11):1170–3.
11. González-Fernández M, Ottenstein L, Atanelov L, Christian AB. Dysphagia after stroke: an overview. Curr Phys Med Rehabil Rep. 2013;1:187–96.
12. Robbins J. The evolution of swallowing neuroanatomy and physiology in humans: a practical perspective. 1999. p. 279–80.
13. Mann G, Hankey GJ, Cameron D. Swallowing function after stroke: prognosis and prognostic factors at 6 months. Stroke. 1999;30(4):744–8.

14. Martino R, Foley N, Bhogal S, Diamant N, Speechley M, Teasell R. Dysphagia after stroke: incidence, diagnosis, and pulmonary complications. Stroke. 2005;36(12):2756–63.
15. Langmore SE, Kenneth SM, Olsen N. Fiberoptic endoscopic examination of swallowing safety: a new procedure. Dysphagia. 1988;2:216–9.
16. Cabré M, Serra-Prat M, Force L, Almirall J, Palomera E, Clavé P. Oropharyngeal dysphagia is a risk factor for readmission for pneumonia in the very elderly persons: observational prospective study. J Gerontol A Biol Sci Med Sci. 2014;69(3):330–7.
17. Altman KW, Yu G-P, Schaefer SD. Consequence of dysphagia in the hospitalized patient: impact on prognosis and hospital resources. Arch Otolaryngol Head Neck Surg. 2010;136(8):784–9.
18. Qureshi AI, Suri MFK, Huang W, Akinci Y, Chaudhry MR, Pond DS, et al. Annual direct cost of dysphagia associated with acute ischemic stroke in the United States. J Stroke Cerebrovasc Dis. 2022;31(5):106407.
19. McHorney CA, Martin-Harris B, Robbins J, Rosenbek J. Clinical validity of the SWAL-QOL and SWAL-CARE outcome tools with respect to bolus flow measures. Dysphagia. 2006;21:141–8.
20. Finizia C, Rudberg I, Bergqvist H, Rydén A. A cross-sectional validation study of the Swedish version of SWAL-QOL. Dysphagia. 2012;27:325–35.
21. Lam PM, Lai CKY. The validation of the Chinese version of the swallow quality-of-life questionnaire (SWAL-QOL) using exploratory and confirmatory factor analysis. Dysphagia. 2011;26:117–24.
22. Lim K-B, Lee H-J, Yoo J, Kwon Y-G. Effect of low-frequency rTMS and NMES on subacute unilateral hemispheric stroke with dysphagia. Ann Rehabil Med. 2014;38(5):592.
23. Fujishima I, Fujiu-Kurachi M, Arai H, Hyodo M, Kagaya H, Maeda K, et al. Sarcopenia and dysphagia: position paper by four professional organizations. Geriatr Gerontol Int. 2019;19(2):91–7.
24. Dg S. Complications and outcome after acute stroke. Does dysphagia matter? Stroke. 1996;27:1200–4.
25. Katzan IL, Cebul RD, Husak S, Dawson N, Baker D. The effect of pneumonia on mortality among patients hospitalized for acute stroke. Neurology. 2003;60(4):620–5.
26. Dávalos A, Ricart W, Gonzalez-Huix F, Soler S, Marrugat J, Molins A, et al. Effect of malnutrition after acute stroke on clinical outcome. Stroke. 1996;27(6):1028–32.
27. Collaboration FT. Poor nutritional status on admission predicts poor outcomes after stroke: observational data from the FOOD trial. Stroke. 2003;34(6):1450–6.
28. Namasivayam-MacDonald AM, Slaughter SE, Morrison J, Steele CM, Carrier N, Lengyel C, et al. Inadequate fluid intake in long term care residents: prevalence and determinants. Geriatr Nurs. 2018;39(3):330–5.
29. Charney P. Nutrition screening vs nutrition assessment: how do they differ? Nutr Clin Pract. 2008;23(4):366–72.
30. Correia MITD. Nutrition screening vs nutrition assessment: what's the difference? Nutr Clin Pract. 2018;33(1):62–72.
31. Wakabayashi H, Matsushima M. Dysphagia assessed by the 10-item eating assessment tool is associated with nutritional status and activities of daily living in elderly individuals requiring long-term care. J Nutr Health Aging. 2016;20(1):22–7.
32. Andrade PA, Santos CA, Firmino HH, Rosa COB. The importance of dysphagia screening and nutritional assessment in hospitalized patients. Einstein (Sao Paulo). 2018;16:eAO4189.
33. Andersen UT, Beck AM, Kjaersgaard A, Hansen T, Poulsen I. Systematic review and evidence based recommendations on texture modified foods and thickened fluids for adults (≥18 years) with oropharyngeal dysphagia. e-SPEN J. 2013;8(4):e127–e34.
34. Philpott H, Garg M, Tomic D, Balasubramanian S, Sweis R. Dysphagia: thinking outside the box. World J Gastroenterol. 2017;23(38):6942.
35. Mari A, Tsoukali E, Yaccob A. Eosinophilic esophagitis in adults: a concise overview of an evolving disease. Korean J Fam Med. 2020;41(2):75.

36. Ala'A AJ, Katzka DA, Castell DO. Approach to the patient with dysphagia. Am J Med. 2015;128(10):1138. e17–23.
37. Kuroda Y, Kuroda R. Relationship between thinness and swallowing function in J apanese older adults: implications for Sarcopenic dysphagia. J Am Geriatr Soc. 2012;60(9):1785–6.
38. Wakabayashi H. Presbyphagia and Sarcopenic dysphagia: association between aging, sarcopenia, and deglutition disorders. J Frailty Aging. 2014;3(2):97–103.
39. Blackburn GL, Thornton PA. Nutritional assessment of the hospitalized patient. Med Clin North Am. 1979;63(5):11103–15.
40. Masiero S, Pierobon R, Previato C, Gomiero E. Pneumonia in stroke patients with oropharyngeal dysphagia: a six-month follow-up study. Neurol Sci. 2008;29:139–45.
41. Saito T, Hayashi K, Nakazawa H, Yagihashi F, Oikawa LO, Ota T. A significant association of malnutrition with dysphagia in acute patients. Dysphagia. 2018;33:258–65.
42. Kalf J, De Swart B, Bloem B, Munneke M. Prevalence of oropharyngeal dysphagia in Parkinson's disease: a meta-analysis. Parkinsonism Relat Disord. 2012;18(4):311–5.
43. Clavé P, De Kraa M, Arreola V, Girvent M, Farre R, Palomera E, et al. The effect of bolus viscosity on swallowing function in neurogenic dysphagia. Aliment Pharmacol Ther. 2006;24(9):1385–94.
44. Logemann JA. Dysphagia: evaluation and treatment. Folia Phoniatr Logop. 1995;47(3):140–64.
45. Cabre M, Serra-Prat M, Palomera E, Almirall J, Pallares R, Clavé P. Prevalence and prognostic implications of dysphagia in elderly patients with pneumonia. Age Ageing. 2010;39(1):39–45.
46. Vickers K, Upton C, Chan D. Swallowing and oropharyngeal dysphagia. Clin Med. 2014;14:2.
47. Attrill S, White S, Murray J, Hammond S, Doeltgen S. Impact of oropharyngeal dysphagia on healthcare cost and length of stay in hospital: a systematic review. BMC Health Serv Res. 2018;18:1–18.
48. Campos SML, Trindade DRP, Cavalcanti RVA, Taveira KVM, Ferreira LMBM, Magalhães Junior HV. Signs and symptoms of oropharyngeal dysphagia in institutionalized older adults: an integrative review. Audiology-communication. Research. 2022;27:e2492.
49. Bours GJ, Speyer R, Lemmens J, Limburg M, de Wit R. Bedside screening tests vs. videofluoroscopy or fibreoptic endoscopic evaluation of swallowing to detect dysphagia in patients with neurological disorders: systematic review. J Adv Nurs. 2009;65(3):477–93.
50. Summers D, Leonard A, Wentworth D, Saver JL, Simpson J, Spilker JA, et al. Comprehensive overview of nursing and interdisciplinary care of the acute ischemic stroke patient: a scientific statement from the American Heart Association. Stroke. 2009;40(8):2911–44.
51. Swan K, Cordier R, Brown T, Speyer R. Psychometric properties of visuoperceptual measures of videofluoroscopic and fibre-endoscopic evaluations of swallowing: a systematic review. Dysphagia. 2019;34:2–33.
52. Johnston BC, et al. Patient-reported outcomes, in Cochrane handbook for systematic reviews of interventions. In: Thomas JPTHJ, editor. Cochrane handbook for systematic reviews of interventions. Cochrane; 2019.
53. Prinsen CA, Vohra S, Rose MR, Boers M, Tugwell P, Clarke M, et al. How to select outcome measurement instruments for outcomes included in a "Core outcome set"–a practical guideline. Trials. 2016;17:1–10.
54. Speyer R. Oropharyngeal dysphagia: screening and assessment. Otolaryngol Clin N Am. 2013;46(6):989–1008.
55. Donovan NJ, Daniels SK, Edmiaston J, Weinhardt J, Summers D, Mitchell PH. Dysphagia screening: state of the art: invitational conference proceeding from the state-of-the-art nursing symposium, international stroke conference 2012. Stroke. 2013;44(4):e24–31.
56. Boaden EL. Improving the identification and management of aspiration after stroke. University of Central Lancashire; 2011.
57. Clavé P, Arreola V, Romea M, Medina L, Palomera E, Serra-Prat M. Accuracy of the volume-viscosity swallow test for clinical screening of oropharyngeal dysphagia and aspiration. Clin Nutr. 2008;27(6):806–15.

58. Ruiz Merino L, Hochsprung A, Garcia Q, editors. Results of the adoption of an inter-disciplinary dysphagia protocol in the kick-off of a new stroke unit in a dedicated ward. INTERNATIONAL JOURNAL OF STROKE. WILEY-BLACKWELL 111 RIVER ST, HOBOKEN 07030–5774. NJ: USA; 2014.
59. Heritage M. Swallowing caseloads. RCSLT. Bulletin. 2003;612:10–1.
60. Cocho D, Sagales M, Cobo M, Homs I, Serra J, Pou M, et al. Lowering bronchoaspiration rate in an acute stroke unit by means of a 2 volume/3 texture dysphagia screening test with pulsioximetry. Neurología (English Edition). 2017;32(1):22–8.
61. Giraldo-Cadavid LF, Leal-Leaño LR, Leon-Basantes GA, Bastidas AR, Garcia R, Ovalle S, et al. Accuracy of endoscopic and videofluoroscopic evaluations of swallowing for oropha-ryngeal dysphagia. Laryngoscope. 2017;127(9):2002–10.
62. Hsiao MY, Wu CH, Wang TG. Emerging role of ultrasound in dysphagia assessment and intervention: a narrative review. Front Rehabil Sci. 2021;2:708102.
63. Hsiao MY, Chang YC, Chen WS, Chang HY, Wang TG. Application of ultrasonog-raphy in assessing oropharyngeal dysphagia in stroke patients. Ultrasound Med Biol. 2012;38(9):1522–8.
64. Omari T, Schar M. High-resolution manometry: what about the pharynx? Curr Opin Otolaryngol Head Neck Surg. 2018;26(6):382–91.
65. Dungan S, Gregorio D, Abrahams T, Harrison B, Abrahams J, Brocato D, et al. Comparative validity of the American speech-language-hearing association's national outcomes measure-ment system, functional oral intake scale, and G-codes to mann assessment of swallowing ability scores for dysphagia. Am J Speech Lang Pathol. 2019;28(2):424–9.
66. Sheppard JJ, Hochman R, Baer C. The dysphagia disorder survey: validation of an assess-ment for swallowing and feeding function in developmental disability. Res Dev Disabil. 2014;35(5):929–42.
67. Everton LF, Benfield JK, Hedstrom A, Wilkinson G, Michou E, England TJ, et al. Psychometric assessment and validation of the dysphagia severity rating scale in stroke patients. Sci Rep. 2020;10(1):7268.
68. Sellers D, Mandy A, Pennington L, Hankins M, Morris C. Development and reliability of a system to classify the eating and drinking ability of people with cerebral palsy. Dev Med Child Neurol. 2014;56(3):245–51.
69. Uhm KE, Kim M, Lee YM, Kim B-R, Kim Y-S, Choi J, et al. The easy dysphagia symptom questionnaire (EDSQ): a new dysphagia screening questionnaire for the older adults. Eur Geriatr Med. 2019;10:47–52.
70. Crary MA, Mann GDC, Groher ME. Initial psychometric assessment of a functional oral intake scale for dysphagia in stroke patients. Arch Phys Med Rehabil. 2005;86(8):1516–20.
71. Steele CM, Namasivayam-MacDonald AM, Guida BT, Cichero JA, Duivestein J, Hanson B, et al. Creation and initial validation of the international dysphagia diet standardisation initia-tive functional diet scale. Arch Phys Med Rehabil. 2018;99(5):934–44.
72. Mann G. MASA: the Mann assessment of swallowing ability. Singular: Thomson Learning. Inc, New York; 2002.
73. Carnaby GD, Crary MA. Development and validation of a cancer-specific swallowing assess-ment tool: MASA-C. Support Care Cancer. 2014;22:595–602.
74. Lambert HC, Gisel EG, Groher ME, Wood-Dauphinee S. McGill Ingestive skills assessment (MISA): development and first field test of an evaluation of functional ingestive skills of elderly persons. Dysphagia. 2003;18:101–13.
75. Antonios N, Carnaby-Mann G, Crary M, Miller L, Hubbard H, Hood K, et al. Analysis of a physician tool for evaluating dysphagia on an inpatient stroke unit: the modified Mann assessment of swallowing ability. J Stroke Cerebrovasc Dis. 2010;19(1):49–57.
76. Hall KM. Overview of functional assessment scales in brain injury rehabilitation. NeuroRehabilitation. 1992;2(4):98–113.
77. Karsten R, Hilgers F, van der Molen L, van Sluis K, Smeele L, Stuiver M. The timed swal-lowing proficiency for eating and drinking (SPEAD) test: development and initial valida-

tion of an instrument to objectify (impaired) swallowing capacity in head and neck cancer patients. Dysphagia. 2021;1-16:1072.

78. Moorhead S, Swanson E, Johnson M. Nursing outcomes classification (NOC)-E-book: nursing outcomes classification. (NOC)-E-Book: Elsevier Health Sciences; 2023.
79. Athukorala RP, Jones RD, Sella O, Huckabee M-L. Skill training for swallowing rehabilitation in patients with Parkinson's disease. Arch Phys Med Rehabil. 2014;95(7):1374–82.
80. Restivo DA, Panebianco M, Casabona A, Lanza S, Marchese-Ragona R, Patti F, et al. Botulinum toxin a for Sialorrhoea associated with neurological disorders: evaluation of the relationship between effect of treatment and the number of glands treated. Toxins (Basel). 2018;10(2)
81. Guigoz Y. The mini nutritional assessment (MNA®) review of the literature-what does it tell us? J Nutr Health Aging. 2006;10(6):466.
82. Cheney DM, Siddiqui MT, Litts JK, Kuhn MA, Belafsky PC. The ability of the 10-item eating assessment tool (EAT-10) to predict aspiration risk in persons with dysphagia. Ann Otol Rhinol Laryngol. 2015;124(5):351–4.
83. Kubota T. Paralytic dysphagia in cerebrovascular disorder-screening tests and their clinical application. Gen Rehabil. 1982;10:271.
84. Tohara H, Saitoh E, Mays KA, Kuhlemeier K, Palmer JB. Three tests for predicting aspiration without videofluorography. Dysphagia. 2003;18:126–34.
85. Lazarus CL, Logemann JA, Rademaker AW, Kahrilas PJ, Pajak T, Lazar R, et al. Effects of bolus volume, viscosity, and repeated swallows in nonstroke subjects and stroke patients. Arch Phys Med Rehabil. 1993;74(10):1066–70.
86. Nishiwaki K, Tsuji T, Liu M, Hase K, Tanaka N, Fujiwara T. Identification of a simple screening tool for dysphagia in patients with stroke using factor analysis of multiple dysphagia variables. J Rehabil Med. 2005;37(4):247–51.
87. Barer DH. The natural history and functional consequences of dysphagia after hemispheric stroke. J Neurol Neurosurg Psychiatry. 1989;52(2):236–41.
88. Borean M, Shani K, Brown MC, Chen J, Liang M, Karkada J, et al. Development and evaluation of screening dysphagia tools for observational studies and routine care in cancer patients. Health Sci Rep [Internet]. 2018 1(7):[e48 p.]. Available from: http://europepmc.org/abstract/MED/30623085, https://onlinelibrary.wiley.com/doi/pdfdirect/10.1002/hsr2.48, https://doi.org/10.1002/hsr2.48, https://europepmc.org/articles/PMC6266365, https://europepmc.org/articles/PMC6266365?pdf=render.
89. Wallace KL, Middleton S, Cook IJ. Development and validation of a self-report symptom inventory to assess the severity of oral-pharyngeal dysphagia. Gastroenterology. 2000;118(4):678–87.
90. Chen AY, Frankowski R, Bishop-Leone J, Hebert T, Leyk S, Lewin J, et al. The development and validation of a dysphagia-specific quality-of-life questionnaire for patients with head and neck cancer: the MD Anderson dysphagia inventory. Arch Otolaryngol Head Neck Surg. 2001;127(7):870–6.
91. Ekberg O, Hamdy S, Woisard V, Wuttge–Hannig A, Ortega P. Social and psychological burden of dysphagia: its impact on diagnosis and treatment. Dysphagia. 2002;17:139–46.
92. McHorney CA, Bricker DE, Kramer AE, Rosenbek JC, Robbins J, Chignell KA, et al. The SWAL-QOL outcomes tool for oropharyngeal dysphagia in adults: I. Conceptual foundation and item development. Dysphagia. 2000;15:115–21.
93. Silbergleit AK, Schultz L, Jacobson BH, Beardsley T, Johnson AF. The dysphagia handicap index: development and validation. Dysphagia. 2012;27:46–52.
94. Woisard V, Andrieux M, Puech M. Validation of a self-assessment questionnaire for swallowing disorders (deglutition handicap index). Rev Laryngol Otol Rhinol (Bord). 2006;127(5):315–25.
95. Nip W, Perry L, McLaren S, Mackenzie A. Dietary intake, nutritional status and rehabilitation outcomes of stroke patients in hospital. J Hum Nutr Diet. 2011;24(5):460–9.
96. Wong MC, Chan KMK, Wong TT, Tang HW, Chung HY, Kwan HS. Quantitative textural and rheological data on different levels of texture-modified food and thickened liquids classi-

fied using the international dysphagia diet standardisation initiative (IDDSI) guideline. Food Secur. 2023;12(20):3765.

97. Garcia JM, Chambers E IV. Managing dysphagia through diet modifications. Am J Nurs. 2010;110(11):26–33.

98. Shimazu S, Yoshimura Y, Kudo M, Nagano F, Bise T, Shiraishi A, et al. Frequent and personalized nutritional support leads to improved nutritional status, activities of daily living, and dysphagia after stroke. Nutrition. 2021;83:111091.

99. Lieber AC, Hong E, Putrino D, Nistal DA, Pan JS, Kellner CP. Nutrition, energy expenditure, dysphagia, and self-efficacy in stroke rehabilitation: a review of the literature. Brain Sci. 2018;8(12):218.

100. Jeejeebhoy KN. Enteral feeding. Curr Opin Clin Nutr Metab Care. 2002;5(6):695–8.

101. Brown B, Roehl K, Betz M. Enteral nutrition formula selection: current evidence and implications for practice. Nutr Clin Pract. 2015;30(1):72–85.

102. Hadde EK, Chen J. Texture and texture assessment of thickened fluids and texture-modified food for dysphagia management. J Texture Stud. 2021;52(1):4–15.

103. Pardoe EM. Development of a multistage diet for dysphagia. J Am Diet Assoc. 1993;93(5):568–71.

104. Hotaling DL. Nutritional considerations for the pureed diet texture in dysphagic elderly. Dysphagia. 1992;7(2):81–5.

105. Chen J, Rosenthal A. Modifying food texture: volume 2: sensory analysis, consumer requirements and preferences: Woodhead publishing; 2015.

106. Layne KA. Feeding strategies for the dysphagic patient: a nursing perspective. Dysphagia. 1990;5(2):84–8.

107. Logemann JA. Factors affecting ability to resume oral nutrition in the oropharyngeal dysphagic individual. Dysphagia. 1990;4(4):202–8.

108. Aguilera JM, Park DJ. Bottom-up approaches in the Design of Soft Foods for the elderly. Nanotechnology in agriculture and food. Science. 2017:153–66.

109. Vivanti AP, Campbell K, Suter M, Hannan-Jones M, Hulcombe J. Contribution of thickened drinks, food and enteral and parenteral fluids to fluid intake in hospitalised patients with dysphagia. J Hum Nutr Diet. 2009;22(2):148–55.

110. Howard MM, Nissenson PM, Meeks L, Rosario ER. Use of textured thin liquids in patients with dysphagia. Am J Speech Lang Pathol. 2018;27(2):827–35.

111. Thomas DR, Cote TR, Lawhorne L, Levenson SA, Rubenstein LZ, Smith DA, et al. Understanding clinical dehydration and its treatment. J Am Med Dir Assoc. 2008;9(5):292–301.

112. Anjo I, Amaral T, Afonso C, Borges N, Santos A, Moreira P, et al. Are hypohydrated older adults at increased risk of exhaustion? J Hum Nutr Diet. 2020;33(1):23–30.

113. Bruno C, Collier A, Holyday M, Lambert K. Interventions to improve hydration in older adults: a systematic review and meta-analysis. Nutrients. 2021;13(10):3640.

114. Taylor KA, Barr SI. Provision of small, frequent meals does not improve energy intake of elderly residents with dysphagia who live in an extended-care facility. J Am Diet Assoc. 2006;106(7):1115–8.

115. Malhi H. Dysphagia: warning signs and management. Br J Nurs. 2016;25(10):546–9.

116. Shune SE, Linville D. Understanding the dining experience of individuals with dysphagia living in care facilities: a grounded theory analysis. Int J Nurs Stud. 2019;92:144–53.

117. Luk JK, Chan DK. Preventing aspiration pneumonia in older people: do we have the 'know-how'? Hong Kong Med J. 2014;20(5):421.

118. Mesioye A, Smith J, Zilberstein M, Hart H, Bush-Thomas P, Ward M, editors. Dysphagia rounds: Interdisciplinary collaboration to improve swallowing safety in a VA community living center. J Am Geriatr Soc; 2018: Wiley 111 River St, Hoboken 07030–5774, NJ USA.

119. Wu X, Yousif L, Miles A, Braakhuis A. Exploring meal provision and mealtime challenges for aged care residents consuming texture-modified diets: a mixed methods study. Geriatrics. 2022;7(3):67.

120. Smith R, Bryant L, Reddacliff C, Hemsley B. A review of the impact of food design on the mealtimes of people with swallowing disability who require texture-modified food. Int J Food Design. 2022;7(1):7–28.
121. Hemsley B, Palmer S, Kouzani A, Adams S, Balandin S. Review informing the design of 3D food printing for people with swallowing disorders: constructive, conceptual, and empirical problems. 2019.
122. Kuhlemeier K, Palmer J, Rosenberg D. Effect of liquid bolus consistency and delivery method on aspiration and pharyngeal retention in dysphagia patients. Dysphagia. 2001;16:119–22.
123. Boczko F, Feightner K. Dysphagia in the older adult: the roles of speech-language pathologists and occupational therapists. Top Geriatr Rehabil. 2007;23(3):220.

Part II

Public Health Nutrition

Essential Micronutrients for a Healthy Life

8

Sabuktagin Rahman, Santhia Ireen, and Amal K. Mitra ⓘ

Learning Objectives

After completing the chapter, you will be able to

- Describe types of vitamins and major micronutrients
- Describe important physiological functions and deficiency symptoms of different vitamins and minerals
- Identify the most important food sources and dietary recommendations for different micronutrients
- Identify the health implications of micronutrients
- Provide a few public health intervention strategies

Introduction

Micronutrients are vitamins and minerals that the body needs in very small amounts. They are indispensable for normal growth and development because they produce hormones, enzymes, and other essential elements [1]. The *Lancet*

S. Rahman
Department of Public Health, Faculty of Arts and Social Sciences, American International University-Bangladesh, Dhaka, Bangladesh
e-mail: sabuktagin@aiub.edu

S. Ireen (✉)
James P. Grant School of Public Health, Brac University, Dhaka, Bangladesh
e-mail: santhia.ireen1@bracu.ac.bd

A. K. Mitra
Department of Public Health, Julia Jones Matthews School of Population and Public Health, Texas Tech University Health Sciences Center, Abilene, TX, USA
e-mail: amal.mitra@ttuhsc.edu

© The Author(s), under exclusive license to Springer Nature Switzerland AG 2025
A. K. Mitra, D. Vanoh (eds.), *Essentials of Clinical and Public Health Nutrition*, Nutrition and Health, https://doi.org/10.1007/978-3-031-95373-6_8

169

Table 8.1 General characteristics of fat-soluble and water-soluble vitamins

	Fat-soluble vitamins Vitamins A, D, E, and K	Water-soluble vitamins B vitamins and vitamin C
Absorption	These vitamins are absorbed like fats—first into lymph and then into the blood.	These vitamins are absorbed directly into the blood.
Transport	The must travel with protein carriers in water body fluids.	They travel freely in watery fluids.
Storage	They are stored in the liver or fatty tissues.	They are mostly not stored in the body.
Excretion	They are not readily excreted and tend to build up in the tissues.	They are readily excreted through urine.
Toxicity	Toxicities are likely from supplements but rarely occur from food.	Toxicities are unlikely but possible from high-dose supplements.
Requirements	They are needed in periodic doses (weeks or months) as the body can draw on its stores.	They are needed in frequent doses (every 1–3 days) because the body does not store them.

Global Health estimates that one of every two preschool-aged children and two of every three women of reproductive age worldwide have at least one micronutrient deficiency. Micronutrient deficiencies are most prevalent among people of developing nations, including those in South Asia and sub-Saharan Africa, but inadequate micronutrients are common also because of the inappropriate selection of food among many people in high-income countries [2]. This section describes different types of vitamins and minerals and their importance in health and well-being.

In general, fat-soluble vitamins act like other lipids: They are absorbed into the lymph, and they travel in the blood with the help of protein carriers. Fat-soluble vitamins can be stored in the liver or in other fatty tissues in the body. Excess amounts of some of these may cause toxicity in the body. Water-soluble vitamins are absorbed directly into the bloodstream, where they travel freely. Most water-soluble vitamins are not stored in the body, and an excess of them is excreted through the urine. Thus, the risk of toxicity is minor for water-soluble vitamins. Table 8.1 depicts the key characteristics of different types of vitamins.

Fat-Soluble Vitamins

Vitamin A

Vitamin A is an essential nutrient necessary for various physiological functions. Vitamin A deficiency is probably the most common cause of preventable blindness among children in developing countries. Three forms of vitamin A are active in the body; retinol (one of the active forms) is stored in the liver. The liver makes retinol available to the bloodstream and thereby to the body's cells. The cells convert retinol into its other two active forms—retinal and retinoic acid—as needed. Preformed vitamin A is found only in animals and a small number of bacteria. β-carotene and some other carotenes from plants that can be oxidized to retinol are known as provitamin A carotenoids. Because relatively few foods are rich sources of retinol, carotenes are nutritionally vital. In developed countries, with a relatively high intake of animal foods, some 20–34% of vitamin A is derived from carotenoids, and more than 70% of provitamin A carotenoids are obtained from food [3]. Because vitamin A cannot be synthesized in the body, it must be provided from the diet in sufficient amounts to meet all the body's physiological needs.

Functions of Vitamin A: A Magic Bullet

Vitamin A is very versatile, playing essential roles in regulating key biological processes, including those involved in gene expression, growth maturation, vision, reproduction, maintaining body linings and skin, immune defenses, and, more broadly, cellular differentiation and proliferation throughout life [4]. Vitamin A is crucial for several key functions: vision, cell growth and differentiation, immune function, reproduction and growth, and delivering antioxidant properties.

Vision

- *Rhodopsin formation*: The most known function of vitamin A is to sustain normal eyesight. Vitamin A in the visual cycle enables vision in low light. Vitamin A is a critical component of rhodopsin, a protein in the retina that absorbs light, and it plays two indispensable roles in vision, namely in the process of light perception at the retina and in the maintenance of a healthy, crystal-clear outer window, the cornea [5]. It also helps in the functioning of the cones in the retina, which are necessary for color vision [5].
- *Preventing night blindness*: Adequate vitamin A intake helps to prevent night blindness and maintain good vision. In the absence of vitamin A, the cornea becomes very dry, thus damaging the retina and cornea [5].

Cell Growth and Differentiation

- *Regulation of gene expression*: All-trans-retinoic acid is an essential signaling molecule in cell differentiation, proliferation, and apoptosis, and it participates in gene transcription, representing the pathways through which vitamin A likely mediates most of its effects on morphogenesis; organogenesis (e.g., lung, heart, vascular and central nervous system, kidney, and limbs); immune function; tissue epithelialization (including the cornea and conjunctival surfaces of the eye); hematopoiesis; and bone growth and development [5, 6]. Over 500 genes are thought to respond to the retinoic acid form of vitamin A through direct or indirect transcriptional mechanisms [7].
- *Epithelial cell health and wound healing*: Vitamin A is involved in the differentiation of epithelial cells, which line the internal and external surfaces of the body. This is crucial for skin health and wound healing [8].

Immune Function
- *Maintaining the immune system*: Vitamin A plays a vital role in maintaining the integrity and function of skin and mucosal cells (barriers to infection), and it supports the production and function of white blood cells [9]. This is why vitamin A is also known as "the anti-infective vitamin." Deficiencies in vitamin A have been linked to an increased susceptibility to skin infection and inflammation [10].

Reproduction and Growth
- *Fetal development*: All-trans-retinoic acid supports both male and female reproduction as well as embryonic development, including the development of the heart, lungs, kidneys, and other organs [11].
- *Growth in children*: It supports the normal growth and development of children [12].

Delivering Antioxidant Properties
- *Neutralizing free radicals*: β-carotene has antioxidant properties that help neutralize free radicals, reducing oxidative stress and potentially lowering the risk of chronic diseases [13].

Vitamin A Deficiency
Vitamin A deficiency results from a dietary intake of vitamin A that is inadequate to satisfy the body's physiological needs. It may be exacerbated by high rates of infection, especially diarrhea and measles. It is common in developing countries but rarely seen in developed countries. A plasma or serum retinol concentration < 0.70 μmol/l indicates subclinical vitamin A deficiency in children and adults, and a concentration of < 0.35 μmol/l indicates severe vitamin A deficiency [14]. The prevalence of serum retinol at 0.70 μmol/l or below can be used to assess the severity of vitamin A deficiency in most age groups as a public health problem.

Dietary Sources of Vitamin A
Vitamin A is found in both animal and plant-based foods, existing in two primary forms: preformed vitamin A (retinol and its esterified form, retinyl ester) from animal sources and provitamin A carotenoids (such as beta-carotene) from plant sources. Vitamin A comes from two key dietary sources: animal sources and plan sources.

Animal sources: Liver (richest source), such as beef liver, chicken liver, and other animal livers; fish oils, such as from cod, halibut, and other fish livers; and dairy products, such as milk, cheese, and butter.
Plant sources: Yellow and dark leafy vegetables and fruits, such as carrots, sweet potatoes, pumpkin, spinach, kale, collard greens, butternut squash, red and orange bell peppers, cantaloupe, tomatoes, and mangoes.

Vitamin A requirements differ by age and for women during pregnancy and lactation. An excess of vitamin A can cause toxicity, especially in infants and very young children. The signs of toxicity include a bulged anterior fontanelle of the skull in infants and convulsions.

Recommended Dietary Allowances [15]
- Birth to 6 months—400 mcg RAE (retinol activity equivalent)
- 7–12 months—500 mcg RAE
- 1–3 years—300 mcg RAE
- 4–8 years—400 mcg RAE
- 9–13 years—600 mcg RAE
- 14–18 years—900 mcg RAE
  - Pregnancy—750 mcg RAE
  - Lactation—1200 mcg RAE
- 19–50 years—900 mcg RAE
  - Pregnancy—770 mcg RAE
  - Lactation—1300 mcg RAE
- 51+ years—900 mcg RAE

Box 8.1 The Health Implications of Vitamin A Deficiency
- Night blindness: Night blindness is one of the earliest signs of vitamin A deficiency.
- Xerophthalmia: This is a severe condition characterized by dryness of the conjunctiva and cornea, which can lead to blindness if untreated.
- Increased infection risk: Deficiency impairs the immune system, increasing susceptibility to infections, particularly in children.
- Growth retardation: Inadequate vitamin A can cause stunted growth in children.
- Maternal health: Vitamin A deficiency during pregnancy can increase the risk of maternal mortality and complications.

Vitamin D

Vitamin D is a fat-soluble vitamin that is crucial for maintaining bone health; supporting the immune system, brain, and nervous system; regulating insulin levels; and supporting lung function and cardiovascular health. Vitamin D can be obtained naturally via exposure to sunlight and through certain foods and supplements.

Functions of Vitamin D
Bone Health
- Calcium absorption: Vitamin D is essential to optimize intestinal calcium and phosphorus absorption for the proper formation of the bone mineral matrix [16].
- Bone mineralization and preventing osteomalacia: Vitamin D is a secosteroid hormone essential for calcium absorption and bone mineralization, which is positively associated with bone mineral density [17], helping to prevent rickets in children and osteomalacia in adults.

Immune Function
- Modulating the immune response: Vitamin D metabolizes enzymes and is present in various immune cells such as antigen-presenting-cells, T cells, B cells, and monocytes. Vitamin D plays a role in modulating the immune system, enhancing the pathogen-fighting effects of monocytes and macrophages—white blood cells that are critical in defending the body against infections [18].
- Reducing inflammation: Vitamin D helps prevent chronic disease and infections by regulating inflammatory responses [19].

Cell Growth and Differentiation
- Gene expression: Vitamin D influences the expression of genes involved in cell growth, differentiation, and apoptosis (programmed cell death), which are important processes in cancer prevention and overall cellular health [19].

Neuromuscular Function
- Muscle health: Vitamin D is important for improving muscle performance and balance and for lowering the risk of falling in older adults [20].

Cardiovascular Health
- Blood pressure regulation: Some studies have suggested that vitamin D may play a role in regulating blood pressure and reducing the risk of hypertension. Vitamin D regulates blood pressure by acting on endothelial cells and smooth muscle cells [21].

Sources of Vitamin D
Sunlight: The skin synthesizes vitamin D when exposed to ultraviolet B rays from sunlight. The amount produced depends on factors like geographic location, skin pigmentation, and time spent outdoors.

Dietary sources: Vitamin D can be obtained from fish such as salmon, mackerel, sardines, tuna; liver, egg yolk, and cod liver oil; and dairy products and fortified foods such as milk, cereals, juice, and margarine.

RDA for Vitamin D
The Recommended Dietary Allowance (RDA) requirements for vitamin D depend on age and the pregnancy and lactation state of women [22].

- Birth to 12 months—400 IU (international unit)
- 1–18 years—600 IU
- 19–70 years—600 IU
- > 70 years—800 IU
- Pregnancy and lactation—600 IU

Box 8.2 The Health Implications of Vitamin D Deficiency
- Rickets: In children, severe vitamin D deficiency can cause rickets, a condition characterized by soft and weakened bones.
- Osteomalacia: In adults, deficiency can lead to osteomalacia, resulting in bone pain and muscle weakness.
- Osteoporosis: Chronic low levels of vitamin D can contribute to osteoporosis, increasing the risk of fractures.
- Increased infection risk: Deficiency has been linked to an increased susceptibility to infections, such as respiratory tract infections.
- Chronic diseases: Low vitamin D levels have been associated with an increased risk of chronic diseases, including certain cancers, cardiovascular diseases, and autoimmune conditions.

Vitamin E

Vitamin E is a group of fat-soluble compounds known as tocopherols and tocotrienols, alpha-tocopherol being the most biologically active form in the human body. It acts primarily as an antioxidant and is essential for various bodily functions [23].

Functions of Vitamin E
Antioxidant Properties
- Free radical scavenging: Vitamin E protects cell membranes from oxidative damage caused by free radicals and reactive oxygen species (ROS), thereby reducing oxidative stress [24].
- Protecting lipids: Vitamin E plays a role in maintaining the integrity of the cell membranes of nerves and muscles (tissues rich in polyunsaturated fatty acids) [25].

Immune Function
- Enhancing the immune response: Vitamin E supports immune function by promoting the activity of immune cells, which helps the body defend against infections and diseases [26].
- Protecting skin and healing wounds: As an antioxidant, vitamin E helps protect skin cells from damage caused by ultraviolet (UV) rays and environmental pollutants. It also promotes wound healing by supporting the growth of new skin cells [27].

Cardiovascular Health
- Protecting blood vessels: Vitamin E may help prevent the oxidation of low-density lipoprotein (LDL) cholesterol ("bad" cholesterol), which is a risk factor for cardiovascular diseases.
- Blood clotting: Vitamin E plays a role in inhibiting platelet aggregation, reducing the risk of blood clots.

Neurological Function
- Protecting nerves: Vitamin E is important for maintaining nerve health and may help protect against neurodegenerative diseases.
- Cognitive function: Some research suggests that vitamin E may support cognitive function and reduce the risk of cognitive decline with aging.

Reproductive Health
- Fertility: Vitamin E is involved in maintaining reproductive health, including the health of sperm and eggs.

Dietary Sources of Vitamin E
Plant-based oils such as wheat germ oil, sunflower oil, safflower oil, and soybean oil; nuts and seeds such as almonds, sunflower seeds, hazelnuts, peanuts, and peanut butter (moderate amounts of vitamin E); leafy green vegetables such as spinach, Swiss chard, and kale; and fortified foods are all dietary sources of vitamin E.

RDA for Vitamin E [28]
As with other fat-soluble vitamins, the RDA for vitamin E depends on age and the pregnancy and lactation state of women.

- 0–6 months—4 mg
- 7–12 month—5 mg
- 1–3 years—6 mg
- 4–8 years—7 mg
- 9–13 years—11 mg
- 14+ years—15 mg
- Pregnancy—15 mg
- Lactation—19 mg

Box 8.3 The Health Implications of Vitamin E Deficiency
- Neurological symptoms: Mild deficiency may result in peripheral neuropathy, characterized by numbness and tingling in the hands and feet.
- Muscle weakness: Severe deficiency can lead to muscle weakness.
- Immune dysfunction: Vitamin E deficiency leads to reduced immune function and increased susceptibility to infections.
- Vision problems: Long-term deficiency may contribute to retinal damage and vision loss.

Vitamin K

Vitamin K is a fat-soluble vitamin that plays a crucial role in blood clotting and bone health. There are two primary forms of vitamin K: vitamin K1 (phylloquinone), which is found in plant sources, and vitamin K2 (menaquinones), which is synthesized by bacteria in the gut and found in fermented foods [29].

Functions of Vitamin K
Blood Clotting
- Coagulation factor synthesis: Vitamin K plays a key role in the synthesis of several proteins involved in blood clotting, including prothrombin and other clotting factors. This role is critical in wound healing and preventing excessive bleeding [29].

Bone Health
- Vitamin K supports bone health by regulating calcium balance in the body by promoting the deposition of calcium into bones and reducing the risk of osteoporosis. It facilitates the activation of osteocalcin, a protein that binds calcium to bones, thereby supporting bone mineralization and strength [30].

Cardiovascular Health
- Vitamin K prevents the calcification of blood vessels and soft tissues, leading to a reduced risk of cardiovascular diseases [31].

Dietary Sources of Vitamin K
Dietary sources of vitamin K1 (phylloquinone) include green leafy vegetables such as kale, spinach, Swiss chard, collard greens, and broccoli and vegetable oils such as soybean oil, canola oil, and olive oil. Dietary sources of Vitamin K2 (menaquinones) include fermented foods such as natto (fermented soybeans), sauerkraut, and certain cheeses (e.g., gouda and brie) and small amounts in animal products such as meat, dairy, and egg yolks.

RDA for Vitamin K [15]
- Birth to 6 months—2 mcg
- 7–12 months—2.5 mcg
- 1–3 years—30 mcg
- 4–8 years—55 mcg
- 9–13 years—60 mcg
- 14–18 years—75 mcg
  - Pregnancy and lactation—75 mcg

- 19+ years
  - Male—120 mcg
  - Female—90 mcg
  - Pregnancy and lactation—90 mcg

Box 8.4 The Health Implications of Vitamin K Deficiency
Increased bleeding risk: Deficiency can lead to impaired blood clotting, resulting in excessive bleeding or easy bruising.
Bone health issues: Insufficient vitamin K may contribute to decreased bone mineral density, potentially increasing the risk of fractures.
Calcification disorders: Inadequate vitamin K levels may contribute to the abnormal calcification of blood.

Water-Soluble Vitamins

Water-soluble vitamins fall under two main categories.

- B complex vitamins: This group includes all the B vitamins, such as thiamin (B_1), riboflavin (B_2), niacin (B_3), pantothenic acid (B_5), pyridoxine (B_6), biotin (B_7), folate, and cobalamin (B_{12}) which play vital roles in energy production, cell metabolism, and the synthesis of neurotransmitters, among other functions.
- Vitamin C (ascorbic acid): Vitamin C is crucial for the synthesis of collagen, the absorption of iron, and the maintenance of the immune system. It also acts as an antioxidant, protecting cells from damage.

Vitamin B Complex

Vitamin B complex refers to a group of eight vitamins. Table 8.2 summarizes the functions, deficiency symptoms, and dietary sources of vitamin B complex.

Vitamin C

Vitamin C, also known as ascorbic acid, is essential for the formation, growth, and repair of connective tissue, bones, and skin. It also maintains the normal function of blood vessels. The role of vitamin C in various physiological functions and overall health could be listed as follows:

- Antioxidant properties: Vitamin C helps to reduce cell damage caused by free radicals and reactive oxygen species. This property helps reduce oxidative stress in the body [33].
- Collagen synthesis: Vitamin C is necessary for the synthesis of collagen, a pro-

Table 8.2 Functions, deficiencies, and dietary sources of vitamin B complex [32]

Vitamin	Functions	Deficiency symptoms	Dietary sources
Thiamin (B$_1$)	Energy production: Thiamin is essential for converting carbohydrates into energy. Nervous system: Thiamin supports the nervous system's functions and muscle contractions.	Beriberi (weakness, nerve damage) Wernicke–Korsakoff syndrome (memory issues, confusion) Fatigue, irritability	Whole grains: enriched or fortified cereals, bread, rice, and pasta Legumes: beans, lentils, and peas Nuts and seeds: sunflower seeds, macadamia nuts Meat: lean cuts of pork, beef, and lamb
Riboflavin (B$_2$)	Energy metabolism: Riboflavin is involved in energy production from carbohydrates, fats, and proteins. Antioxidant properties: It has antioxidant properties, protecting cells from oxidative stress and maintains healthy skin, healthy eyes, and a healthy nervous system.	Cracked lips, sore throat Skin disorders (sensitivity to light) Swelling of mouth and throat	Dairy products: milk, yogurt, cheese Meat: beef, lamb, pork Eggs: particularly the yolk Leafy green vegetables
Niacin (B$_3$)	Energy production: Niacin is a component of coenzyme A, which is essential for energy metabolism. Synthesis of hormones and cholesterol: It plays a role in the synthesis of steroid hormones and cholesterol.	Pellagra: dermatitis, diarrhea, dementia (can lead to death if untreated)	Meat: chicken, turkey, lean cuts of beef Fish: tuna, salmon, swordfish. Whole grains: brown rice, barley, whole wheat Legumes: peanuts, lentils, peas
Pantothenic acid (B$_5$)	Energy production: Pantothenic acid is a component of coenzyme A, which is essential for energy metabolism. Synthesis of hormones and cholesterol: It plays a role in the synthesis of steroid hormones and cholesterol.	Fatigue, irritability, numbness, muscle cramps	Animal products: chicken, beef, pork, eggs Whole grains: brown rice, whole wheat Legumes: lentils, chickpeas Vegetables: avocadoes, sweet potatoes

(continued)

Table 8.2 (continued)

Vitamin	Functions	Deficiency symptoms	Dietary sources
Pyridoxine (B$_6$)	Amino acid metabolism: Pyridoxine is involved in the metabolism of amino acids (building blocks of proteins). Neurotransmitter production: Pyridoxine aids in the production of neurotransmitters such as serotonin and dopamine.	Microcytic anemia (fatigue, weakness) Depression, confusion Weakened immune response	Meat: chicken, turkey, pork Fish: tuna, salmon Bananas: particularly rich in pyridoxine Potatoes: especially in the skin
Biotin (B$_7$)	Metabolism: Biotin is essential for carbohydrate, fat, and protein metabolism. Hair, skin, and nail health: It is often associated with promoting healthy hair, skin, and nails.	Dermatitis: skin rashes, hair loss Neurological symptoms: depression, lethargy, hallucinations	Egg yolks: rich sources of biotin Nuts: almonds, peanuts. Whole grains: oats, barley. Vegetables: sweet potatoes, spinach
Folate (B$_9$)	DNA synthesis and cell division: Folate is essential for the synthesis and repair of DNA. It is particularly important during infancy, adolescence, and pregnancy, when rapid cell division takes place. Red blood cell formation: Folate is necessary for the production of red blood cells (erythropoiesis). Amino acid metabolism: Folate is involved in the metabolism of amino acids. It plays a role in the conversion of homocysteine into methionine, which is important for cardiovascular health. Neurological function: Folate plays a role in neurotransmitter synthesis and supports cognitive function. Folic acid levels are crucial for proper neurological function and development. Fetal development: Folic acid is critical during pregnancy for the prevention of neural tube defects (such as spina bifida) in a developing fetus.	Megaloblastic anemia: Deficiency can lead to the production of large, immature red blood cells that do not function properly. Neural tube defects (NTDs): Deficiency during early pregnancy causes serious birth defects affecting the brain, spine, or spinal cord of the developing fetus. Increased risk of cardiovascular disease: Deficiency is associated with low methionine levels, which may increase the risk of cardiovascular diseases.	Leafy green vegetables: spinach, kale, collard greens, broccoli Legumes: lentils, chickpeas, black beans Fruits: oranges, bananas, avocadoes Fortified grains: fortified breakfast cereals, fortified breads and pasta Liver and other organ meats

(continued)

Table 8.2 (continued)

Vitamin	Functions	Deficiency symptoms	Dietary sources
Cobalamin (B$_{12}$)	DNA synthesis: Vitamin B$_{12}$ is necessary for DNA synthesis and red blood cell formation. Nervous system function: Vitamin B$_{12}$ supports nerve cell function and the production of myelin, which insulates nerve fibers.	Pernicious anemia Neurological disturbances: numbness and tingling in the hands and feet, difficulty walking, muscle weakness, memory loss, confusion, mood changes (irritability, depression)	Animal products: beef, chicken, fish Dairy products: milk, cheese, yogurt Eggs: particularly the yolk Fortified foods: breakfast cereals, nutritional yeast

tein that forms the structural basis of skin, ligaments, tendons, and blood vessels. It plays a crucial role in wound healing and maintaining skin elasticity.
- Immune function: Vitamin C supports the epithelial barrier's function against pathogens and promotes the oxidant scavenging activity of the skin. It also enhances the function of various immune cells, such as neutrophils, lymphocytes, and phagocytes, leading to microbial killing [34]. It helps the body defend against infections by viruses.
- Iron absorption: Vitamin C is a powerful enhancer of nonheme iron (iron from plant-based sources) absorption and can reverse the inhibiting effect of such substances as tea and calcium/phosphate. This is particularly important for individuals who consume a vegetarian or vegan diet because plant-based iron is less readily absorbed than iron from animal sources [35].
- Neurotransmitter synthesis: Vitamin C is involved in the synthesis of neurotransmitters such as serotonin, which plays a role in mood regulation and cognitive function.

Vitamin C Deficiency
There are several major diseases and conditions that may occur as a results of vitamin C deficiency.

- Impaired immune function: This weakens the immune response and increases susceptibility to infections.
- Skin lesions: Dry skin, rough skin, and prematurely aged skin are due to impaired collagen synthesis.
- Scurvy: Severe vitamin C deficiency can lead to scurvy, characterized by fatigue, swollen and bleeding gums, joint pain, and poor wound healing.

RDA for Vitamin C [28]
- 1–3 years—15 mg
- 4–8 years—25 mg
- 9–13 years—45 mg

- 14–18 years
  - Male—75 mg
  - Female—65 mg
- 19+ years
  - Male—90 mg
  - Female—75 mg
  - Pregnancy—85 mg
  - Lactation—120 mg

Dietary Sources of Vitamin C

Fruits such as oranges, lemons, limes, grapefruits, kiwi, pineapple, strawberries, raspberries, blueberries, Indian gooseberry (amloki, *Phyllanthus emblica*), guava, papaya, mango, cantaloupe, and watermelon and vegetables such as bell peppers, green chilies, broccoli and brussels sprouts (rich sources of vitamin C), cauliflower, spinach, kale, cabbage, tomatoes, and cabbage are all dietary sources of vitamin C.

Minerals

Minerals are inorganic elements such as calcium, phosphorus, potassium, sodium, iodine, iron, zinc, and so forth. The carbon atoms in all carbohydrates, fats, proteins, and vitamins combine with oxygen to form carbon dioxide, which disappears in the air. The hydrogen and oxygen of those compounds unite to form water. When this water evaporates, the ashes left behind are minerals [32]. Minerals help to build tissues, regulate body fluids, or assist in various body functions. Like vitamins, they are required in small quantities and are vital to the body. Minerals can be classified into two groups: major minerals and trace minerals.

1. Major minerals or macrominerals: These are required in large amounts. These include calcium, phosphorus, potassium, sulfur, sodium, chloride, and magnesium.
2. Trace minerals: These are required in small quantities. Trace minerals that are key to human health include iron, zinc, copper, iodine, and selenium.

Calcium and Phosphorus

Calcium is by far the most abundant mineral in the body. At birth, the body contains about 26 to 30 g of calcium. This amount rises quickly after birth, reaching about 1200 g in women and 1400 g in men by adulthood [22]. Nearly 99% of the body's calcium is stored in the bones and the teeth, giving them structure and hardness. The majority of calcium in these tissues is present as hydroxyapatite, which is a complex of calcium phosphate, $C_{10}(PO_4)_6(OH)_2$. The remaining 1% is distributed in the intravascular, interstitial, and intracellular fluids (where plasma calcium is tightly regulated at 2.5 mmol/l). Bone calcium serves as a bank to maintain the calcium level in body fluid even if the slightest drop in blood calcium level occurs.

Body phosphorus is also largely associated with the bones; approximately 85% of the 500–700 g in the body is found in the skeleton as insoluble calcium salt. The remaining 15% is found in the cell membrane and soft tissues as organic phosphate. This phosphate pool plays a role in the dynamic equilibrium through the gut, kidney, bones, and other tissues (Yano & Sugimoto, 2009).

The major function of both calcium and phosphorus is to form hydroxyapatite, a major inorganic bone component. Approximately 60% of bone weight is due to the presence of calcium-rich mineral deposits. Calcium phosphate salts crystallize on a foundation material composed of the protein collagen. The resulting hydroxyapatite crystals invade the collagen and gradually lend more and more rigidity to maturing bones. The acquisition of bone mineral continues throughout childhood and adolescence, reaching a lifetime maximum in early adulthood. Adolescence is a particularly critical time for bone mineral accretion given that more than half of the calcium in bones is normally acquired during the teen years [36]. Teeth are formed in a similar way—hydroxyapatite crystals form on a collagen matrix to create the dentin that gives strength to the teeth.

Functions (Table 8.3)

Table 8.3 Functions of calcium and phosphorus

Calcium	Phosphorus
Mineralizes bones and forms teeth	Forms and maintains bones and teeth
Regulates the transport of ions across cell membranes and is particularly important in nerve transmission	Produces energy (as a component of adenosine triphosphate, or ATP, the energy currency of cells)
Helps maintain normal blood pressure	Performs DNA and RNA synthesis (as a part of the genetic material)
Plays an essential role in the clotting of blood	
Is essential for muscle contraction and therefore for the heartbeat	Regulates the acid–base balance in the body
	Provides cell membrane structure (as a component of phospholipids)
Facilitates the secretion of hormones, digestive enzymes, and neurotransmitters	Activates enzymes and hormones (as part of phosphorylation processes)

Health Implications of Calcium and Phosphorus Deficiency (Table 8.4)

Table 8.4 Health implications of calcium and phosphorus deficiency

Calcium	Phosphorus
Osteoporosis: weakening of bones, increased risk of fractures, especially in older adults	Bone pain and weakness: similar to calcium deficiency, leading to weak and fragile bones
Osteopenia: lower bone density, a precursor to osteoporosis	Rickets: in children, similar to calcium deficiency, causing soft and weak bones
Rickets: softening of bones in children, leading to deformities (bowed legs)	Osteomalacia: softening of bones in adults, leading to bone pain and fractures
Tetany: muscle cramps, spasms, and numbness due to low calcium levels affecting nerve function	Muscle weakness: due to impaired energy production and muscle function
Dental problems: weak and brittle teeth, increased risk of cavities	Respiratory issues: difficulty breathing due to weakened muscles
Heart issues: abnormal heart rhythms and possible cardiovascular issues	Impaired growth: especially in children, due to insufficient bone and tissue development

RDA for Calcium and Phosphorus [37] (Table 8.5)

Table 8.5 Recommended daily allowance for calcium and phosphorus

Age group	Calcium (mg/day)	Phosphorus (mg/day)
Infants (0–6 months)	200	100
Infants (7–12 months)	260	275
Children (1–3 years)	700	460
Children (4–8 years)	1000	500
Children (9–18 years)	1300	1250
Adults (19–50 years)	1000	700
Adults (51–70 years)	1000 (men)	700
	1200 (women)	
Adults (> 70 years)	1200	700
Pregnancy (14–18 years)	1300	1250
Pregnancy (19–50 years)	1000	700
Lactation (14–18 years)	1300	1250
Lactation (19–50 years)	1000	700

Dietary Sources of Calcium and Phosphorus (Table 8.6)

Table 8.6 Dietary sources of calcium and phosphorus

Calcium	Phosphorus
Dairy products: milk, cheese, yogurt	Meat and poultry: chicken, turkey, beef, pork
Leafy green vegetables: kale, spinach, broccoli, collard greens	Fish: salmon, cod, tuna
	Dairy products: milk, cheese, yogurt
Fortified foods: juice, cereals, fortified plant-based milk (almond milk, soy milk)	Legumes and nuts: lentils, chickpeas, almonds, peanuts
Fish with edible bones: sardines, canned salmon	Whole grains: whole wheat bread, brown rice, oatmeal
Nuts and seeds: almonds, sesame seeds	Eggs: egg yolks
Other sources: tofu (especially if made with calcium sulfate), rhubarb	Processed foods (with added phosphates): processed cheese, packaged baked goods

Sodium and Potassium

Sodium and potassium are essential minerals and electrolytes that play crucial roles in maintaining various physiological processes in the human body. Their balance is particularly important for cardiovascular health, nerve function, muscle function, and fluid balance.

Functions of Sodium
Fluid and Electrolyte Balance
- Regulating blood volume and pressure: Sodium helps regulate blood volume and pressure by controlling the amount of water retained in the body [38].
- Osmotic balance: Sodium maintains osmotic pressure, ensuring proper fluid distribution between cells and their surroundings [39].

Nerve and Muscle Function
- Nerve impulse transmission: Sodium ions are crucial for the generation and transmission of nerve signaling.
- Muscle contraction: Sodium works with potassium and calcium to facilitate muscle contraction.

Acid–Base Balance
- Sodium bicarbonate acts as a buffer to maintain the body's pH balance.

Box 8.5 The Health Implications of Excess Sodium
- Hypertension: Excessive sodium consumption (> 5 g of sodium per day) has been linked to the onset of hypertension and cardiovascular complications [40].
- Kidney function: High sodium intake can lead to impaired function and fluid retention.
- Bone health: Excessive sodium can increase calcium loss, potentially affecting bone health.

Functions of Potassium

Fluid and Electrolyte Balance

- Cellular function: Potassium is crucial for maintaining intracellular fluid balance.
- Osmotic pressure: Potassium helps regulate osmotic pressure within cells.

Nerve and Muscle Function

- Nerve impulse transmission: Potassium ions are essential for the proper functioning of nerve cells and the transmission of electrical signals.
- Muscle contraction: Potassium is vital for normal muscle contraction, including the heart muscle, reducing the risk of arrhythmias.

Cardiovascular Health

- Blood pressure regulation: Potassium helps counteract the effects of sodium, promoting vasodilation and reducing blood pressure.
- Heart health: Adequate potassium levels support regular heart function and reduce the risk of cardiovascular diseases.

Sodium–Potassium Interactions

- The balance between sodium and potassium is critical for maintaining health. They maintain complementary roles in blood pressure regulation and the balance of eletrolytes.

Blood Pressure Regulation

- Sodium–potassium ratio: A high sodium-to-potassium ratio is associated with increased blood pressure and cardiovascular risk. Increasing potassium intake while reducing sodium can help lower blood pressure.
- Dietary approaches: Diets rich in potassium (fruits, vegetables, and whole grains) and low in sodium are recommended for cardiovascular health.

Electrolyte Balance

- Cellular function: Sodium is primarily extracellular, whereas potassium is intracellular. Their gradients are maintained by the sodium–potassium pump, essential for cellular function and nerve impulse transmission.

RDA for Sodium and Potassium [38, 41] (Table 8.7)

Table 8.7 Recommended daily allowance for sodium and potassium

Age group	Sodium (mg/day)	Potassium (mg/day)
Infants (0–6 months)	110 (adequate intake, or AI)	400 (AI)
Infants (7–12 months)	370 (AI)	860 (AI)
Children (1–3 years)	1000 (AI)	2000 (AI)
Children (4–8 years)	1200 (AI)	2300 (AI)
Children (9–13 years)	1500 (AI)	2300 (AI)
Adolescents (14–18 years)	1500 (AI)	2300 (AI)
Adults (19–50 years)	1500 (AI)	2600 (AI) (women)
		3400 (AI) (men)
Adults (51–70 years)	1300 (AI)	2600 (AI)
Adults (> 70 years)	1200 (AI)	2600 (AI)
Pregnancy (14–50 years)	1500 (AI)	2900 (AI)
Lactation (14–50 years)	1500 (AI)	2800 (AI)

Essential Trace Minerals

Iron

Functions of Iron in Human Health
Oxygen Transport
- Hemoglobin: Iron is a key component of hemoglobin, the protein in red blood cells that carries oxygen from the lungs to tissues and organs throughout the body.
- Myoglobin: Iron is also a component of myoglobin, a protein that provides oxygen to the muscles.

Energy Production
- Cellular respiration: Iron is involved in the electron transport chain within mitochondria, playing a crucial role in energy production through cellular respiration.

Enzyme Function
- Cofactor: Iron acts as a cofactor for various enzymes involved in metabolic processes, including DNA synthesis and repair, and the metabolism of amino acids, lipids, and carbohydrates.

Immune System
- Immune function: Iron is essential for the proliferation and maturation of immune cells, particularly lymphocytes, which are important for the body's immune response.

Cognitive Function
- Brain health: Adequate iron levels are important for cognitive function, neurodevelopment, and the production of neurotransmitters.

Iron Deficiency and Health Implications
Iron Deficiency Anemia
- Symptoms: Fatigue, weakness, pale skin, shortness of breath, dizziness, and cognitive impairment.
- Causes: Inadequate dietary intake, poor absorption, blood loss, or increased iron requirements (e.g., pregnancy).

Impaired Cognitive and Physical Development
- Children: Iron deficiency in children can lead to developmental delays, behavioral disturbances, and impaired cognitive performance.

Weakened Immune System
- Infection risk: Iron deficiency can compromise the immune system, making the body more susceptible to infections.

RDA for Iron [15]
- Infants (< 1 year)—11 mg
- 1–3 years—7 mg
- 4–8 years—10 mg
- 9–13 years—8 mg
- 14–18 years
  - Male—11 mg
  - Female—15 mg
- 19–50 years
  - Male—8 mg
  - Female—18 mg
  - Pregnancy—27 mg
  - Lactation—9 mg

Zinc

Zinc is an essential mineral that plays a crucial role in human health. It is involved in numerous hysiological processes and is necessary for the proper functioning of our bodies.

Functions of Zinc
Immune function: Zinc is vital for a healthy immune system. It helps support the development and function of immune cells, such as T cells and natural killer cells, which play crucial roles in fighting off infections and diseases.

Box 8.6 The Health Implications of Zinc Deficiency

Zinc deficiency can lead to a variety of symptoms and health issues. This box lists some common symptoms that may occur in individuals with zinc deficiency.

- Impaired immune function: One of the most noticeable symptoms of zinc deficiency is a weakened immune system, leading to frequent infections, slow wound healing, and increased susceptibility to illnesses.
- A loss of appetite: A decrease in appetite can be a symptom of zinc deficiency. This may result in weight loss and a lack of interest in eating.
- Hair loss: Zinc is important for the health of hair follicles. A deficiency in zinc can lead to hair loss or thinning hair.
- Skin problems: Zinc plays a role in maintaining the health of the skin. Zinc deficiency may manifest as skin rashes, acne, dry or flaky skin, and slow wound healing.
- Delayed growth and development: In children, zinc deficiency can impair normal growth and development. It may result in stunted growth, delayed sexual maturation, and poor wound healing.
- Cognitive and behavioral changes: Zinc is involved in brain function and neurotransmitter regulation. A deficiency may contribute to cognitive impairment, poor memory, difficulty concentrating, and mood disturbances.
- Changes in taste and smell: Zinc is important for the proper functioning of taste and smell receptors. A deficiency can lead to a decrease in the ability to taste or smell.

- Growth and development: Zinc is necessary for normal growth and development in children. It is involved in the production of proteins and DNA, which are essential for proper cell division and growth.
- Wound healing: Zinc is involved in the process of wound healing. It helps to promote cell growth, collagen synthesis, and tissue repair, making it important for the healing of wounds and injuries.
- Taste and smell: Zinc is necessary for the proper functioning of taste and smell receptors. A deficiency in zinc can lead to a decreased sense of taste and smell.
- Cognitive function: Zinc is involved in brain development and function. It plays a role in neurotransmitter signaling and helps support cognitive processes such as learning and memory.
- Reproduction: Zinc is important for reproductive health in both men and women. It is involved in the production of genetic material and hormone synthesis, which are essential for fertility and reproduction.

Dietary Sources of Zinc
- Meat: red meat, such as beef, lamb, and pork
- Poultry: chicken and turkey
- Seafood: shellfish—especially oysters—and crab, shrimp, salmon, and sardines
- Legumes: chickpeas, lentils, and beans
- Nuts and seeds: cashews, almonds, peanuts, pumpkin seeds, and sesame seeds
- Dairy products: milk, cheese, and yogurt
- Whole grains: wheat, quinoa, and oats

RDA for Zinc [15]
- Infants (< 1 year)—3 mg
- 1–3 years—3 mg
- 4–8 years—5 mg
- 9–13 years—8 mg
- 14–18 years
  - Male—11 mg
  - Female—9 mg

- 19+ years
  - Male—11 mg
  - Female—8 mg
  - Pregnancy—12 mg
  - Lactation—13 mg

Iodine

Functions of Iodine
Iodine has many important functions in human health.

- Thyroid function: Iodine is a key component of thyroid hormones, including thyroxine (T4) and triiodothyronine (T3). These hormones are responsible for regulating the body's metabolism, energy production, and growth. Adequate iodine intake is necessary for the proper functioning of the thyroid gland.
- Brain development: Iodine is particularly important during pregnancy and infancy for proper brain development. Insufficient iodine intake during these critical periods can lead to cognitive impairments, including a lower intelligence quotient (IQ) and developmental delays.
- Energy metabolism: Thyroid hormones, which require iodine, help regulate the body's energy metabolism. They affect the breakdown of nutrients, such as carbohydrates, fats, and proteins, for energy production.
- Pregnancy and fetal development: Sufficient iodine intake is crucial during pregnancy to support the healthy development of the fetus. Iodine deficiency during pregnancy can lead to complications, such as miscarriage, stillbirth, or impaired neurological development in the baby.

- Breast health: Iodine is also important for breast health. It is concentrated in breast tissue and is involved in maintaining the structure and function of the mammary glands.

Iodine-Deficiency Diseases
- Goiter: This is an enlargement of the thyroid gland, which can cause a visible swelling in the neck.
- Hypothyroidism: This is a condition characterized by low levels of thyroid hormones, leading to symptoms like fatigue, weight gain, and depression.
- Cretinism: Severe iodine deficiency during pregnancy can result in cretinism, a condition causing stunted physical and mental growth in children.
- Impaired cognitive function: Iodine deficiency, especially in pregnant women and young children, can lead to a lower IQ and cognitive impairments.
- Increased risk of stillbirth and miscarriages: Inadequate iodine levels during pregnancy can increase the risk of adverse pregnancy outcomes.

RDA for Iodine [15]
- Infants (< 1 year)—130 mcg
- 1–3 years—90 mcg
- 4–8 years—90 mcg
- 9–13 years—120 mcg
- 14–18 years—150 mcg
- 19+ years—150 mcg
  - Pregnancy—220 mcg
  - Lactation—290 mcg

Dietary Sources of Iodine
- Seaweed: Seaweed is one of the richest sources of iodine. Different types of seaweed, such as kelp, kombu, and wakame, can provide varying amounts of iodine.
- Iodized salt: This is salt fortified with iodine.
- Dairy products: Milk, cheese, and yogurt can be good sources of iodine, especially if they have been fortified with iodine.
- Fish and seafood: Some fish and seafood are naturally rich in iodine, including cod, tuna, lobster, shrimp.
- Grains: Some grains may be fortified with iodine, such as bread and breakfast creals.
- Nuts and seeds: Some seeds and needs contain idione, such as pumpkin seeds and sunflower seeds.

Multiple Micronutrient Deficiency: A Major Public Health Issue

Multiple micronutrient deficiencies are significant public health problems in developing countries, affecting millions of people, particularly women and children. These deficiencies can have severe consequences on health, development, and

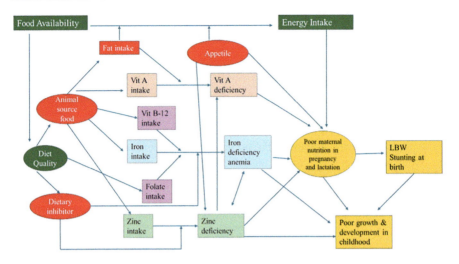

Fig. 8.1 Sources, intake levels, and health outcomes of micronutrient deficiencies

productivity. The most common micronutrient deficiencies are due to a lack of iron, vitamin A, iodine, zinc, and folate. The mechanisms of micronutrient decficiencies are illustrated in Fig. 8.1.

Causes of Deficiencies
- Inadequate dietary intake: Many populations in developing countries rely on staple foods that are low in essential vitamins and minerals.
- Poor absorption: Conditions such as intestinal infections and chronic diseases can impair the body's ability to absorb nutrients.
- Increased needs: Pregnant and lactating women and growing children have higher micronutrient requirements.
- Food insecurity: Economic constraints and a lack of access to diverse foods contribute to inadequate nutrient intake.

Intervention Strategies
A food-based approach to combat multiple micronutrient deficiencies involves promoting dietary diversity and emphasizing the consumption of nutrient-rich foods. The following section features key strategies for addressing multiple micronutrient deficiencies through food.

Promoting Dietary Diversity
Encouraging individuals to consume a variety of foods from different food groups, such as those below, ensures that they receive a wide range of essential nutrients.

- Fruits and vegetables: Encourage the daily consumption of a colorful variety of fruits and vegetables because different colors indicate different nutrient profiles.

- Whole grains: Include whole grains such as brown rice, whole wheat bread, oats, and quinoa, which provide essential vitamins and minerals.
- Protein sources: Include a variety of lean meats, poultry, fish, eggs, legumes (beans and lentils), and nuts and seeds to ensure an adequate intake of iron, zinc, and B vitamins.
- Dairy or dairy alternatives: Incorporate dairy products or fortified plant-based alternatives to obtain calcium, vitamin D, and other nutrients.

Food Fortification
Fortifying commonly consumed staple foods with essential micronutrients, such as those below, can help address widespread deficiencies.

- Fortified staple foods: Fortify commonly consumed foods such as flour, rice, salt, and cooking oils with essential micronutrients like iron, folic acid, vitamin A, and iodine.
- Fortified breakfast cereals: Promote the consumption of fortified cereals that provide a range of vitamins and minerals.

Sustainable Agriculture and Food Systems: Biofortification
Support sustainable agricultural practices that enhance the nutrient content of crops and improve access to nutrient-rich foods:

- Biofortification: Promote the cultivation and consumption of biofortified crops that are naturally enriched with key vitamins and minerals.
- Local food production: Encourage local food production and the consumption of seasonal fruits and vegetables to ensure freshness and nutrient density.

Addressing Specific Population Needs
Interventions must be tailored to address specific population groups at higher risk of micronutrient deficiencies.

- Pregnant women and lactating women: Promote the consumption of iron-rich foods, folic acid, and calcium to support maternal and fetal health.
- Infants and young children: Encourage breastfeeding and introduce nutrient-dense complementary foods rich in iron, zinc, vitamin A, and vitamin C.
- Adolescents: Focus on meeting increased nutrient needs during growth spurts through a balanced diet.

Nutrition Education
Educate communities about the importance of balanced nutrition and how to incorporate nutrient-dense foods into their diets.

- Nutrition counseling: Provide nutrition education and counseling to promote healthy eating habits and increase awareness of nutrient-rich food choices.
- Cooking demonstrations: Conduct cooking demonstrations that showcase affordable and locally available nutrient-dense foods and recipes.

Policy and Advocacy
Advocate for policies and programs that support access to nutrient-rich foods and fortification initiatives.

- Food policy: Support policies that promote nutrition-sensitive agriculture, food fortification, and dietary diversity.
- Public health campaigns: Launch public health campaigns to raise awareness about the importance of diverse diets and micronutrient-rich foods.

Further Practice

1. Fat-soluble vitamins include which of the following?
    a. Vitamin A
    b. Vitamin D
    c. Vitamin E
    d. Vitamin K
    e. All of the above

2. Rhodopsin is needed for dentin formation in teeth.
   True/false

3. _____ is called the anti-infective vitamin.

4. A serum level of retinol that is below which of the following volumes indicates subclinical vitamin A deficiency?

    a. 0.25 μmol/l
    b. 0.35 μmol/l
    c. 0.70 μmol/l
    d. 0.90 μmol/l

5. Which of the following vitamins supports the immune function of the human body?

    a. Vitamin A
    b. Vitamin C
    c. Vitamin D
    d. All of the above

6. Which one of the following vitamins aids in blood clotting?

    a. Vitamin A
    b. Vitamin B
    c. Vitamin D
    d. Vitamin E
    e. Vitamin K

7. Trace amounts of which mineral(s) are required for the human body to function?

   a. Iron
   b. Zinc
   c. Copper
   d. Selenium
   e. All of the above

8. Sodium regulates blood volume and water retention in the human body.
   True/false

9. Sodium bicarbonate acts as a buffer to maintain blood pH.
   True/false

10. Potassium is necessary for maintaining intracellular fluid balance.
    True/false

11. An adequate level of which of the following aids in cognitive function?

    a. Iron
    b. Magnesium
    c. Copper
    d. Vitamin B complex

12. Zinc deficiency can cause xerophthalmia.
    True/false

Answer Keys

1 e; 2. False; 3. Vitamin A; 4 c; 5 d; 6 e; 7 e; 8 True; 9. True; 10. True; 11 a; 12. False

---

References

1. Shenkin A. Micronutrients in health and disease. Postgrad Med J. 2006;82(971):559–67. https://doi.org/10.1136/pgmj.2006.047670.
2. Stevens GA, Beal T, Mbuya MNN, Luo H, Neufeld LM. Micronutrient deficiencies among preschool-aged children and women of reproductive age worldwide: a pooled analysis of individual-level data from population-representative surveys. Lancet Glob Health. 2022;10(11):e1590–9. https://doi.org/10.1016/s2214-109x(22)00367-9.
3. Van Loo-Bouwman CA, Naber TH, Schaafsma G. A review of vitamin A equivalency of β-carotene in various food matrices for human consumption. Br J Nutr. 2014;111(12):2153–66. https://doi.org/10.1017/s0007114514000166.
4. Perrotta S, Nobili B, Rossi F, Di Pinto D, Cucciolla V, Borriello A, et al. Vitamin A and infancy. Biochemical, functional, and clinical aspects. Vitam Horm. 2003;66:457–591. https://doi.org/10.1016/s0083-6729(03)01013-6.
5. Sajovic J, Meglič A, Glavač D, Markelj Š, Hawlina M, Fakin A. The role of Vitamin A in retinal diseases. Int J Mol Sci. 2022;23(3):1014. https://doi.org/10.3390/ijms23031014.
6. Blomhoff R, Blomhoff HK. Overview of retinoid metabolism and function. J Neurobiol. 2006;66(7):606–30. https://doi.org/10.1002/neu.20242.

7. Balmer JE, Blomhoff R. Gene expression regulation by retinoic acid. J Lipid Res. 2002;43(11):1773–808. https://doi.org/10.1194/jlr.r100015-jlr200.
8. Penkert RR, Jones BG, Häcker H, Partridge JF, Hurwitz JL. Vitamin A differentially regulates cytokine expression in respiratory epithelial and macrophage cell lines. Cytokine. 2017;91:1–5. https://doi.org/10.1016/j.cyto.2016.11.015.
9. Roche FC, Harris-Tryon TA. Illuminating the role of Vitamin A in skin innate immunity and the skin microbiome: a narrative review. Nutrients. 2021;13(2):302. https://doi.org/10.3390/nu13020302.
10. Szymański Ł, Skopek R, Palusińska M, Schenk T, Stengel S, Lewicki S, et al. Retinoic acid and its derivatives in skin. Cells. 2020;9(12):2660. https://doi.org/10.3390/cells9122660.
11. Clagett-Dame M, Knutson D. Vitamin A in reproduction and development. Nutrients. 2011;3(4):385–428. https://doi.org/10.3390/nu3040385.
12. Awasthi S, Awasthi A. Role of vitamin a in child health and nutrition. Clin Epidemiol Glob Health. 2020;8(4):1039–42. https://doi.org/10.1016/j.cegh.2020.03.016.
13. Bohn T, Böhm V, Dulińska-Litewka J, Landrier JF, Bánáti D, Kucuk O, et al. Is vitamin A an antioxidant? Int J Vitam Nutr Res. 2023;93(6):481–2. https://doi.org/10.1024/0300-9831/a000752.
14. WHO. Serum retinol concentrations for determining the prevalence of vitamin A deficiency in populations. Vitamin and Mineral Nutrition Information System WHO/NMH/NHD/MNM/11.3. 2011.
15. IOM. Dietary reference intakes for Vitamin A, Vitamin K, Arsenic, Boron, Chromium, Copper, Iodine, Iron, Manganese, Molybdenum, Nickel, Silicon, Vanadium, and Zinc. Retrieved from Washington DC. 2001.
16. Khazai N, Judd SE, Tangpricha V. Calcium and vitamin D: skeletal and extraskeletal health. Curr Rheumatol Rep. 2008;10(2):110–7. https://doi.org/10.1007/s11926-008-0020-y.
17. Laird E, Ward M, McSorley E, Strain JJ, Wallace J. Vitamin D and bone health: potential mechanisms. Nutrients. 2010;2(7):693–724. https://doi.org/10.3390/nu2070693.
18. Prietl B, Treiber G, Pieber TR, Amrein K. Vitamin D and immune function. Nutrients. 2013;5(7):2502–21. https://doi.org/10.3390/nu5072502.
19. Ismailova A, White JH. Vitamin D, infections and immunity. Rev Endocr Metab Disord. 2022;23(2):265–77. https://doi.org/10.1007/s11154-021-09679-5.
20. Dawson-Hughes B. Vitamin D and muscle function. J Steroid Biochem Mol Biol. 2017;173:313–6. https://doi.org/10.1016/j.jsbmb.2017.03.018.
21. de la Guía-Galipienso F, Martínez-Ferran M, Vallecillo N, Lavie CJ, Sanchis-Gomar F, Pareja-Galeano H. Vitamin D and cardiovascular health. Clin Nutr. 2021;40(5):2946–57. https://doi.org/10.1016/j.clnu.2020.12.025.
22. IOM. Dietary Reference Intakes for Calcium and Vitamin D. Retrieved from Washington, DC. 2011.
23. Traber MG. In: ME SMS, Ross AC, Caballero B, Cousins R, editors. Modern nutrition in health and disease. 10th ed. Baltimore: Lippincott Williams & Wilkins; 2006.
24. Khallouki F, Owen RW, Akdad M, Bouhali BE, Silvente-Poirot S, Poirot M. Chapter 3 – Vitamin E: an overview. In: Patel VB, editor. Molecular Nutrition. Academic Press; 2020. p. 51–66.
25. Wang X, Quinn PJ. Vitamin E and its function in membranes. Prog Lipid Res. 1999;38(4):309–36. https://doi.org/10.1016/s0163-7827(99)00008-9.
26. Lee GY, Han SN. The role of vitamin E in immunity. Nutrients. 2018;10(11):1614. https://doi.org/10.3390/nu10111614.
27. Hobson R. Vitamin E and wound healing: an evidence-based review. Int Wound J. 2016;13(3):331–5. https://doi.org/10.1111/iwj.12295.
28. IOM. Dietary Reference Intakes: Vitamin C, Vitamin E, Selenium, and Carotenoidsexternal link disclaimer. Retrieved from Washington, DC. 2000.
29. Mladěnka P, Macáková K, Kujovská Krčmová L, Javorská L, Mrštná K, Carazo A, et al. Vitamin K – Sources, physiological role, kinetics, deficiency, detection, therapeutic use, and

toxicity. Nutr Rev. 2022;80(4):677–98. https://doi.org/10.1093/nutrit/nuab061.

30. Rodríguez-Olleros Rodríguez C, Díaz Curiel M. Vitamin K and bone health: a review on the effects of Vitamin K deficiency and supplementation and the effect of non-Vitamin K antagonist Oral anticoagulants on different bone parameters. J Osteoporos. 2019;2019:2069176. https://doi.org/10.1155/2019/2069176.

31. Shea MK, Berkner KL, Ferland G, Fu X, Holden RM, Booth SL. Perspective: evidence before enthusiasm-a critical review of the potential cardiovascular benefits of Vitamin K. Adv Nutr. 2021;12(3):632–46. https://doi.org/10.1093/advances/nmab004.

32. Sizer FS, Whitney E. Nutrition: concepts and controversies. 11th ed. Thomson Wadsworth; 2008.

33. Padayatty SJ, Katz A, Wang Y, Eck P, Kwon O, Lee JH, et al. Vitamin C as an antioxidant: evaluation of its role in disease prevention. J Am Coll Nutr. 2003;22(1):18–35. https://doi.org/10.1080/07315724.2003.10719272.

34. Carr AC, Maggini S. Vitamin C and immune function. Nutrients. 2017;9(11):1211. https://doi.org/10.3390/nu9111211.

35. Lynch SR, Cook JD. Interaction of vitamin C and iron. Ann N Y Acad Sci. 1980;355:32–44. https://doi.org/10.1111/j.1749-6632.1980.tb21325.x.

36. Bachrach LK. Bone mineralization in childhood and adolescence. Curr Opin Pediatr. 1993;5(4):467–73. https://doi.org/10.1097/00008480-199308000-00017.

37. IOM. Dietary Reference Intakes for Calcium, Phosphorus, Magnesium, Vitamin D, and Fluoride. Retrieved from Washington DC. 1997. https://www.ncbi.nlm.nih.gov/books/NBK109809/

38. Grillo A, Salvi L, Coruzzi P, Salvi P, Parati G. Sodium intake and hypertension. Nutrients. 2019;11(9) https://doi.org/10.3390/nu11091970.

39. Agrawal V, Agarwal M, Joshi SR, Ghosh AK. Hyponatremia and hypernatremia: disorders of water balance. J Assoc Physicians India. 2008;56:956–64.

40. Strazzullo P, D'Elia L, Kandala NB, Cappuccio FP. Salt intake, stroke, and cardiovascular disease: meta-analysis of prospective studies. BMJ. 2009;339:b4567. https://doi.org/10.1136/bmj.b4567.

41. Stallings VA, Harrison M, Oria M (eds). Dietary Reference Intakes For Sodium and Potassium. The National Academies Press, Washington, D.C.. 2019. Availavle online: chrome-extension://efaidnbmnnnibpcajpcglclefindmkaj/https://www.ncbi.nlm.nih.gov/books/NBK538102/pdf/Bookshelf_NBK538102.pdf. Accessed 25 Jan 2025.

Tender Beginning: Nutrition for Infants and Young Children

9

Malay Kanti Mridha

Malay Kanti Mridha

Learning Objectives

After completing this chapter, you will be able to

- Describe the importance of early-life nutrition for health and well-being
- List the evidence-based interventions necessary to ensure optimal nutrition during early life
- Provide practical guidelines for implementing evidence-based interventions for fetal life and early life at the national and individual levels
- Explain the research gaps relevant to early-life interventions

Introduction

Nutrition during pregnancy and early life affects health and development throughout the life course. Malnutrition during the first 1000 days of life (i.e., from conception to the end of the second year) has health and development consequences during early and adult life. Malnutrition during fetal life is a risk factor for intrauterine growth retardation (IUGR, defined as birthweight below the tenth percentile for the age of gestation) and can cause stillbirth, premature birth, increased morbidity, hypoxic brain injury, retinopathy, and mortality as short-term complications [1]. The long-term complications of IUGR include impaired physical growth, motor incompetence, neurological dysfunction, poor school attainment, behavioral problems, low cognitive scores, poor work capacity, cerebral palsy, poor social competence, and poor perceptual performance [1]. Fetal malnutrition and IUGR can lead to low birth weight (LBW, defined as birth weight < 2500 g irrespective of the age of gestation)

M. K. Mridha (✉)
BRAC James P. Grant School of Public Health, BRAC University, Dhaka, Bangladesh
e-mail: malay.mridha@bracu.ac.bd

© The Author(s), under exclusive license to Springer Nature
Switzerland AG 2025
A. K. Mitra, D. Vanoh (eds.), *Essentials of Clinical and Public Health Nutrition*,
Nutrition and Health, https://doi.org/10.1007/978-3-031-95373-6_9

[2]. LBW babies are also at risk of impaired motor and cognitive development and of behavioral and psychological problems [2, 3]. The Developmental Origins of Health and Disease (DOHaD) hypothesis proposes that fetal malnutrition leads to cardiovascular, endocrine, or metabolic changes due to fetal programming and epigenetic modification and ultimately increases the risk of insulin resistance, type-2 diabetes, hypertension, hyperlipidemia [2, 4, 5], mental health disorders, renal diseases, liver diseases, ischemic heart diseases, stroke, obesity, reactive airway diseases, Parkinsonism, immune dysfunction, osteoporosis, and Alzheimer diseases [6]. Malnutrition during fetal and early life propagates the intergenerational cycle of malnutrition [7]. An LBW baby may remain stunted, wasted, or underweight during their childhood and adolescence and may have malnourished children during adulthood, and this cycle may continue from generation to generation [8]. Therefore, to break the intergenerational cycle of malnutrition, a life-course approach is necessary. Though an ideal life-course approach should start during the preconception period because the nutrition status of a mother determines her pregnancy outcomes [4], a more practical start point could focus on improving nutrition during the first 1000 days.

Evidence-Based Interventions to Ensure Optimal Nutrition During Fetal and Early Life

Fetal and early-life nutrition during the first 1000 days has received renewed attention over the past decades. In 2008 and 2013, the *Lancet* published two series dedicated to maternal and child nutrition [8–10]. These series summarized the effects of evidence-based interventions for the prevention and control of maternal and child malnutrition. The global nutrition community also redefined malnutrition as a combination of undernutrition, overnutrition, and micronutrient deficiency [2]. In 2021, *Lancet* authors revisited the evidence base for the interventions aimed at improving maternal and child nutrition. Apart from the *Lancet* initiative, the Department for Nutrition for Health and Development at the World Health Organization (WHO) initiated a project named the e-Library of Evidence for Nutrition Actions (eLENA), which aims to help countries successfully implement and scale up nutrition interventions by informing as well as guiding policy development and program design [7]. The following section lists key evidence-based interventions from the 2021 *Lancet* publication and eLENA that are recommended to deliver during pregnancy and early childhood to optimize fetal and early-life nutrition [11]. Importantly, eLENA interventions are grouped into three categories: category (1) includes interventions that are approved by the WHO guideline review committee or endorsed by the World Health Assembly; category (2) includes interventions that are supported by systematic reviews but have not been approved by an WHO guideline review committee; and category (3) includes interventions with limited evidence and for which systematic reviews have yet to be conducted. The *Lancet* categorized the interventions into four types: (1) Strong evidence for implementation, (2) moderate evidence for implementation, (3) weak evidence for implementation, and (4) emerging evidence. These evidence-based interventions are grouped under maternal interventions during pregnancy (Table 9.1), child interventions (Table 9.2), and other interventions (Table 9.3) (i.e., interventions that are not directly specific to mothers or children but that have effects on their nutritional status).

Table 9.1 Maternal interventions

Intervention	1. Lancet 2.eLENA 3. Both	Lancet/ eLENA category
Assessment for nutrition-related disorders during pregnancy: An assessment of anemia and diabetes should be carried out on all people during their pregnancy.	2	NA/1
Balanced energy and protein supplementation during pregnancy: In undernourished populations, balanced energy and protein dietary supplementation (supplements with < 25% of total energy from protein) are recommended for pregnant people to reduce the risk of stillbirths and neonates who are small for gestational age.	3	2/1
Breastfeeding education for increased breastfeeding duration: Where facilities provide antenatal care, pregnant people and their families should be counseled about the benefits and management of breastfeeding.	3	1/1
Calcium supplementation during pregnancy to reduce the risk of pre-eclampsia: Calcium supplementation (1.5–2.0 g of oral elemental calcium) is recommended for pregnant people with low dietary calcium intake.	3	2/1
Daily iron and folic acid supplementation during pregnancy: Daily oral iron and folic acid supplementation with 30 mg to 60 mg of elemental iron and 400 μg (0.4 mg) of folic acid is recommended for pregnant people to prevent maternal anemia, puerperal sepsis, low birth weight, and preterm birth.	2	1
Deworming in pregnant people: Preventive chemotherapy (deworming), using single-dose albendazole (400 mg) or mebendazole (500 mg), is recommended as a public health intervention for pregnant people, after the first trimester, who live in areas where both (1) the baseline prevalence of hookworm and/or *T. trichiura* infection is 20% or higher among pregnant people and (2) where anemia is a severe public health problem, with a prevalence of 40% or higher among pregnant people, to reduce the worm burden of hookworm and *T. trichiura* infection.	2	NA/1
Complementary feeding education without food provision in food-secure and food-insecure populations: Education on complementary feeding should be provided to all pregnant people irrespective of their food-security status.	1	2/NA
Intermittent iron and folic acid supplementation during pregnancy: Intermittent oral iron and folic acid supplementation with 120 mg of elemental iron and 2800 μg (2.8 mg) of folic acid once weekly is recommended for pregnant people to improve maternal and neonatal outcomes if daily iron is not acceptable due to side effects and in populations with an anemia prevalence among pregnant people of less than 20%.	2	NA/1

(continued)

Table 9.1 (continued)

Intervention	1. Lancet 2.eLENA 3. Both	Lancet/ eLENA category
Intermittent iron and folic acid supplementation during pregnancy in malaria-endemic areas: In malaria-endemic areas, iron and folic acid supplementation programs should be implemented in conjunction with adequate measures to prevent, diagnose, and treat malaria during pregnancy.	2	NA/1
Intermittent preventive treatment to reduce the risk of malaria during pregnancy: In malaria-endemic areas in Africa, intermittent preventive treatment with sulfadoxine–pyrimethamine (SP-IPTp) is recommended for all pregnant people in their first or second pregnancy. Dosing should start in the second trimester, and doses should be given at least 1 month apart, with the objective of ensuring that at least three doses are received.	2	NA/1
Iodine supplementation in pregnant and lactating women: The WHO and the United Nations International Children's Emergency Fund (UNICEF) recommend iodine supplementation for pregnant and lactating people in countries where less than 20% of households have access to iodized salt until the salt iodization program has been scaled up.	2	NA/2
Iron supplementation with or without folic acid to reduce the risk of postpartum anemia: Oral iron supplementation, either alone or in combination with folic acid, may be provided to postpartum people for 6–12 weeks following delivery to reduce the risk of anemia in settings where gestational anemia is a public health concern (i.e., a 20% or higher population prevalence of gestational anemia).	3	NA/1
Iron supplementation with or without folic acid, which aims to reduce the risk of postpartum anemia in malaria-endemic areas: In malaria-endemic areas, the provision of iron and folic acid supplements should be implemented in conjunction with measures to prevent, diagnose, and treat malaria. In areas using sulfadoxine–pyrimethamine, high doses of folic acid should be avoided because they may interfere with the efficacy of this antimalarial drug.	2	NA/1
Multiple micronutrient supplementation in pregnancy: Antenatal multiple micronutrient supplements that include iron and folic acid are recommended in the context of rigorous research.	3	1/1
Nutrition counseling during pregnancy: Counseling about healthy eating and keeping physically active during pregnancy is recommended for pregnant people to stay healthy and to prevent excessive weight gain during pregnancy.	1	1
Periconceptional folic acid supplementation, which aims to prevent neural tube defects: All potentially pregnant people, from the moment they begin trying to conceive until 12 weeks of gestation, should take a folic acid supplement (400 µg of folic acid daily).	2	NA/ 2
Restricting caffeine intake during pregnancy: For pregnant people with a high daily caffeine intake (more than 300 mg per day), lowering daily caffeine intake during pregnancy is recommended to reduce the risk of pregnancy loss and low-birth-weight neonates.	2	NA/1

(continued)

Table 9.1 (continued)

Intervention	1. Lancet 2.eLENA 3. Both	Lancet/ eLENA category
Support for mothers after childbirth: All mothers should be supported in the following: (1) initiating early and uninterrupted skin-to-skin contact and breastfeeding as soon as possible after childbirth; (2) establishing breastfeeding and managing common breastfeeding problems; (3) expressing breast milk as a means of maintaining lactation in the event of their being temporarily separated from their infants; (4) practicing responsive feeding as part of nurturing care; (5) recognizing their infants' cues for feeding, closeness, and comfort and enabling them to respond accordingly to these cues with a variety of options; and (6) discouraging them from giving any food or fluids other than breast milk to their children before the children have reached 6 months of age unless otherwise medically indicated.	2	NA/1
Vitamin A supplementation during pregnancy: Vitamin A supplementation is recommended only for pregnant people who live in areas where vitamin A deficiency is a severe public health problem ($\geq$ 5% of women in a population have a history of night blindness in their most recent pregnancy in the previous 3–5 years that ended in a live birth, or if $\geq$ 20% of pregnant people have a serum retinol level < 0.70 μmol/l), to prevent night blindness.	2	NA/1

Source: World Health Organization and the Lancet

Table 9.2 Child interventions

Intervention	1. Lancet 2.eLENA 3. Both	Lancet/ eLENA category
Appropriate complementary feeding: Infants should be exclusively breastfed for the first 6 months of life to achieve optimal growth, development, and health. Thereafter, to meet their evolving nutritional requirements, infants should receive nutritionally adequate and safe complementary foods while continuing to breastfeed them for up to 2 years or beyond.	3	1/2
Exclusive and continued breastfeeding: Infants should be exclusively breastfed for the first 6 months of life to achieve optimal growth, development, and health. Thereafter, to meet their evolving nutritional requirements, infants should receive nutritionally adequate and safe complementary foods while continuing to breastfeed for up to 2 years or beyond.	2	NA/1
Daily iron supplementation in children 24–59 months of age: Daily iron supplementation is recommended as a public health intervention in preschool-age children aged 24–59 months living in settings where the prevalence of anemia in infants and young children is 40% or higher, the aim being to increase hemoglobin concentrations and improve iron status.	2	NA/1

(continued)

Table 9.2 (continued)

Intervention	1. Lancet 2.eLENA 3. Both	Lancet/ eLENA category
Daily iron supplementation in children 6–23 months of age: Daily iron supplementation is recommended as a public health intervention in infants and young children aged 6–23 months living in settings where the prevalence of anemia is 40% or higher in this age group, the aim being to prevent iron deficiency and anemia.	2	NA/1
Daily iron supplementation in children and adolescents 5–12 years of age: Daily iron supplementation is recommended as a public health intervention in school-age children aged 60 months (i.e. 5 years) and older living in settings where the prevalence of anemia in infants and young children is 40% or higher, the aim being to prevent iron deficiency and anemia.	2	NA/1
Breastfeeding of low-birth-weight infants: LBW infants who are able to breastfeed should be put to the breast as soon as possible after birth when they are clinically stable and should be exclusively breastfed until 6 months of age. This recommendation does not address sick LBW infants or infants with birth weights less than 1.0 kg.	2	NA/1
Alternate feeding method for low-birth-weight infants unable to fully breastfeed: LBW infants who need to be fed by an alternative oral feeding method should be fed with a cup (or palladai, which is a cup with a beak) or a spoon.	2	NA/1
Demand feeding for low-birth-weight infants: LBW infants who are fully or mostly fed via an alternative oral feeding method should be fed according to the infants' hunger cues (demand feeding), except when the infant remains asleep beyond 3 h since the last feed. This recommendation does not address sick LBW infants or infants with birth weights less than 1.0 kg.	2	NA/1
Donor human milk for low-birth-weight infants: LBW infants, including those with very low birth weight, who cannot be fed their mother's milk should be fed donor human milk. This recommendation is relevant for settings where safe and affordable milk-banking facilities are available or can be set up.	2	NA/1
Delayed cord clamping for the prevention of iron deficiency anemia in infants: Delayed umbilical cord clamping (no earlier than 1 min after birth) is recommended for improved maternal and infant health and nutrition outcomes.	3	1/1
Deworming in children: Preventive chemotherapy (deworming), using annual or biannual single-dose albendazole (400 mg) or mebendazole (500 mg), is recommended as a public health intervention for all young children 12–23 months of age, preschool children 1–4 years of age, and school-age children 5–12 years of age (in some settings up to 14 years of age) living in areas where the baseline prevalence of any soil-transmitted infection is 20% or higher among children to reduce the worm burden of soil-transmitted helminth infection.	2	NA/1
The early initiation of breastfeeding to promote exclusive breastfeeding: All mothers should be supported to initiate breastfeeding as soon as possible after birth, within the first hour after delivery. Mothers should receive practical support to enable them to initiate and establish breastfeeding and manage common breastfeeding difficulties.	2	NA/1

(continued)

Table 9.2 (continued)

Intervention	1. Lancet 2.eLENA 3. Both	Lancet/ eLENA category
Emollient use (i.e., coconut oil or sunflower oil) for preterm and low-birth-weight newborns: The use of emollients (e.g., coconut oil or sunflower oil) in some settings is recommended to improve skin integrity and prevent infections.	1	4/NA
Feeding infants unable to breastfeed directly in care facilities: (1) Mothers should be discouraged from giving any food or fluids other than breast milk to their infants unless medically indicated. If expressed, breast milk or other feeds are medically indicated for term infants; feeding methods such as cups, spoons, or feeding bottles and teats may be used during their stay at the facility. (2) For preterm infants who are unable to breastfeed directly, non-nutritive sucking and oral stimulation may be beneficial until breastfeeding has been established. If expressed breast milk or other feeds are medically indicated for preterm infants, feeding methods such as cups or spoons are preferable to feeding bottles and teats.	2	NA/1
Feeding very low-birth-weight infants: (1) VLBW infants who cannot be fed their mother's milk or donor human milk should be given preterm infant formula if they fail to gain weight despite adequate feeding with standard infant formula; (2) VLBW infants who are fed their mother's milk or donor human milk should not be routinely given bovine milk–based human-milk fortifier (this recommendation is relevant for resource-limited settings); (3) VLBW infants who fail to gain weight despite adequate breast-milk feeding should be given human-milk fortifiers, preferably those that are human milk based; (4) VLBW infants should be given 10 ml/kg per day of enteral feeds, preferably expressed breast milk, starting from the first day of life, where the remaining fluid requirement is met by using intravenous fluids (this recommendation is relevant for resource-limited settings); (5) for VLBW infants who need to be given intragastric tube feeding, the intragastric tube may be placed via either the oral route or the nasal route depending on the preferences of healthcare providers. In VLBW infants who need to be fed via an alternative oral feeding method or given intragastric tube feeds, feed volumes can be increased by up to 30 ml/kg per day with careful monitoring for feed intolerance.	2	NA/ 1
The identification and management of severe acute malnutrition in children 6–59 months of age in the health facility and in the community: In community settings, trained community health workers and community members should measure the mid-upper arm circumference of infants and children who are 6–59 months of age, whereas in primary healthcare facilities and hospitals, healthcare workers should assess the mid-upper arm circumference or the weight-for-height/weight-for-length status. In both settings, infants and children should be examined for bilateral pitting edema.	2	NA/1
The identification and management of severe acute malnutrition in children 0–5 months: Infants who are under 6 months of age with severe acute malnutrition should be identified and managed. Depending on complications, some of them will need hospitalization.	2	NA/1

(continued)

Table 9.2 (continued)

Intervention	1. Lancet 2.eLENA 3. Both	Lancet/ eLENA category
Intermittent iron supplementation in preschool and school-age children: In settings where the prevalence of anemia in preschool (24–59 months) or school-age (5–12 years) children is 20% or higher, intermittent iron supplementation is recommended as a public health intervention to improve iron status and reduce the risk of anemia.	2	NA/1
Intermittent iron supplementation in preschool and school-age children in malaria-endemic areas: In settings where the prevalence of anemia in preschool (24–59 months) or school-age (5–12 years) children is 20% or higher, the WHO recommends the intermittent use of iron supplements as a public health intervention to improve iron status and reduce the risk of anemia among children. In malaria-endemic areas, the provision of iron supplements should be implemented in conjunction with measures to prevent, diagnose, and treat malaria.	2	NA/1
Kangaroo mother care, which reduces morbidity and mortality in low-birth-weight infants: Kangaroo mother care is recommended for the routine care of newborns weighing 2000 g or less at birth and should be initiated in healthcare facilities as soon as the newborns are clinically stable.	3	1/1
Kangaroo mother care for term newborn babies: Kangaroo mother care is also beneficial for healthy newborn babies in terms of weight gain and exclusive breastfeeding.	1	3/NA
Managing HIV-infected children under 5 years of age with severe acute malnutrition: Children under 5 years of age with severe acute malnutrition who are HIV infected should be managed with the same therapeutic feeding approaches as those for children with severe acute malnutrition who are not HIV infected.	2	NA/1
Managing infants under 6 months of age with severe acute malnutrition: Feeding approaches for infants who are under 6 months of age with severe acute malnutrition should prioritize establishing, or re-establishing, effective exclusive breastfeeding by the mother or other caregiver.	2	NA/1
Micronutrient supplementation for children with severe acute malnutrition: All severely malnourished children should receive adequate vitamins and minerals. For this reason, commercially available therapeutic milks, ready-to-use therapeutic foods, and rehydration solutions for malnourished children contain a mix of minerals and vitamins. Ready-made vitamin and mineral mixes can also be used in the preparation of local therapeutic foods and rehydration solutions.	2	NA/1

(continued)

Table 9.2 (continued)

Intervention	1. Lancet 2.eLENA 3. Both	Lancet/ eLENA category
Micronutrient supplementation in low-birth-weight and very low-birth-weight infants: (1) VLBW infants should be given vitamin D supplements at a dose ranging from 400 IU to 1000 IU per day until 6 months of age; (2) VLBW infants who are fed their mother's milk or donor human milk should be given daily calcium (120–140 mg/kg per day) and phosphorus (60–90 mg/kg per day) supplementation during their first months of life; (3) VLBW infants fed their mother's milk or donor human milk should be given 2–4 mg/kg per day of iron supplementation starting at 2 weeks until 6 months of age; and (4) daily oral vitamin A and zinc are not needed for LBW children.	2	NA/1
Mother's milk for low-birth-weight infants: LBW infants, including those with very low birth weight, should be fed their mother's milk (this recommendation does not apply to sick LBW infants or infants with birth weights less than 1.0 kg).	2	NA/1
Multiple micronutrient powders for the point-of-use fortification of foods consumed by children 2–12 years of age: In populations where the prevalence of anemia in school-age children is 20% or higher, the point-of-use fortification of foods with iron-containing micronutrient powders is recommended in children aged 2–12 years to improve iron status and reduce anemia.	3	2/1
Multiple micronutrient powders for the point-of-use fortification of foods consumed by children 6–23 months of age: In populations where the prevalence of anemia in children under 2 years of age or under 5 years of age is 20% or higher, the point-of-use fortification of complementary foods with iron-containing micronutrient powders is recommended in infants and young children aged 6–23 months to improve iron status and reduce anemia.	3	2/1
Small-quantity lipid-based nutrient supplements for growth in children: Small-quantity lipid-based nutrient supplements are recommended for all children to prevent stunting and being underweight.	1	1/NA
Nutritional care for HIV-infected children: Children (6 months–14 years) living with HIV should be assessed, classified, and managed according to a nutrition care plan to cover their nutrient needs associated with the presence of HIV and nutritional status and to ensure appropriate growth and development.	2	NA/2
Probiotics for preterm and low-birth-weight newborns: Small studies have shown beneficial effects but the use of probiotics for preterm and LBW babies is still controversial.	1	4/NA
Reducing the consumption of sugar-sweetened beverages to reduce the risk of childhood overweight and obesity: The WHO recommends a reduced intake of free sugars throughout the life course.	2	NA/2
Reducing free sugar intake in children to reduce the risk of noncommunicable diseases: The WHO recommends reducing the intake of free sugars to less than 5% of total energy intake.	2	NA/1
Reducing sodium intake to control blood pressure in children: The WHO recommends a reduction in sodium intake to control blood pressure in children aged 2–15 years.	2	NA/1

(continued)

Table 9.2 (continued)

Intervention	1. Lancet 2.eLENA 3. Both	Lancet/ eLENA category
Standard formula for low-birth-weight infants following hospital discharge: LBW infants, including those with VLBW, who cannot be fed their mother's milk or donor human milk should be fed standard infant formula from the time of discharge until 6 months of age.	2	NA/1
Supplementary foods for the management of moderate acute malnutrition in children aged 6–59 months: Infants and children aged 6–59 months with moderate acute malnutrition need to consume nutrient-dense foods to meet their extra needs for weight and height gain and functional recovery.	2	NA/1
Ready-to-use supplementary food for the management of acute malnutrition: Ready-to-use supplementary food should be promoted to treat children with severe acute malnutrition in all settings.	1	1/NA
Therapeutic feeding for children 6–59 months of age with severe acute malnutrition and acute or persistent diarrhea: Ready-to-use therapeutic food (RUTF) can be given in the same way as it can for children without diarrhea whether or not they are being managed as inpatients or outpatients.	2	NA/1
Transition feeding for children 6–59 months of age with severe acute malnutrition: In settings where RUTF is provided in the rehabilitation phase (following formula 75 (F-75) in the stabilization phase), once children have been stabilized, have an appetite, and have had their edema reduced, they should transition from F-75 to RUTF over 2–3 days, as tolerated.	2	NA/1
Treatment of hypothermia and hypoglycemia in children with severe acute malnutrition: The treatment or prevention of hypoglycemia and hypothermia should be included in the initial treatment that a severely malnourished child receives when first admitted to hospital.	2	NA/1
The use of antibiotics in the outpatient management of children 6–59 months of age with severe acute malnutrition: Children who are 6–59 months of age with uncomplicated severe acute malnutrition who do not need to be admitted and who are managed as outpatients should be given a course of oral antibiotics, such as amoxicillin.	2	NA/1
Vitamin A supplementation in children 6–59 months of age with severe acute malnutrition: Children who are 6–59 months of age with severe acute malnutrition should receive the daily recommended nutrient intake of vitamin A throughout the treatment period. Children with severe acute malnutrition should be provided with about 5000 IU of vitamin A daily, either as an integral part of therapeutic foods or as part of a multi-micronutrient formulation.	3	1/1
Vitamin A supplementation in infants and children 6–59 months of age: In settings where vitamin A deficiency is a public health problem (the prevalence of night blindness is 1% or higher in children 24–59 months of age or where the prevalence of vitamin A deficiency (serum retinol 0.70 μmol/l or lower) is 20% or higher in infants and children 6–59 months of age), high-dose vitamin A supplementation is recommended in infants and children 6–59 months of age.	3	1/1

(continued)

Table 9.2 (continued)

Intervention	1. Lancet 2.eLENA 3. Both	Lancet/ eLENA category
Zinc supplementation in the management of diarrhea: Mothers, other caregivers, and healthcare workers should provide children with 20 mg per day of zinc supplementation for 10–14 days (10 mg per day for infants under the age of 6 months).	3	1/2
Supplementing with zinc to prevent diarrhea and reduce diarrhea incidence: Preventive zinc supplementation for diarrhea needs further exploration in at-risk populations.	1	2/NA

Source: The World Health Organization and the *Lancet*

Table 9.3   Other interventions

Interventions	1. Lancet 2.eLENA 3. Both	Lancet/ eLENA category
The biofortification of staple crops: Such biofortification includes the iron biofortification of rice, beans, sweet potato, cassava, and legumes; the zinc biofortification of wheat, rice, beans, sweet potato, and maize; the provitamin A biofortification of sweet potato, maize, and cassava; and the amino acid and protein biofortification of sorghum and cassava.	2	NA/3
Creating an environment in healthcare facilities that supports breastfeeding: (1) Facilities providing maternity and newborn services should have a clearly written breastfeeding policy that is routinely communicated to staff and parents; (2) health facility staff who provide infant feeding services, including breastfeeding support, should have sufficient knowledge, competence, and skills to support people engaging in breastfeeding; (3) as part of protecting, promoting, and supporting breastfeeding, discharge from facilities providing maternity and newborn services should be planned for and coordinated so that parents and their infants have access to ongoing support and appropriate care; (4) facilities providing maternity and newborn services should enable mothers and their infants to remain together and practice rooming in throughout the day and night, though this may not apply in circumstances when infants need to be moved for specialized medical care; and (5) where facilities provide antenatal care, pregnant people and their families should be counseled about the benefits and management of breastfeeding.	2	NA/1
Family planning and birth spacing: Birth spacing has beneficial effects on both maternal and child outcomes.	1	1/NA
Food distribution program during pregnancy: A general food distribution program with or without education on nutrition positively affects child outcomes, including birth weight and birth length.	1	3/NA

(continued)

Table 9.3 (continued)

Interventions	1. Lancet 2.eLENA 3. Both	Lancet/ eLENA category
The fortification of maize flour and corn meal: (1) the fortification of maize flour and corn meal with iron is recommended to prevent iron deficiency in populations, particularly vulnerable groups such as children and women, and (2) the fortification of maize flour and corn meal with folic acid is recommended to reduce the risk of births with neural tube defects.	3	1/1
The fortification of rice: (1) The fortification of rice with iron is recommended as a public health strategy to improve the iron status of populations living in settings where rice is a staple food; (2) the fortification of rice with vitamin A may be used as a public health strategy to improve vitamin A nutrition of populations; and (3) the fortification of rice with folic acid may be used as a public health strategy to improve the folate nutritional status of populations.	3	1/1
The fortification of wheat flour: Wheat flour fortification should be considered when industrially produced flour is regularly consumed by large population groups in a country.	3	1/2
Implementing the Baby-Friendly Hospital Initiative: The Baby-Friendly Hospital Initiative is a global effort to implement practices that protect, promote, and support breastfeeding. It aims to ensure that all maternity facilities become centers of breastfeeding support.	2	NA/2
Insecticide-treated bednets for the control of malaria: Insecticide-treated bednets can reduce child mortality and *P. falciparum* malaria, which have effects on child nutrition.	3	1/2
The iodization of salt for the prevention and control of iodine-deficiency disorders: All food-grade salt used in household and food processing should be fortified with iodine as a safe and effective strategy for the prevention and control of iodine-deficiency disorders in populations living in stable and emergency settings.	2	NA/1
Reducing the impact of marketing foods and nonalcoholic beverages to children: The WHO has developed a set of 12 recommendations, endorsed by the World Health Assembly, aimed at reducing the impact of marketing foods high in saturated fats, trans-fatty acids, free sugars or salt to children.	2	NA/1
The regulation of marketing breast-milk substitutes: The International Code of Marketing of Breast-Milk Substitutes advocates that infants be breastfed. If they are not breastfed, the code also advocates that infants be fed safely on the best available nutritional alternative. Breast-milk substitutes should be available when needed but should not be promoted.	2	NA/1
Water, sanitation, and hygiene interventions to prevent diarrhea: Access to safe drinking water, access to improved sanitation facilities, and hand washing with soap at critical times (e.g., after toilet use and before the preparation of food).	3	2/2
The use of ferritin concentrations to assess iron status in individuals and populations: Ferritin concentration is a good marker of iron stores and should be used to diagnose iron deficiency in otherwise apparently healthy individuals, including women and children.	2	NA/1

Source: The World Health Organization and the *Lancet*

Evidence-based interventions during pregnancy include macronutrient, micronutrient, behavior change communication, counseling, and other health interventions (e.g., caffeine reduction and deworming). Many of these interventions are obviously missing from the *Lancet* list of interventions, and the eLENA list is more comprehensive. Moreover, the category of evidence differs between the two sources.

The evidence-based interventions for children are mainly about feeding practices (breastfeeding and complementary feeding), micronutrient or single nutrient supplementation, and health interventions (e.g., delayed cord clamping, emollient use, and kangaroo mother care). Again, some interventions are highly recommended by eLENA by not so by the *Lancet* and vice versa.

Implementation of Evidence-Based Interventions to Ensure Optimal Nutrition During Fetal and Early Life

The evidence-based nutrition mentioned above can be delivered at the global, regional, national, community, household, and individual levels. Specific considerations are required for the implementation and scaling-up of these interventions by level. However, due to the lack of space allocated for this chapter, we describe the steps of implementing these interventions only at the national and individual levels.

Implementation of Evidence-Based Interventions at the National Level

The steps that are needed to implement evidence-based nutrition interventions at the national level require several steps. Because every country is different in terms of the status of early-life nutrition, there is no one-size-fits-all strategy. However, here, we try to describe the general steps that are applicable to most countries.

Step 1: Carry out a comprehensive assessment on national needs, existing policies, and strategies.

The first steps should be a comprehensive assessment of national needs, existing policies, strategies, programs, and research. A situation analysis should be carried out to gather data and information. The methods for this step can include literature review (both academic and gray) and interviews with the relevant policymakers. The primary goal of this assessment is to identify gaps in the policies and strategies for the effective implementation of interventions for improving fetal and early-life nutrition.

Step 2: Develop a strong evidence base for fetal and early-life nutrition interventions.

The list of evidence-based interventions given earlier needs to be contextualized for each country depending on the findings from Step 1 because all the interventions may not be required or feasible for implementation. Accordingly, a country-specific list of evidence-based interventions can be developed from this step. This list of evidence can guide the required revision or development of nutrition policies, strategies, and programs for improving fetal and early-life nutrition.

Step 3: Carry out a landscape analysis on existing programs, research, and stakeholders.

After the development of a country-specific list of evidence-based interventions, the next step is to assess the existing programs, research, and stakeholders. A landscape analysis will scan the existing programs, research, and relevant stakeholders and identify the availability of resources, gaps, strengths, opportunities, and risks. Importantly, a comprehensive understanding of the fetal and early-life nutrition research landscape is often missing. The primary objective of this step is to understand who the key actors of nutrition programs and research are, what they are doing, what their future plans are, and which resources they have allocated and will allocate in the future.

Step 4: Revise or develop a multisectoral strategy for improving fetal and early-life nutrition.

Evidence-based nutrition interventions are broadly divided into two categories depending on the types of determinants of malnutrition they are addressing: nutrition-specific interventions and nutrition-sensitive interventions. The nutrition-specific interventions address the immediate determinants of malnutrition (e.g., food intake and nutrition care practices), and nutrition-sensitive interventions address the underlying determinants (e.g., the availability of nutrition, health, water, sanitation services, and a food system) [2]. The delivery of both nutrition-sensitive interventions and nutrition-specific interventions cannot be completed through the health or nutrition sector only. Accordingly, a multisectoral strategy involving health, nutrition, agriculture, food, and other relevant sectors is necessary for implementing evidence-based interventions to improve fetal and early-life nutrition. Many countries in the world already have multisectoral strategies, but the target populations and objectives for these strategies differ. For example, if the strategy is based on a life-course approach, efforts can be directed toward revising the fetal and early-life nutrition component of the strategy. If the country lacks a multisectoral strategy, a new strategy should be developed due to the growing evidence of the impacts of multisectoral approaches on nutrition [3].

Step 5: Mobilize available resources.

The implementation of multisectoral strategies for improving fetal and early-life nutrition will not be possible without the adequate allocation of resources (i.e., financial, human, capital, and technology). Although financial resources are always emphasized and are required to mobilize other forms of resources, the development and deployment of human resources, the procurement of capital resources, and figuring out the right mix of technology always take time, and those reasons support why time should be considered as a nonrenewable resource. Mobilizing each type of resource is a complex issue and should be based on cost-effectiveness or cost–benefit analysis data whenever possible.

Step 6: Implement interventions and operations research.

Step 6 involves the implementation of evidence-based interventions with the help of the resources mentioned above. Countries usually adopt various approaches to implement interventions. For example, piloting and refining a package of interventions may precede deciding on the final package and scaling up nationwide. Moreover, a country can decide to develop different packages of interventions for different geographical areas depending on the data, information, stakeholders, and resource availability. The efficiency of the delivery of interventions will need to be increased on a continual basis, and therefore, operations research should be coupled with the delivery of interventions.

Step 7: Engage in monitoring and evaluation.

A predefined monitoring and evaluation framework should be present to capture the status of the progress made toward improving fetal and early-life nutrition interventions. Again, a monitoring and evaluation plan for a multisectoral nutrition strategy is a complex issue and needs buy-in from every sector from the beginning of implementation.

Step 8: Revise the intervention package and sustain it.

Because we live in an ever-changing world, the evidence, resource availability, and stakeholders will continue to change. Accordingly, the interventions package needs to be revised, and new efforts are needed to address resource scarcity. However, the primary goal of this step should be to sustain the interventions by making changes.

The approaches to implement evidence-based nutrition interventions at the individual level are quite different from those at the national level. Although the individual-level interventions are part of national programs, every parent and family member has a responsibility to learn about and implement these interventions.

Implementation of Evidence-Based Interventions for Mothers

The evidence-based interventions for mothers include food-based interventions (e.g., balanced energy, balanced protein, and caffeine restriction), nutrient supplementation (e.g., iron, folic acid, calcium, iodine, vitamin A, and multiple micronutrients), communication-based interventions (e.g., education for breastfeeding and for complementary feeding and nutrition counseling), deworming, and an assessment of health conditions (e.g., diabetes). The successful implementation of these interventions requires not only awareness about and education for mothers but also support from their partner and other family members. The implementation of evidence-based interventions also requires that resources be spent by mothers and their families. For example, the family may need to buy nutrient supplements (if the supplements are unavailable from the national health and nutrition programs), spend time on education and communication, and spend time and money on availing themselves of health and nutrition services.

During pregnancy, adequate maternal nutrition is necessary to ensure the healthy growth and development of the fetus and to facilitate the growth and deposition of maternal tissues. The fetal demands for nutrients are high due to the rapid growth from a unicellular zygote to a fully formed human baby. The embryonic and fetal stages of life are unique due to the total dependence on the maternal supply of nutrients. Therefore, maternal undernutrition during pregnancy may lead to miscarriage, intrauterine growth retardation, premature birth, stillbirths, low birth weight, and birth defects [2, 5]. Malnutrition at the embryonic and fetal stages increases the risk of health conditions in the later stages of life too [3]. Pregnancy also comes with increased energy and nutrient demand for the changes in the breast and uterine tissues, increased body mass, and the formation of the placenta [7, 12]. Over the course of pregnancy, a pregnant person will gain 12.5 kg of weight on average, and optimal weight gain during pregnancy is an important determinant of pregnancy outcomes [12].

During pregnancy, a pregnant person can suffer from nausea, vomiting, hyperemesis, pregnancy-induced hypertension, gestational diabetes, anemia, or micronutrient deficiency, and all these conditions have health and nutrition consequences on the pregnant person and their baby. Accordingly, ensuring optimal nutrition during pregnancy at an individual level through the practice of evidence-based intervention is an important step for a proper start to human life. Table 9.4 gives a snapshot of the daily macro- and micronutrient requirements of pregnant and lactating people. In the table, a comparison is made with the daily requirement of nonpregnant and nonlactating people so that readers can easily identify the additional needs during pregnancy and lactation.

Box 9.1 Practical Tips to Follow During Pregnancy and Lactation
1. Consume a balanced diet that contains whole grains, healthy fats, healthy protein, fruits and vegetables, and dairy, and eat small, frequent meals.
2. Take vitamin and mineral supplements (e.g., folic acid, iron, calcium, iodine etc.).
3. Consume additional calories each day during the second (300 additional calories) and third (450 additional calories) trimesters of pregnancy and 500 additional calories during lactation.
4. Stay hydrated by drinking 8–10 glasses of water per day.
5. Avoid harmful substances (e.g., alcohol, tobacco, and recreational drugs).
6. Limit sugar-sweetened beverages, processed foods, caffeine, fried snacks, food with excessive salt etc.
7. Monitor weight gain.

Table 9.4 Dietary reference intakes (DRIs): recommended dietary allowances and adequate intakes of minerals, vitamins, water, and macronutrients for non-pregnant and nonlactating people and for pregnant and lactating people

Life stage									
	Nonpregnant, nonlactating (years)			Pregnancy (years)			Lactation (years)		
Nutrient	14–18	19–30	31–50	14–18	19–30	31–50	14–18	19–30	31–50
Minerals									
Calcium (mg/d)	1300	1000	1000	1300	1000	1000	1300	1000	1000
Chromium (µg/d)	24*	25*	25*	29*	30*	30*	44*	45*	45*
Copper (µg/d)	890	900	900	1000	1000	1000	1300	1300	1300
Fluoride (mg/d)	3*	3*	3*	3*	3*	3*	3*	3*	3*
Iodine (µg/d)	150	150	150	220	220	220	290	290	290
Iron (mg/d)	15	18	18	27	27	27	10	9	9
Magnesium (mg/d)	360	310	320	400	350	360	360	310	320
Manganese (mg/d)	1.6*	1.8*	1.8*	2.0*	2.0*	2.0*	2.6*	2.6*	2.6*
Molybdenum (µg/d)	43	45	45	50	50	50	50	50	50
Phosphorus (mg/d)	1250	700	700	1250	700	700	1250	700	700
Selenium (µg/d)	55	55	55	60	60	60	70	70	70
Zinc (mg/d)	9	8	8	12	11	11	13	12	12
Potassium (mg/d)	2300*	2600*	2600*	2600*	2900*	2900*	2500*	2800*	2800*
Sodium (mg/d)	1500*	1500*	1500*	1500*	1500*	1500*	1500*	1500*	1500*
Chloride (g/d)	2.3*	2.3*	2.3*	2.3*	2.3*	2.3*	2.3*	2.3*	2.3*
Vitamins									
Vitamin A (µg/d)	700	700	700	750	770	770	1200	1300	1300
Vitamin C (mg/d)	65	75	75	80	85	85	115	120	120
Vitamin D (µg/d)	15	15	15	15	15	15	15	15	15
Vitamin E (mg/d)	15	15	15	15	15	15	19	19	19

(continued)

Table 9.4 (continued)

Nutrient	Life stage								
	Nonpregnant, nonlactating (years)			Pregnancy (years)			Lactation (years)		
	14–18	19–30	31–50	14–18	19–30	31–50	14–18	19–30	31–50
Vitamin K (µg/d)	75*	90*	90*	75*	90*	90*	75*	90*	90*
Thiamin (mg/d)	1	1.1	1.1	1.4	1.4	1.4	1.4	1.4	1.4
Riboflavin (mg/d)	1	1.1	1.1	1.4	1.4	1.4	1.6	1.6	1.6
Niacin (mg/d)	14	14	14	18	18	18	17	17	17
Vitamin B6 (mg/d)	1.2	1.3	1.3	1.9	1.9	1.9	2	2	2
Folate (µg/d)	400	400	400	600	600	600	500	500	500

Source: Food and Nutrition Board, National Academies
*AI adequate intake, *ND* not detected

8. Consult with your healthcare providers for antenatal checkups, common pregnancy discomfort, and complications.
9. Monitor the reactions of your baby.
10. Reduce stress and get adequate rest.

Implementation of Evidence-Based Interventions for Children

The evidence-based interventions for children include feeding practices (e.g., breastfeeding, complementary feeding, specific feeding approaches for LBW and VLBW children, and avoiding food with high amounts of salt and sugar), nutrient supplementation (e.g., iron and multiple micronutrients), and specific health interventions (e.g., delayed cord clamping, deworming, the use of emollients, special food to treat severe or moderate acute malnutrition, and zinc for the treatment of diarrhea). Table 9.5 provides a summary of the macro- and micronutrient requirements for infants and children, including older children.

Table 9.5 Dietary reference intakes (DRIs): recommended dietary allowances and adequate intakes of minerals, vitamins, water, and macronutrients for infants and children

Nutrients	Infants (months)		Children (years)	
	0–6	7–12	1–3	4–8
Minerals				
Calcium (mg/d)	200	260	700	1000
Chromium (µg/d)	0.2*	5.5*	11*	15*
Copper (µg/d)	200*	220*	340	440
Fluoride (mg/d)	0.01*	0.5*	0.7*	1*
Iodine (µg/d)	110*	130*	90	90
Iron (mg/d)	0.27*	11	7	10
Magnesium (mg/d)	30*	75*	80	130
Manganese (mg/d)	0.003*	0.6*	1.2*	1.5*
Molybdenum (µg/d)	2*	3*	17	22
Phosphorus (mg/d)	100*	275*	460	500
Selenium (µg/d)	15*	20*	20	30
Zinc (mg/d)	2*	3	3	5
Potassium (mg/d)	400*	860*	2000*	2300*
Sodium (mg/d)	110*	370*	800*	1000*
Chloride (g/d)	0.18*	0.57*	1.5*	1.9*
Vitamins				
Vitamin A (µg/d)	400*	500*	300	400
Vitamin C (mg/d)	40*	50*	15	25
Vitamin D (µg/d)	10*	10*	15	15
Vitamin E (mg/d)	4*	5*	6	7
Vitamin K (µg/d)	2.0*	2.5*	30*	55*
Thiamin (mg/d)	0.2*	0.3*	0.5	0.6
Riboflavin (mg/d)	0.3*	0.4*	0.5	0.6
Niacin (mg/d)	2*	4*	6	8

(continued)

Table 9.5 (continued)

Nutrients	Infants (months)		Children (years)	
	0–6	7–12	1–3	4–8
Vitamin B6 (mg/d)	0.1*	0.3*	0.5	0.6
Folate (μg/d)	65*	80*	150	200
Vitamin B12 (μg/d)	0.4*	0.5*	0.9	1.2
Pantothenic acid (mg/d)	1.7*	1.8*	2*	3*
Biotin (μg/d)	5*	6*	8*	12*
Choline (mg/d)	125*	150*	200*	250*
Water and macronutrients				
Total water (L/d)	0.7*	0.8*	1.3*	1.7*
Carbohydrate (g/d)	60*	95*	130	130
Total fiber (g/d)	ND	ND	19*	25*
Fat (g/d)	31*	30*	ND	ND
Linoleic acid (g/d)	4.4*	4.6*	7*	10*
α-Linolenic acid (g/d)	0.5*	0.5*	0.7*	0.9*
Protein (g/d)	9.1*	11	13	19

Source: Food and Nutrition Board, National Academies
*AI adequate intake, *ND* not detected

Again, successful implementation at the individual level requires a double-pronged approach by involving both health and nutrition service providers and mothers and other family members [13]. Accordingly, capacity strengthening and resource mobilization are needed for both health and nutrition service providers and the mobilization of resources. For example, to implement breastfeeding and complementary feeding interventions, the self-efficacy and skills of mothers need to be improved through antenatal and postnatal counseling; through awareness campaigns; by ensuring that a breastfeeding-friendly environment is available at home and the workplace; by demonstrating breastfeeding techniques and ways to overcome breastfeeding difficulties; and by addressing individual-, family-, and community-level barriers. The delivery of micronutrient supplementation, therapeutic food, and other health commodities needs a well-developed health and nutrition system with skilled human resources and the necessary supplies.

Box 9.2 Practical Tips to Follow to Ensure Optimal Child Health and Nutrition
1. Engage in exclusively breastfeeding and complementary feeding.
2. Monitor the growth and development of the child.
3. Once solid and semi-solid food are introduced, ensure adequate hydration with safe water.
4. Stay hydrated by drinking 8–10 glasses of water per day.

(continued)

5. Limit or avoid sugar-sweetened beverages, processed foods, caffeine, fried snacks, food with excessive salts, etc.
6. Ensure immunization and timely healthcare seeking.
7. Teach your child good hygiene practices.
8. Avoid the use of any screen and make sure that the child gets the recommended sleep (12–16 h/day for infants, 11–14 h/day for toddlers, and 10–13 h/day for preschoolers).
9. Ensure that the child receives early stimulation and has a safe environment for social, emotional, and cognitive development.
10. Monitor the child's physical development and their achievement of motor milestones.

Implementation of the Other Evidence-Based Interventions Affecting Maternal and Child Nutrition

The biofortification, food fortification, and system-level interventions (e.g., water, sanitation, and hygiene interventions, hospital initiatives, the introduction of biomarkers, and family planning) that have indirect effects on individual maternal and early-life nutrition are dependent on national programs and regulations.

Research and Program Gaps Relevant to Fetal and Early-Life Interventions and Recommended Ways to Address These Gaps

Fetal and early-life nutrition is a highly researched topic. In 2022, Landry et al. [14] reported that between 2018 and 2020, the US National Institutes of Health (NIH) allocated USD 794,727,173 to fund projects focused on nutrition and early life. The authors of this paper also identified 13 broad areas of research gaps (beverage consumption; breastfeeding duration; breastfeeding intensity, proportion, and amount; breastfeeding never versus ever; complementary foods; dietary patterns; folic acid supplementation; eating frequency; iron supplementation; the maternal diet of food allergens; omega-3-fatty acid supplementation; seafood supplementation; and vitamin D supplementation) and reported that the NIH funded 235 research projects, costing USD 115,312,940, to address these research gaps [3]. Despite the ongoing and previous studies in the area of early-life nutrition, several research gaps persist. Although a detailed description of these gaps is beyond the scope of this chapter, the following list briefly describes some of the research gaps [10, 15].

• Preconception nutrition and its effects on early-life nutrition: Only limited evidence is available on the impact of nutrition during the preconception period on early-life nutrition and child development.

- Intergenerational effects of under- and overnutrition: The role of maternal under- and overnutrition on fetal programming and the effect of fetal programming on the growth and development of offspring in early and later life are understood to a limited degree.
- Nutrition during adolescence and early-life nutrition: Given the rise of adolescent pregnancies, insufficient evidence is available on how nutrition during adolescence affects the early-life nutrition of children born to adolescent mothers.
- The long-term effects of supplementation: The use of food supplements and micronutrient supplements is not new, but the long-term effects of such supplementation on growth and development have yet to be fully understood.
- Paternal well-being and early-life nutrition: One of the less-researched areas is the effect of paternal nutrition on the health and well-being of offspring. Limited evidence is available on the effects of the preconception nutrition of the father on the nutrition of offspring.
- Micronutrient deficiencies and ways to combat them: Micronutrient deficiencies have been well researched. However, context-specific interventions still need to be developed and implemented to address all forms of micronutrient deficiencies in both developing and developed countries.
- The effects of maternal mental health on early-life nutrition: The mental health of mothers affects the nutrition and well-being of children in various ways. However, more research is needed in this area.
- The possible role of digital tools in supporting and monitoring maternal and child nutrition: The use of digital technologies to improve knowledge and skills and to support mothers to ensure optimal nutrition for them and their children and monitoring maternal and child nutrition all need more research.
- Preventing preterm birth and low birth weights: Preterm births and low birth weights may have unwanted consequences, including morbidity and mortality. However, more studies are needed to find ways to further reduce preterm births and low birth weights.
- Male involvement in maternal and child nutrition: The role of male partners and ways to successfully engage them in maternal and child nutrition is still an under-researched topic.
- Climate change and its impacts on maternal and early-life nutrition: Climate change affects health and nutrition in many ways. Our understanding of how climate change affects maternal and early-life nutrition and ways to combat the effects of climate change on maternal and early-life nutrition need to be further improved.
- The variability of breast-milk composition and its effects on child growth and development: Breast-milk composition varies depending on the population and maternal diet and nutrition. However, this variability and its long-term effects on early- and later-life nutrition are understood to only a limited degree.
- Complementary feeding: More evidence is needed on the timing and sequence of introducing different types of complementary foods to address difficulties such as intolerance, food-related morbidities, and food allergies.

- The long-term effects of early-life under- and overnutrition: Early-life under- and overnutrition affects future health and well-being in many ways. Although some of the pathways of early-life undernutrition and noncommunicable diseases are now known, little is understood about ways to prevent the epigenetic changes responsible for diseases in later life and about the ways to prevent or delay the gene expression responsible for the onset of noncommunicable diseases.
- Early-life nutrition and neurodevelopment: The link between early-life nutrition and long-term emotional, social, and cognitive development needs further exploration.
- Early-life nutrition and the gut microbiome: How the gut microbiome is shaped by early-life nutrition and how the gut microbiome affects the growth, neurodevelopment, and immunity of children are understood to only a limited degree.

Conclusion

Fetal and early-life nutrition is a strong determinant of health, well-being, and productivity not only during childhood but also across the lifespan. The first 1000 days (i.e., conception to second birthday) is already known to be a window of opportunity to maximize the potential for growth and development. Accordingly, early-life nutrition is crucial for the development of the brain and other organs, cognitive development, strengthening the immune function, reducing the risk of noncommunicable diseases, and, more importantly, breaking the cycle of malnutrition and poverty. The evidence gap reveals that many evidence-based interventions exist to optimize early-life nutrition. Given the importance of early-life nutrition, all the nations of the world must invest adequate resources to ensure early-life nutrition for all children.

Further Practice

1. Pregnant people are advised to drink _____ glasses of water per day.

   A. 6–7
   B. 8–10
   C. 2–5
   D. 10–20
   E. 14–17

2. What is the recommended daily sleeping time for an infant?

   A. 12–16 hours
   B. 5–7 hours
   C. 8–9 hours
   D. 5–9 hours
   E. 6–9 hours

3. What is the folate requirement during pregnancy?

    A. 400 ug
    B. 300 ug
    C. 500 ug
    D. 600 ug
    E. 1000 ug

4. What is the iron requirement during pregnancy?

    A. 10 mg
    B. 20 mg
    C. 17 mg
    D. 15 mg
    E. 27 mg

5. Pregnant people require additional calories.

True/false

6. Caffeine does not need to be limited during pregnancy.

True/false

7. The additional calories needed in each trimester of pregnancy are different.

True/false

8. What is the iodine requirement during lactation?

    A. 130 ug
    B. 140 ug
    C. 250 ug
    D. 290 ug
    E. 300 ug

9. The sodium requirement during pregnancy and lactation is _____ mg/day.

    A. 2300 mg
    B. 1500 mg
    C. 2400 mg
    D. 3000 mg
    E. 1300 mg

10. Iodine deficiency can be prevented by iodizing salt.

True/false

11. Children under the age of 6 months must be supplemented with 20 mg of _____to prevent diarrhea.

    A. Iodine
    B. Sodium
    C. Zinc
    D. Potassium
    E. Iron

12. Sugar intake among children must be limited to less than ____% of energy intake.

    A. 10
    B. 5
    C. 15
    D. 20
    E. 8

13. Delayed cord clamping is recommended to improve maternal and infant health.

True/false

14. Donor human milk is not recommended to be used for low-birth-weight infants if their mother's milk is not available.

True/false

15. Exclusive breastfeeding refers to providing breast milk to children up to ____ months of age.

    A. 4
    B. 5
    C. 6
    D. 2
    E. 3

Answer Keys

1. B, 2. A, 3. D, 4. E, 5. True, 6. False, 7. True, 8. D, 9. B, 10. True, 11. C, 12. B, 13. True, 14. False, 15. C.

References

1. Jang DG, Jo YS, Lee SJ, Kim N, Lee GS. Perinatal outcomes and maternal clinical charac-teristics in IUGR with absent or reversed end-diastolic flow velocity in the umbilical artery. Arch Gynecol Obstet. 2011;284(1):73–8. https://doi.org/10.1007/s00404-010-1597-8. Epub 2010 Jul 24

2. Sharma D, Shastri S, Sharma P. Intrauterine growth restriction: antenatal and postnatal aspects. Clin Med Insights Pediatr. 2016;10:67–83. https://doi.org/10.4137/CMPed.S40070. PMID: 27441006; PMCID: PMC4946587

3. Cosmi E, Fanelli T, Visentin S, Trevisanuto D, Zanardo V. Consequences in infants that were intrauterine growth restricted. J Pregnancy. 2011;2011:364381. https://doi.org/10.1155/2011/364381. Epub 2011 Mar 20. PMID: 21547088; PMCID: PMC3087146

4. Arlinghaus KR, Truong C, Johnston CA, Hernandez DC. An intergenerational approach to break the cycle of malnutrition. Curr Nutr Rep. 2018 Dec;7(4):259–67. https://doi.org/10.1007/s13668-018-0251-0.

5. Anil KC, Basel PL, Singh S. Low birth weight and its associated risk factors: health facility-based case-control study. PLoS One. 2020;15(6):e0234907. https://doi.org/10.1371/journal.pone.0234907. PMID: 32569281; PMCID: PMC7307746

6. World Health Organization. P07: disorders related to short gestation and low birth weight, not elsewhere classified. In: International statistical classification of diseases and health related problems. Geneva: World Health Organization; 2010.

7. Langley-Evans SC. Nutrition in early life and the programming of adult disease: a review. J Hum Nutr Diet. 2015;28(Suppl 1):1–14. https://doi.org/10.1111/jhn.12212. Epub 2014 Jan 31

8. Black RE, Allen LH, Bhutta ZA, Caulfield LE, de Onis M, Ezzati M, Mathers C, Rivera J, Maternal and Child Undernutrition Study Group. Maternal and child undernutrition: global and regional exposures and health consequences. Lancet. 2008 Jan 19;371(9608):243–60. https://doi.org/10.1016/S0140-6736(07)61690-0.

9. Bhutta ZA, Ahmed T, Black RE, et al. What works? Interventions for maternal and child undernutrition and survival. Lancet. 2008;371:417–40.

10. Bhutta ZA, Das JK, Rizvi A, et al. Evidence-based interventions for improvement of maternal and child nutrition: what can be done and at what cost? Lancet. 2013;382:452–77.

11. Keats EC, Das JK, Salam RA, Lassi ZS, Imdad A, Black RE, Bhutta ZA. Effective interventions to address maternal and child malnutrition: an update of the evidence. Lancet Child Adolesc Health. 2021;5(5):367–84. https://doi.org/10.1016/S2352-4642(20)30274-1. Epub 2021 Mar 7. PMID: 33691083

12. Most J, Dervis S, Haman F, Adamo KB, Redman LM. Energy intake requirements in pregnancy. Nutrients. 2019;11(8):1812. https://doi.org/10.3390/nu11081812. PMID: 31390778; PMCID: PMC6723706

13. Escher NA, Andrade GC, Ghosh-Jerath S, Millett C, Seferidi P. The effect of nutrition-specific and nutrition-sensitive interventions on the double burden of malnutrition in low-income and middle-income countries: a systematic review. Lancet Glob Health. 2024;12(3):e419–32. https://doi.org/10.1016/S2214-109X(23)00562-4. Epub 2024 Jan 29. PMID: 38301666; PMCID: PMC7616050

14. Landry MJ, Ruiz LD, Gibbs K, Radtke MD, Lerman J, Vargas AJ. Perspective: early-life nutrition research supported by the US National Institutes of Health from 2018 to 2020. Adv Nutr. 2022;13(5):1395–401. https://doi.org/10.1093/advances/nmac044. PMID: 35438148; PMCID: PMC9526875

15. Ruducha J, Bhatia A, Mann C, Torlesse H. Multisectoral nutrition planning in Nepal: evidence from an organizational network analysis. Matern Child Nutr. 2022;18(Suppl 1):e13112. https://doi.org/10.1111/mcn.13112. Epub 2021 Mar 4. PMID: 33661554; PMCID: PMC8770655

Nutrition Approaches for Adolescents and Older Adults

10

Holly Huye, Desiree Ratcliffe,
and Teresa Walker-Cartwright

Learning Objectives

After completing this chapter, you will be able to

- Identify two nutritional issues in adolescence
- Describe the components of MyPlate
- List the food group amounts for adolescents based on a 2200-calorie diet
- Describe two healthy breakfast ideas for adolescents
- Discuss two physiological changes in older adulthood
- Discuss the importance of three nutrient needs and their corresponding food sources for older adults
- List the food group amounts for older adults based on a 1600-calorie diet
- Identify two ways to support older adults in achieving a healthy diet

Nutritional Approaches for Adolescents

The youth of today are the future adults of tomorrow. Although adolescence can be an exciting time of making new friends and exploring interests and hobbies, it can also be a stressful time. Adolescents experience uncomfortable growth periods, academic expectations, peer and parental pressures, and transitions from elementary school to high school, among others. Adolescence is a transformative period in which nutrition is essential for future health in adulthood. This section of the

H. Huye (✉) · D. Ratcliffe · T. Walker-Cartwright
School of Kinesiology and Nutrition, The University of Southern Mississippi,
Hattiesburg, MS, USA
e-mail: Holly.Huye@usm.edu; Desiree.Ratcliffe@usm.edu; Teresa.Cartwright@usm.edu

© The Author(s), under exclusive license to Springer Nature
Switzerland AG 2025
A. K. Mitra, D. Vanoh (eds.), *Essentials of Clinical and Public Health Nutrition*,
Nutrition and Health, https://doi.org/10.1007/978-3-031-95373-6_10

chapter provides an overview of the nutritional requirements for adolescents, common nutritional problems that adolescents experience, and strategies that can help adolescents develop healthy eating habits.

Nutrient Requirements During Adolescence

Dietary needs for the adolescent population differ from those of other life stages due to the significant growth that takes place starting from childhood. After infancy, adolescence is the most rapidly growing stage in the human lifespan [1]. The World Health Organization (WHO) defines the adolescent age to be between 10 and 19 years of age [2]. To meet adolescent changes in development, the Food and Nutrition Board of the National Research Council established Recommended Dietary Allowances (RDAs) for selected nutrients during each life stage, including adolescents [3]. Table 10.1 shows the requirements for children in early adolescence (9–13 years), in which the nutrient values do not differ between boys and girls in this age group. Table 10.1 also shows the requirements for teens in middle to late adolescence (14–18 years). The nutrient values for late adolescence are increased compared to those for early adolescence and can differ between male teens and female teens. This is in part due to the increase in lean body mass, particularly for male teens, and marks the beginning of the menstruation period in female teens, who require additional iron [4].

Dietary Guidelines for Americans and MyPlate

Every 5 years, the US Department of Agriculture (USDA) and Health and Human Services (HHS) work together to update and release the Dietary Guidelines for

Table 10.1 Essential RDAs for adolescents

RDAs for adolescents (9–13 years)		RDAs for adolescents (14–18 years)	
Nutrient	Male and female	Male	Female
Protein, g	34	52	46
Vitamin A, mcg	600	900	700
Vitamin B6, mg	1.0	1.3	1.2
Folate, mcg	300	400	400
Vitamin C, mg	45	75	65
Vitamin D, mcg	15	15	15
Vitamin E, mg	11	15	15
Calcium, mg	1300	1300	1300
Magnesium, mg	240	410	360
Iron, mg	8	11	15
Zinc, mg	8	11	9
Potassium, mg	4500	4700	4700
Sodium, mg	1500	1500	1500

Americans (DGA) [5]. The DGA is used by healthcare professionals, policymakers, and nutrition educators and is meant to offer guidance on adequate dietary intake to promote health and prevent disease. The most recent DGA was published in 2020 and includes four key recommendations: (1) Follow a healthy diet for your life stage; (2) tailor nutritious food and beverage choices to your taste preferences, culture, and budget; (3) meet your dietary needs in each food group with foods that are high in nutrients and low in calories; and (4) decrease your intake of foods and beverages that are high in added sugars, saturated fat, and sodium and decrease your consumption of alcoholic beverages.

To meet the dietary recommendations through intake alone, adolescents are advised to eat a balanced diet that includes a variety of foods from each food group, most days of the week. MyPlate was launched in 2011 as a visual representation of the DGA. The graphic uses colors to show what and how much to eat from each of the food groups, including fruits, vegetables, grains, protein, and dairy (Fig. 10.1). According to MyPlate, the estimated average energy requirements during adolescence are 2200 calories per day but can vary depending on age, sex, and activity level [6]. Recommendations for carbohydrate, protein, and fat consist of 45–65% of total calories from carbohydrate, 10–35% of total calories from protein, and 20–35% of total calories from fat (USDA and HHS, 2020). The results of the National Health and Nutrition Examination Survey (NHANES) between 2001 and 2014 indicated that adolescents in the United States typically consume twice the amount of protein that is recommended for their age group [7]. Similarly, the results from the more recent NHANES (2017–2020) indicated that adolescents consumed 5.6 times more protein from animal sources than from plant sources [8]. Plant proteins are lower in saturated fats and rich in vitamins, minerals, and antioxidants, all of which can lower the risk of chronic disease. During these formative years, establishing healthy dietary habits can have a positive impact on adulthood. Although protein intake is more than adequate for this population, intake in other food groups is not being met consistently for optimal nutrition status. Figure 10.2 illustrates the serving amounts recommended from each food group to create a healthy diet plan.

Older adolescents (ages 14–18) consume only half the recommended amounts of fruits and vegetables [11]. High intakes of ultra-processed foods such as artificially sweetened and sugar-sweetened beverages, calorie-dense (energy-dense) packaged snacks (e.g., chips, cookies, and breakfast bars), and processed protein foods (e.g.,

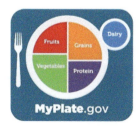

Fig. 10.1 MyPlate graphic [9]

Food Group Amounts for 2,200 Calories a Day for Ages 14+ Years

Fruits	Vegetables	Grains	Protein	Dairy
2 cups	**3 cups**	**7 ounces**	**6 ounces**	**3 cups**
Focus on whole fruits	Vary your veggies	Make half your grains whole grains	Vary your protein routine	Move to low-fat or fat-free dairy milk or yogurt (or lactose-free dairy or fortified soy versions)
Focus on whole fruits that are fresh, frozen, canned, or dried.	Choose a variety of colorful fresh, frozen, and canned vegetables—make sure to include dark green, red, and orange choices.	Find whole-grain foods by reading the Nutrition Facts label and ingredients list.	Mix up your protein foods to include seafood; beans, peas, and lentils; unsalted nuts and seeds; soy products; eggs; and lean meats and poultry.	Look for ways to include dairy or fortified soy alternatives at meals and snacks throughout the day.

Fig. 10.2 Food group amounts for adolescents 14 years and older [10]

 CALCIUM functions: keeps teeth and bones strong, secretes hormones and enzymes, supports blood vessel health. Food sources: seeds, milk, yogurt, sardines, salmon, fortified cereal, and plant-based milk

 VITAMIN D functions: supports healthy immune function, helps your body absorb calcium and phosphorus, reduces growth of cancer cells. **Food sources:** salmon, mushroom, milk, fortified soy, cheese, almond, and oat milks, ready-to-eat fortified cereal, sardines, egg, tuna fish canned (light)

 MAGNESIUM functions: regulates muscle and nerve function, regulates blood sugar, maintains healthy heartbeat, protects teeth and bones. **Food sources:** pumpkin seeds, chia seeds, spinach, almonds, cashews, peanuts, peanut butter, black beans, soymilk, potatoes, yogurt

 IRON functions: transports oxygen to all parts of the body, produces hormones, supports immune system, prevents infections, improves cognitive functions. **Food sources:** oysters, clams, white beans, beef liver, spinach, tofu, dark chocolate, cocoa, chickpeas, sardines, tomatoes, beef, potatoes

Fig. 10.3 Vitamin and mineral functions. (*Source*: National Institutes of Health: Office of Dietary Supplements [14])

breaded chicken nuggets, deli meats, and hot dogs) can result in poor diet quality and inadequate amounts of key nutrients [12, 13].

The latest results from the Healthy Eating Index (HEI) of 2020 (HEI-2020), which measures dietary intake from vegetables, fruits, grains, dairy, and protein foods (on a scale of 0–100) and compares findings to the recommended intake ranges provided by Dietary Guidelines for Americans (DGA), revealed that the average intake of people aged 2–18 years falls short in every food category, with a mean score of 54 [5]. Whole grains, dairy, and vegetables had the lowest scores in the HEI-2020. These food groups include those key nutrients previously mentioned that are crucial for healthy development during adolescence. Figure 10.3 lists the functions and food sources of the vital nutrients required for proper physiological and cognitive functioning in adolescents.

The NHANES data indicated improvement in the intake of added sugars from 2001 to 2018. When comparing the dietary record surveys taken during nine 2-year cycles, adolescents significantly reduced their added sugar intake, from 18.4% to 14.3% [15]. This decline may be due to a reduced intake of sugar-sweetened beverages. Although researchers are seeing some positive progression in nutritional choices during adolescence, intakes of added sugars still exceed the DGA recommendations. Dietary interventions still need to increase the intake of fruit, vegetables, whole grains, and beans/legumes to decrease the incidence of nutritional issues in adolescents.

Common Nutritional Issues Among All Adolescents

Because adolescence is a time of intense growth, this population's dietary habits and nutrient intake directly affect their health status. Malnutrition and overnutrition affect the development of multiple physiological systems. Adolescent eating patterns have bearing on bone health, eating disorders, nutrient deficiencies like iron-deficiency anemia, and obesity.

Disordered eating behaviors can occur during adolescence. Behaviors identified with anorexia nervosa and bulimia nervosa can be conceived during this growth stage, though diagnosis is more common in young women [16]. Up to 50% of women diagnosed with anorexia nervosa will develop the bone disease osteoporosis [17]. Osteoporosis is typically an adult condition; however, the amount of calcium found in adolescent bones will determine a person's risk of developing osteoporosis later in life. Between 40% and 60% of bone mineral mass is estimated to accumulate during the adolescent period [18]. Bone mineral density is determined primarily by genetics; however, up to 20% of peak bone mass is affected by environmental and lifestyle conditions [19]. Adolescents are at a higher risk of bone-related diseases because the majority of this population is not consuming a diet with adequate amounts of fruits, vegetables, and whole grains; thus, bone-building vitamins and minerals, including calcium, vitamin D, phosphorus, and magnesium, are insufficient to support maximum bone mineralization. Meeting the daily requirements shown in Table 10.1 can reduce adolescents' risk of developing osteoporosis and other bone-related injuries.

Globally, according to estimates, 1 in 4 adolescents suffer from iron-deficiency anemia (IDA) [20]. Adolescents with IDA have no obvious symptoms aside from appearing pallid and feeling lethargic. Symptoms such as a rapid heart rate and dizziness do not appear until iron levels are critically low [21]. In most cases, IDA can be resolved by increasing the intake of iron-containing foods (as shown in Fig. 10.2) or supplementing with iron under medical supervision. If unresolved, low iron stores can interfere with cognition, growth, and immune health [20].

A nutrition-driven problem that has been a public health crisis for decades is obesity. The WHO [22] estimated that 160 million children and adolescents aged 5–19 years were classified as obese in 2022. One measurement used to diagnose overweight and obesity in adolescents is body mass index (BMI). Americans are more sedentary today compared to 30 years ago. Also, the adolescent population spends more time indoors and on electronic devices and less time outdoors [23]. A decrease in physical activity and consuming a diet high in saturated fats and trans fats leads to high cholesterol and obesity in all life stages; however, the habits adopted in adolescence carry into adulthood when growth halts and metabolism declines, raising the risk of obesity if healthy eating habits are not a priority in the formative years of life.

Establishing Health Eating Habits in Adolescents

Healthy People 2030 is a health and disease prevention initiative with goals and objectives that aim to bring awareness to the nation's health issues over a 10-year period [24]. Nutrition goals target amounts for fruits, vegetables, whole grains, vitamin D, calcium, potassium, sodium, added sugars, and saturated fats, reflecting the Dietary Guidelines for Americans. Schools, community outreach programs, and public health organizations that support well-being and nutrition can use Healthy People 2030 as a resource guide to design programs with the aim of promoting these goals for this population. Table 10.2 highlights four goals for nutrition and healthy eating for which tracking data indicate that they are "getting worse" compared to the baseline and target data.

The change in food portion sizes and the uptake of fast food differ from years past and are leading contributors to the rise in overweight and obesity in the United States and around the world. In the early 2000s, the standard portion size of French fries was 2.4 oz, containing 210 calories; today, weighing in at 6.9 oz, the standard portion size contains 610 calories [25]. To control for the Unites States' "supersize" food craze and to remain relevant, utilizing online tools to learn about healthy eating can help bridge the gap between adolescents who need to know more about proper nutrition and reaching this audience in an engaging way, by using technology. The free Start Simple with MyPlate app (scan the quick-response (QR) code) was created with adolescents in mind, allowing users to set goals within food groups and monitor progress in real time and rewarding users by letting them earn badges when

Table 10.2 Healthy People 2030 nutrition and healthy eating goals with a "getting worse" status

Goal	Baseline data	Target	Current data
Increase whole grain consumption	0.46 oz per equivalents per 1000 calories	0.62 oz per equivalents per 1000 calories	0.41 oz per equivalents per 1000 calories
Reduce the consumption of saturated fat	11.4% of calories	8.4% of calories	11.9% of calories
Increase the consumption of calcium (mg)	1077 mg	1184 mg	1047 mg
Increase the consumption of potassium (mg)	2517 mg	2769 mg	2463 mg

goals have been met [6]. Parents and caregivers can also jump on board and begin the MyPlate healthy eating challenge with their adolescent. The MyPlate.gov website offers tips for grocery shopping and includes printer-friendly materials that teens can access to support their journey to healthy eating behaviors. See Box 10.1 for healthy eating habits.

Box 10.1 Healthy Eating Habits Checklist and Easy Breakfast Ideas
Healthy eating habits

- Eat a balanced breakfast with protein.
- Drink ~8 glasses of water per day.
- Avoid skipping meals.
- Limit fried foods to once a week.
- Make half your plate fruit and/or vegetables.
- Have regular sit-down meals with family/friends.

Easy on-the-go breakfast ideas

- Whole wheat toast with peanut butter, banana, and honey
- Scrambled egg, cheese, and salsa wrapped in a flour tortilla
- Smoothie made with frozen strawberries, Greek yogurt, maple syrup, and vanilla almond milk
- Yogurt and sliced fruit in waffle ice cream cone

Social support can also be lifechanging for adolescents in terms of their mental and social well-being [26]. When a person feels seen, supported, and encouraged, it yields success in all areas of their life, especially for an adolescent who relies on their peers, parents, and/or community supporters to influence their decisions and actions.

Summary

Healthy eating is essential across all life stages. Adolescents face many challenges in developing healthy habits due to the stressors faced during this transformative growth period. However, by using the evidence-based nutrition recommendations discussed in this section and having healthy role models to follow, adolescents can lead a healthy lifestyle that will benefit them in adulthood as well as in *older* adulthood.

Nutritional Approaches for Older Adults

Would you like to live to be 100 years old? A person who lives to be 100 years old is referred to as a centenarian. When asked this question, most people would answer yes, but they would likely want to add "as long as I am free of disease and have no disabilities." Most people want to enjoy a long life, avoiding disease and disability and keeping their cognitive abilities intact. However, no matter what we do, we cannot avoid getting older. The cells of the body are programmed to die, a process known as apoptosis. Even though aging is inevitable, certain lifestyle choices can be made to slow the aging process and allow for aging successfully.

The concept of successfully aging is multifactorial and includes physical, mental, and social aspects with a primary outcome of longevity [27]. To successfully age, one should be free of disease and disability and be able to function physically and cognitively, develop healthy relationships, and engage in productive activity [28]. One sign of successful aging is the ability to perform the activities of daily living (ADLs), which include daily tasks of self-care such as bathing, dressing, cooking, and caring for oneself. If an individual maintains the ability to perform ADLs, they are thought to be less dependent on others and are typically allowed to live independently longer.

This section of the chapter includes aging statistics, the physiology of aging, common nutrition-related issues for older adults, and strategies for maintaining optimal nutrient intake in older adulthood. It will focus on nutrition and the impact that it has on the aging process.

Statistics on Aging

If you look back over a century ago, to 1900, the life expectancy at birth for men was 46 years, and for women, it was 48 years [29]. Since then, life expectancy has increased considerably. According to data compiled in 2022 by the National Center for Health Statistics, life expectancy at birth is now 77.5 years for the total US population (Fig. 10.4) [30]. Additionally, data from the Administration on Aging indicates that approximately 17% of the US population is 65 years or older, which is expected to grow to 22% by 2040 [31]. The data indicate that Americans are maintaining a higher quality of life for longer (longevity).

Possible reasons for longevity include genetics, an educated population, improved food safety practices, medical advances, improved access to healthcare, and better lifestyle practices, such as physical activity, nutritious food consumption, and stress management [32]. Specifically, diet and nutrition play key roles in one's quality of life and can impact how long a person will live. However, according to the Centers for Disease Control and Prevention (CDC) [33], the majority of those 65 years and older die from chronic conditions. The six of the top ten causes of death for this age group include heart disease, cancer, stroke, Alzheimer disease, diabetes, and kidney diseases, most of which have modifiable risk factors such as dietary patterns [34]. Dietary choices such as nutrient-dense foods that are high in fiber and rich in

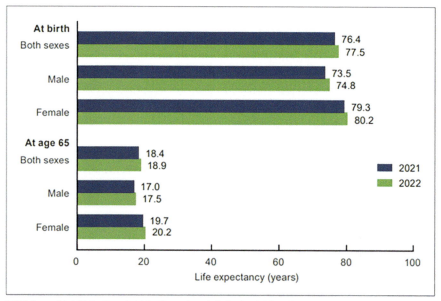

NOTE: Access data table for Figure 1 at: https://www.cdc.gov/nchs/data/databriefs/db492-tables.pdf#1.
SOURCE: National Center for Health Statistics, National Vital Statistics System, mortality data file.

Fig. 10.4. Life expectancy at birth and age 65 divided according to sex: United States, 2021 and 2022

antioxidants can impact and slow the progression of disease. Consuming healthy fats (monounsaturated fat) may decrease the risk of death from certain diseases, such as dementia from Alzheimer disease [35]. Brain physiology changes as one ages, which may lead to declining function. These physiological alterations may negatively impact function and occur in almost all the body tissues and systems as an individual ages. Tessier et al. (2024) found that the consumption of olive oil can lower the risk of dementia-related death by 28% [35]. With age comes numerous other physiological changes occurring in the body that are of concern.

Common Physiological Changes in Older Adults

Typically, age is noticed on the outside; however, as the years go by, the body is aging on the inside as well. As age increases, the organs get older and become more vulnerable to decline and possibly to disease. Overall health and nutrition status can be negatively impacted by some of the normal alterations that occur with aging. Physiological changes can include body composition disturbances that may result in a decreased percentage of muscle or lean tissue and an increase in fat tissue, which increases with age. For example, sarcopenia is a progressive loss of muscle mass, which negatively impacts strength and function. This decline in lean tissue is another normal part of the aging process [36].

A decline in brain function can weaken the thirst response, which causes older adults to drink less, leading to dehydration and, ultimately, to constipation and/or urinary tract infections (UTI). A UTI is the most commonly diagnosed infection in older adults, especially in women [37]. Older adults may drink less fluids because of increased incontinence or the inability to control urination and/or defecation. The dietary recommendation to prevent UTI is adequate fluid intake. The general rule is to divide your body weight (in pounds) by three and drink that amount of fluid in ounces [38]. Men 51 years and older should drink 13 cups of fluids daily, and women in this age bracket should aim to consume at least 9 cups per day. Adequate fluid intake is an important part of a healthy diet and is needed to maintain optimal health.

Changes in the gastrointestinal (GI) tract may also occur with age. The GI tract is where nutrients are broken down, absorbed, and utilized. These changes may begin in the mouth with a reduction in saliva, causing a type of dry mouth known as xerostomia. A decline in the amount of hydrochloric acid produced (achlorhydria) can occur in the stomach, which can reduce the body's ability to digest the food consumed. If food is not appropriately digested, the nutrients cannot be released and cannot be absorbed. When the amount of acid produced declines, the amount of other digestive chemicals, such as intrinsic factors, also declines. Intrinsic factors are needed for the absorption of vitamin B_{12}, and when it is decreased, the risk for pernicious anemia increases.

Decreased sensory abilities such as hearing, vision, smell, and taste may result in a lack of appetite (anorexia), a decrease in oral intake, and ultimately an inadequate number of nutrients being provided to the body [39]. These changes can weaken the immune response and potentially lead to malnutrition, which is a growing issue for older adults. Holly Kellner Greuling, a registered dietitian-nutritionist (RDN) with the Administration on Aging, estimates most older Americans are malnourished due to inadequate nutrition [40].

Nutrients of Concern for Older Adults

Several nutrients are of concern for older adults due to the physiological changes discussed above or inadequate intake. Table 10.3 shows which nutrients are of concern and why they are necessary and shows the best food sources that can be consumed to obtain these nutrients [41].

Recommendations for a Healthy Diet and Physical Activity

Older adults are not meeting the DGA recommendations for most food groups and are exceeding recommendations for added sugars, saturated fats, and sodium [42]. The DGA recommends a healthy dietary pattern that includes increasing the consumption of a variety fruits and vegetables as well as whole grains and dairy and decreasing the consumption of refined sugars, saturated fats, and sodium [5]. Specifically, adults 60 and over should consume adequate amounts of protein to

Table 10.3. Key nutrient needs for older adults and food sources

Nutrient	Why it is needed	Food sources
Vitamin A from beta-carotene found in food, not from supplements	Vision, a healthy immune system, and healthy skin. Caution: High doses of vitamin A from supplements in the body can be toxic and unhealthy for the bones.	Beta-carotene is found in orange foods such as carrots, cantaloupe, and sweet potatoes.
Vitamin B_{12}	Less acid and intrinsic factor in the stomach decreases the ability to absorb B_{12} in food.	Vitamin B_{12} is found in fortified cereals and soy milk. Add a B_{12} supplement if unable to consume adequate amounts in food.
Vitamin D	A decreased ability to make the active form of vitamin D in the body decreases the ability to absorb both calcium and phosphorus, which can lead to osteoporosis.	Vitamin D is found in fortified dairy products such as milk and yogurt as well as fortified cereals. Add a vitamin D supplement if unable to consume adequate amounts in food.
Calcium	Older adults are at a higher risk for dietary calcium deficiency and osteoporosis.	Consume 3 servings of dairy foods daily as well as calcium-fortified foods. Add a calcium supplement if unable to consume adequate amounts in food.
Fiber	It helps with normal bowel movements and can assist with naturally lowering cholesterol levels.	Fiber is found in whole wheat breads and cereals, brown rice, vegetables, and whole fruits.
Iron	Older adults are at a higher risk for anemias.	Iron is found in lean meat, fish, poultry, and iron-enriched grains and cereals. Add vitamin C-containing foods to iron-rich meals to enhance iron absorption.
Zinc	Older adults may have a suppressed immune response and suppressed appetite.	Zinc is found in lean meats, poultry, legumes, nuts, and zinc-fortified cereals.
Nutrient-dense food	Older adults have a lower metabolic rate, which reduces daily calorie needs.	These are foods that are low in added sugar and saturated fat and high in protein, fiber, vitamins, and/or minerals.
Water	Older adults have a diminished thirst mechanism, a decreased ability of the kidneys to concentrate urine, and an increased risk of dehydration.	Drink water and low-fat or skim milk with and between meals.

prevent the loss of muscle tissue, fluids to prevent dehydration, and vitamin B_{12} to promote absorption. Choosing appropriate portion sizes of nutrient-dense foods will help keep older adults satiated (see Table 10.4).

Food should always be the first choice to meet nutritional needs; however, if a person is unable to adequately meet their nutritional needs with food alone, oral nutrition supplements may be encouraged [43]. Older adults should consult

Table 10.4. Healthy dietary pattern for adults ages 60 and older (1600–2000 calories/day)

Calorie level of pattern	1600	2000
Food group		
Vegetables (cup eq/day)[a]	2	2 ½
Fruits (cup eq/day)[a]	1 ½	2
Whole grains (ounce eq/day)[b]	3	3
Dairy (cup eq/day)[c]	3	3
Protein foods (ounce eq/day)[d]	5	5 ½
Oils (grams/day)	22	27

Note: *eq* equivalent
[a] 1 cup of raw or cooked vegetables or fruit; 1 cup of vegetable or fruit juice; 2 cups of leafy greens
[b] ½ cup of cooked rice, pasta, or cereal; 1 medium slice of bread, tortilla; 1 ounce of ready-to-eat cereal
[c] 1 cup of milk, yogurt, or fortified soymilk; 1 ½ ounces of natural cheese
[d] 1 ounce of lean meats, poultry, or seafood; 1 egg; ¼ cup of cooked beans or tofu; 1 tablespoon of nut or seed butter; ½ ounce of nuts or seeds
Source: Adapted from the 2020–2025 Dietary Guidelines for Americans [5]

their physician and pharmacist before taking dietary and/or herbal supplements to prevent interactions between other medications. A registered dietitian-nutritionist should be consulted to avoid unwanted side effects from food/drug interactions.

Staying physically active as an older adult is essential for overall health and vitality, reducing stress and reducing the risk of chronic diseases like cardiovascular disease and type 2 diabetes [5]. To attain the most health benefits from physical activity, an adult is recommended to participate in moderate-intensity aerobic activity for 150 to 300 min per week. To help prevent the loss of muscle mass, individuals are recommended to engage in activities that make their muscles work harder than usual at least 2 days each week.

Exercise has not only been shown to reduce the risk of developing certain medical conditions, but it is linked to increased longevity. The results of a systematic review indicated a 30% to 35% reduction in early death for participants who were physically active compared to inactive participants [44]. Finding ways to be physically active throughout the day can provide long-lasting health benefits, especially when done with friends or family members.

Supporting Older Adults to Achieve a Healthy Diet

As a person ages, their need for support in performing activities for daily living and/or for optimal mental health increases [45]. Types of support may include support for meal preparation, transportation, or medical care and emotional, social, or financial support, and it may come from family, friends, neighbors, or other people within their community [46]. According to the Elder Care Alliance, spending time with others may increase one's physical and mental quality of life [47]. Staying connected to other people may reduce the risk of certain health conditions, improve memory, increase longevity, and reduce stress, anxiety, and depression. Consuming a variety of foods from each food group is a key factor in promoting adequate intake and reducing the risk of malnutrition. Sharing meals with others helps increase appetite and one's enjoyment of food while also improving mental health and well-being [48]. Congregate meal settings provided by the Older Americans Act are opportunities for older adults to socialize and eat a healthy meal [49]. Older adults may experience chewing and swallowing difficulties, which should be considered. Foods should be prepared with appropriate textures that are appealing and enjoyable to eat to promote intake.

Additional resources to improve dietary intake for older adults include food assistance programs such as home-delivered meals, the Supplemental Nutrition Assistance Program, the Child and Family Care Program, and the Seniors Farmers Market Program [5]. These programs offer financial support and access to healthy meals, snacks, and fruits and vegetables within older adults' communities.

Summary

Aging is a normal part of living; however, certain lifestyle considerations need to be taken into account, and resources are available to minimize the negative outcomes of aging and promote successful aging. Following the recommendations for a healthy diet, adequately meeting nutrient and fluid needs, adding daily physical activity, and seeking out and fostering relationships to increase social support are ways that older adults can achieve physical and mental well-being in their elder years. Small changes over time can make substantial differences, and the time is never too late to begin implementing changes.

Further Practice

1. *Why do nutrient values increase for males and females during late adolescence?*
2. List the food group amounts for fruits, vegetables, and protein for adolescents on a 2200-calorie diet.
3. Describe the complications associated with iron-deficiency anemia?
4. What is the measurement used to classify overweight and obese in adolescents?
5. List two tips from the healthy eating habits checklist for adolescents.
6. List three reasons why people are living longer.
7. List three physiological changes that naturally occur as a person ages and potential outcomes of those changes.
8. Plant proteins are higher in saturated fats and contain fewer vitamins, minerals, and antioxidants.
   True/false
9. Eating disorders are typically diagnosed in adolescence.
   True/false
10. The Start Simple with MyPlate app is a free online resource to assist with meal planning.
    True/false

11. Disability is always a part of the aging process.
    True/false
12. One reason why people gain weight as they age is that the thirst mechanism is enhanced, which can lead to the overconsumption of water.
    True/false
13. Older adults should refrain from physical activity to decrease the risk of sarcopenia.
    True/false
14. Iron is not a nutrient of concern for older adults, because they are at a lower risk for anemias.
    True/false
15. Calcium is a nutrient of concern for older adults because they are at higher risk of osteoporosis.
    True/false

Answer Key

1. Male teens increase in lean body mass and female teens begin menstruating, which requires an increase in iron.
2. 2 cups of fruit, 3 cups of vegetables, and 6 ounces of protein
3. Iron-deficiency anemia interferes with growth, cognitive function, and immune health.
4. Body mass index (BMI)
5. Any of the following is correct:
   • Eat a balanced breakfast with protein.
   • Drink ~8 glasses of water per day.
   • Avoid skipping meals.
   • Limit fried foods to once a week.
   • Make half your plate fruit and/or vegetables.
   • Have regular sit-down meals with family/friends.
6. Any of the following is correct:
   • An educated population
   • Improved food safety practices
   • Medical advances
   • Improved access to healthcare
   • Better lifestyle practices such as physical activity, nutritious food consumption, and stress management
7. Any of the following is correct:
   • Sarcopenia is a progressive loss of muscle mass, which negatively impacts strength and function.
   • Decline in brain function can weaken the thirst response, which causes older adults to drink less, leading to dehydration and, ultimately, to constipation and/or urinary tract infections.
   • Changes in the gastrointestinal (GI) tract may also occur. These changes may begin in the mouth with a reduction in saliva, causing a type of dry mouth known as xerostomia.

- A decline in the amount of hydrochloric acid produced (achlorhydria) can occur in the stomach, which can reduce the body's ability to digest the food consumed.
- When the amount of acid produced declines, the amount of other digestive chemicals, such as intrinsic factor, also declines. Intrinsic factor is needed for the absorption of vitamin B_{12}, and when it decreases, the risk for pernicious anemia increases.
- Decreased sensory abilities such as hearing, vision, smell, and taste may result in a lack of appetite (anorexia), a decrease in oral intake, and ultimately an inadequate amount of nutrients being provided to the body. These changes can weaken the immune response and potentially lead to malnutrition.

8. False
9. False
10. True
11. False
12. False
13. False
14. False
15. True

Glossary[1]

Achlorhydria (a″klor-hi'dre-ah) The absence of hydrochloric acid (HCL) from gastric juice, which is associated with pernicious anemia, stomach cancer, and pellagra

Activities of daily living (ADLs) Everyday routines generally involving functional mobility and personal care, such as bathing, dressing, toileting, and meal preparation

Anorexia (an″o-rek'se-ah) A lack or loss of appetite

Anorexia nervosa (an″o-rek'se-ah nûr-vō'sə) An eating disorder characterized by a fear of becoming fat, a distorted body image, and excessive dieting that leads to emaciation

Apoptosis (ap-op-to-sis) Preprogrammed cell death—which eventually results in a decreased number of viable cells, leading to organ system failure and eventually death

Body mass index A measurement of the relative percentages of fat and muscle mass in the human body, in which weight in kilograms is divided by height in meters squared, and the result is used as an index of obesity

Bone mineral density A measurement corresponding to the mineral density of bone, used to diagnose osteopenia and osteoporosis

---

[1] Definitions are from https://www.thefreedictionary.com/ unless otherwise indicated.

Bulimia nervosa (bŏo-lē′mē-ə nûr-vō′sə) An eating disorder characterized by repeated and secretive episodic bouts of eating large amounts of food over a short period of time (binge eating), followed by self-induced vomiting (purging)

Constipation (kŏn′stə-pā′shən) An acute or chronic condition in which bowel movements occur less often than usual or consist of hard, dry stools that are painful or difficult to pass

Dehydration (dē′hī-drā′shən) A loss of water and salts essential for normal body functions

Dementia (dĭ-mĕn′shə) A loss of cognitive abilities, including memory, concentration, communication, planning, and abstract thinking, resulting from brain injury or from a disease such as Alzheimer disease or Parkinson disease; it is sometimes accompanied by emotional disturbance and personality changes

Dietary Guidelines for Americans (DGA) The recommendations of the US Department of Agriculture and Health and Human Services for dietary intakes to reduce chronic diseases related to food intake (e.g., heart disease, diabetes, and obesity)

Incontinence (ĭn-kŏn′tə-nəns) An inability to control excretory functions

Intrinsic factor A glycoprotein that is secreted by the gastric mucous membrane and is essential for the absorption of vitamin B_{12} in the intestines

Iron-deficiency anemia An anemia that is due to iron deficiency, which is characterized by the production of small red blood cells

Lean body mass The total mass of the body excluding neutral lipid storage; in essence, it is the fat-free mass of the body

Longevity (lŏn-jĕv′ĭ-tē, lôn-) The length or duration of life or viability

Monounsaturated fat (mon′ō-ŭn-sach′ŭr-ā-tĕd fat) A type of unsaturated fat that may help to reduce blood cholesterol levels

Malnutrition (măl′nōō-trĭsh′ən, -nyōō-) A condition that develops when the body does not get the right amount of the vitamins, minerals, and other nutrients that it needs to maintain healthy tissues and organ function

Moderate-intensity aerobic exercise Defined as any activity that increases the heartbeat to faster than 50% to 60% of normal, such as brisk walking or fast dancing (https://health.clevelandclinic.org/what-does-moderate-exercise-mean-anyway).

Osteoporosis (ŏs′tē-ō-pə-rō′sĭs) A disease characterized by a decrease in bone mass and density, occurring especially in postmenopausal women, resulting in a predisposition to fractures

Overnutrition An excessive supply of nutrients, which hinders growth and metabolism

Pernicious anemia (per-nish′us ah-ne′me-ah) A disease in which the red blood cells (RBCs) form abnormally due to an inability to absorb vitamin B_{12}

Physiology (fiz″e-ol′o-je) All the functions of a living organism and any of its parts

Recommended Dietary Allowances (RDAs) The levels of intake of essential nutrients that, on the basis of scientific knowledge, are judged by the Food and Nutrition Board to be adequate to meet the known nutrient needs of practically all healthy people (https://www.ncbi.nlm.nih.gov/books/NBK234926/)

Sarcopenia (sahr′kō-pē′nē-ă) Progressive reduction in muscle cross section and mass with aging

Septicemia (sep″tĭ-se′me-ah) The presence of infective agents or their toxins in the bloodstream, popularly known as blood poisoning

Urinary tract infection The invasion and multiplication of microorganisms that lead to an infection of the urinary tract

Xerostomia (zîr′ə-stō′mē-ə) Abnormal mouth dryness

References

1. Taghizadeh Maghaddam H, Shahinfar S, Bahreini A, Abbasi MA, Fazli F, Saeidi M. Adolescence health: the needs, problems and attention. Int J Pediatr. 2016;4(2):1423–38. https://doi.org/10.22038/ijp.2016.6569.
2. World Health Organization. Adolescent Health. n.d.. https://www.who.int/health-topics/adolescent-health/#tab=tab_1alth (who.int)
3. Institute of Medicine, Food and Nutrition Board. *National Research Council (US) Subcommittee on the Tenth Edition of the Recommended Dietary Allowances*. National Academies Press; 1989.
4. Mesias M, Seiquer I, Navarro MP. Iron nutrition in adolescence. Crit Rev Food Sci Nutr. 2013;53(11):1226–37. https://doi.org/10.1080/10408398.
5. U.S. Department of Agriculture and U.S. Department of Health and Human Services. Dietary guidelines for Americans, 2020–2025. 9th ed. https://www.dietaryguidelines.gov/
6. U.S. Department of Agriculture Food and Nutrition Service. Start simple with MyPlate plan. 2021, July. https://myplate-prod.azureedge.us/sites/default/files/2023-04/2000-calories-ages-9-13-years.pdf
7. Berryman CE, Lieberman HR, Fulgoni VL, Pasiakos SM. Protein intake trends and conformity with the dietary reference intakes in the United States: analysis of the national health and nutrition examination survey, 2001–2014. Am J Clin Nutr. 2018;*108*:405–13. https://doi.org/10.1093/ajcn/nqy/088.
8. Wambogo EA, Ansai N, Terry A, Fryar C, Ogden C. Dairy, meat, seafood, and plant sources of saturated fat: United States, ages two years and over, 2017–2020. J Nutr. 2023;153:2689–98. https://doi.org/10.1016/j.tjnut.2023.06.040.
9. U.S. Department of Agriculture. USDA MyPlate. n.d.. https://www.myplate.gov/resources/graphics/myplate-graphics
10. U.S. Department of Agriculture. MyPlate plan. n.d.. https://www.myplate.gov/myplate-plan/results/2200-calories-ages-9-13
11. Wambogo EA, Ansai N, Ahluwalia N, Ogden C. Fruit and vegetable consumption among children and adolescents in the United States, 2015–2018. National Center for Health Statistics Data Brief (No. 391). 2020, November. https://www.cdc.gov/nchs/products/index.htm.
12. Fryar C, Carroll MD, Ahluwalia N, Ogden C. Fast food intake among children and adolescents in the United States, 2015–2018. National Center for Health Statistics Data Brief (No. 375). 2020, August. https://www.cdc.gov/nchs/products/index.htm.
13. Rosinger A, Herrick K, Gahche J, Park S. Sugar-sweetened beverage consumption among U.S. youth, 2011–2014. National Center for Health Statistics Data Brief (No. 271). 2017, January. https://www.cdc.gov/nchs/products/index.htm.
14. National Institutes of Health, Office of Dietary Supplements. Dietary supplement fact sheets. n.d.. https://ods.od.nih.gov/factsheets/list-all/
15. Ricciuto L, Fulgoni VL, Gaine PC, Scott MO, DiFrancesco L. Trends in added sugars intake and sources among US children, adolescents, and teens using NHANES 2001–2018. J Nutr. 2022;152(2):568–78. https://doi.org/10.1093/jn/nxab395.

16. Das JK, Salam RA, Thornburg KL, Prentice AM, Campisi S, Lassi ZS, Koletzko B, Bhutta ZA. Nutrition in adolescents: physiology, metabolism, and nutritional needs. Ann N Y Acad Sci. 2017;1393(1):21–33. https://doi.org/10.1111/nyas.13330.

17. Mehler PS. Clinical guidance on osteoporosis and eating disorders: the NEDA continuing education series. Eat Disord. 2019;27:471–81. https://doi.org/10.1080/10640266.2019.1642031.

18. Golden NH, Abrams SA, Committee on Nutrition. Optimizing bone health in children and adolescents. Pediatrics. 2014;134(4):e1229–43. https://doi.org/10.1542/peds.2014-2173.

19. Ambrosio MR, Aliberti L, Gagliardi I, Franceschetti P, Zatelli MC. Bone health in adolescence. Minerva Obstet Gynecol. 2021;73(6):662–77. https://doi.org/10.23736/S2724-606X.20.04713-9.

20. Gillespie B, Katageri G, Salam S, Ramadurg U, Patil S, Mhetri J, Charantimath U, Goudar S, Dandappanavar A, Karadiguddi C, Mallapur A, Vastrad P, Roy S, Peerapur B, Anumba D. Attention for and awareness of anemia in adolescents in Karnataka, India: A qualitative study. PLoS One. 2023;18(4):e0283631. https://doi.org/10.1371/journal.pone.0283631.

21. Touhy PC, Albertini LW, Thompson LA. What parents should know about iron deficiency anemia in children. JAMA Pediatr. 2023;177(6):651. https://jamanetwork.com/journals/jamapediatrics/fullarticle/2804208

22. World Health Organization. Obesity and overweight. 2024, March 1. https://www.who.int/news-room/fact-sheets/detail/obesity-and-overweight

23. LeBlanc AG, Gunnell KE, Prince SA, Saunders TJ, Barnes JD, Chaput JP. The ubiquity of the screen: an overview of the risks and benefits of screen time in our modern world. Transl J ACSM. 2017;2(17):104–13. https://doi.org/10.1249/TJX.0000000000000039.

24. Office of Disease Prevention and Health Promotion. Nutrition and healthy eating. Healthy people 2030. U.S. Department of Health and Human Services. n.d.. https://health.gov/healthypeople/objectives-and-data/browse-objectives/nutrition-and-healthy-eating

25. National Institutes of Health. Take charge of your health: a guide for teenagers. National Institute of Diabetes and Digestive and Kidney Diseases; n.d.. https://www.niddk.nih.gov/health-information/weight-management/take-charge-health-guide-teenagers

26. Pudel A, Gurung B, Khanal GP. Perceived social support and psychological wellbeing among Nepalese adolescents: the mediating role of self-esteem. BMC Psychol. 2020;8:43. https://doi.org/10.1186/s40359-020-00409-1.

27. Urtamo A, Jyväkorpi SK, Strandberg TE. Definitions of successful ageing: a brief review of a multidimensional concept. Acta Biomedica. 2019, May 23;90(2):359–63. https://doi.org/10.23750/abm.v90i2.8376.

28. Strawbridge WJ, Wallhagen MI, Cohen RD. Successful aging and well- being: compared with Rowe and Kahn. Gerontologist. 2002;42(6):727–33. https://doi.org/10.1093/geront/42.6.727.

29. NCHS: A Blog of the National Center for Health Statistics. Life expectancy in the U.S., 1900–2018. Centers for Disease Control and Prevention; 2020. https://blogs.cdc.gov/nchs/2020/11/20/7035/

30. Kochanek MA, Murphy SL, Xu J, Arias E. Mortality in the United States, 2022. National Center for Health Statistics Data Brief (No. 492). 2024. https://www.cdc.gov/nchs/products/databriefs/db492.htm#

31. Administration on Aging. 2023 Profile of older Americans. Administration for Community Living. 2024, May. Accessed 31 May 2024 from https://acl.gov/aging-and-disability-in-america/data-and-research/profile-older-americans

32. World Health Organization. World report on ageing and health. World Health Organization; 2015. https://iris.who.int/handle/10665/186463

33. CDC, National Center for Health Statistics (updated 2024, May) https://www.cdc.gov/nchs/fastats/older-american-health.htm

34. Cena H, Calder PC. Defining a healthy diet: Evidence for the role of contemporary dietary patterns in health and disease. Nutrients. 2020;12(2):334. https://doi.org/10.3390/nu12020334.

35. Tessier AJ, Cortese M, Yuan C. Consumption of olive oil and diet quality and risk of dementia-related death. J Am Med Assoc. 2024;7(5):e2410021. https://doi.org/10.1001/jamanetworkopen.2024.10021.

36. Sato PHR, Ferreira AA, Rosado EL. The prevalence and risk factors for sarcopenia in older adults and long living older adults. Arch Gerontol Geriatr. 2020;89:104089. https://doi.org/10.1016/j.archger.2020.104089.

37. Rowe TA, Juthani-Mehta M. Diagnosis and management of urinary tract infection in older adults. Infect Dis Clin North Am. 2014;28(1):75–89. https://doi.org/10.1016/j.idc.2013.10.10.004.

38. National Council on Aging. How to stay hydrated for better health. 2024. https://www.ncoa.org/article/how-to-stay-hydrated-for-better-health

39. Volkert D, Beck AM, Cederholm T, Cereda E, Cruz-Jentoft A, Goisser S, de Groot L, Großhauser F, Kiesswetter E, Norman K, Pourhassan M. Management of malnutrition in older patients—current approaches, evidence and open questions. J Clin Med. 2019;8(7):974. https://doi.org/10.3390/jcm8070974.

40. Greuling HK. Combatting senior malnutrition. Administration for community living; 2020. https://acl.gov/news-and-events/acl-blog/combatting-senior-malnutrition

41. Bernstein M, Munoz N. Position of the academy of nutrition and dietetics: food and nutrition for older adults: promoting health and wellness. J Acad Nutr Diet. 2012;112:1255–77.

42. Centers for Disease Control and Prevention Average Intakes: analysis of What We Eat in America, NHANES 2015–2016, day 1 dietary intake data, weighted. Recommended Intake Ranges: Healthy U.S.-Style Dietary Patterns.

43. Nieuwenhuizen WF, Weenen H, Rigby PM, Hetherington MM. Older adults and patients in need of nutrition support: review of current treatment options and factors influencing nutritional intake. Clin Nutr. 2010;29:160–9.

44. Reimers CD, Knapp G, Reimers AK. Does physical activity increase life expectancy? A review of the literature. J Aging Res. 2012;2012:243958. https://doi.org/10.1155/2012/243958.

45. Ashida S, Heaney CA. Differential associations of social support and social connectedness with structural features of social networks and the health status of older adults. J Aging Health. 2008;20(7):872–93. https://doi.org/10.1177/0898264308322462.

46. Cross CJ, Chatters LM, Taylor RJ, Nguyen AW. Instrumental social support exchanges in African American extended families. J Fam Issues. 2018;39(13):3535–63. https://doi.org/10.1177/0192513X18783805.

47. Elder Care Alliance. The importance of socialization in aging. 2017. https://eldercarealliance.org/blog/importance-of-socialization-in-aging/

48. Herman CP. The social facilitation of eating. A review. Appetite. 2015;86:61–73.

49. Administration for Community Living. Health, Wellness, and Nutrition. 2020. https://acl.gov/programs/health-wellness

Maternal Nutrition for Healthy Pregnancy, Including the Conception, Antenatal, and Postnatal Periods

11

Harit Agroia ⓘ

Learning Objectives

Upon completion of this chapter, students will be able to

1. Understand the role of essential nutrients in a healthy pregnancy and fetal development
2. Identify the requirements for essential nutrients during pregnancy to ensure maternal health and fetal development
3. Identify the dietary guidelines required for a healthy pregnancy for people with comorbid conditions or high-risk pregnancies
4. Learn the importance of nutrition therapy during breastfeeding and lactation
5. Discuss barriers and challenges to healthy nutrition during pregnancy and the short- and long-term impact on outcomes
6. Discuss major public health educational initiatives and interventions that aim to improve maternal nutrition

Introduction

In the United States, one in every five pregnant people report going to bed hungry at night. Given that the United States is a developed country with comparatively greater resources and economic prosperity than other countries, this statistic points to the continued need to address disparities among populations who may face unique barriers and challenges in accessing healthy food options during pregnancy; these barriers may range from financial constraints to

H. Agroia (✉)
San Jose State University, San Jose, CA, USA

© The Author(s), under exclusive license to Springer Nature
Switzerland AG 2025
A. K. Mitra, D. Vanoh (eds.), *Essentials of Clinical and Public Health Nutrition*,
Nutrition and Health, https://doi.org/10.1007/978-3-031-95373-6_11

transportation-related issues like proximity to supermarkets and whole food retailers in order to access a wider range of healthy food options. Malnourished pregnant people may overall face higher reproductive risks that affect them directly, such as an increased risk for early death during or following delivery [1]. One in three women in the United States are also overweight, which may further be indicative of the sparse availability of healthy food options, thereby increasing the likelihood of unhealthy and energy-dense food consumption, such as foods high in carbohydrates, sodium, and cholesterol. Nutrient-poor foods that are high in fats and carbohydrates are known to be linked to inflammatory processes that can be detrimental to a child's neurological development, which can lead to challenges later in life, such as depression, anxiety, attention deficit hyperactivity disorder, or autism spectrum disorder [2–4]. These foods can also cause deficiencies in other essential micronutrients [2, 5, 6] and lead to a condition called hidden hunger, where the human body simply is not able to receive the nutrients that it needs to function at normal energy levels [7]. Recent research suggests that young pregnant people have been more vulnerable to this condition and could specifically develop deficiencies in iron, iodine, and vitamin D, which are all connected to pregnancy-related complications [7]. Instead of consuming nutrient-rich foods, consuming a much higher degree of ultra-processed foods can even cause oxidative stress among pregnant people [8]. A large proportion of pregnant people also experience physical health-related challenges during pregnancy, such as energy or nutrient deficiencies, anemia, poor weight gain, or comorbid conditions such as infectious diseases [1].

Regarding maternal nutrition, these factors are of concern because healthy nutrition during pregnancy has an impact both on the mother and on fetal growth and development [1, 9]; for example, if a pregnant person does not maintain a healthy pregnancy, then their babies could be prone to developmental challenges [9] and chronic disease that may emerge during infancy but persist throughout childhood and the later years of their life. Such challenges may also include prematurity and undernutrition in the infant [1]. Babies born to mothers that did not maintain essential nutrients during pregnancy may further be susceptible to a host of other diseases, such as diseases related to the cardiovascular system, metabolic system, and more. Therefore, pregnant people must take the necessary vitamins and nutrients, maintain a balanced diet, take prenatal vitamin supplements regularly, and monitor their health in partnership with their medical provider during pregnancy. This will not only keep pregnant people healthy, but also contribute to broader improvements in health outcomes related to pregnancy [1]. The goal of this chapter is to discuss how pregnant people can eat well during pregnancy, understand how consuming essential nutrients will help meet the extra needs of their body during pregnancy, and ways that these nutrients support fetal growth and development while maintaining a healthy weight [10].

Role of Nutrients for a Healthy Pregnancy

The term *maternal nutrition* is used to describe the nutritional needs of pregnant people during all phases of their journey to childbirth, including the conception, antenatal, and postnatal periods [1]. Many of those of childbearing age experience nutrient deficiencies, which then lead to adverse health outcomes [1]. Research suggests that nutrition before pregnancy is just as critical for fetal development and the child's long-term health as nutrition during pregnancy [2, 11–14]. This is because the embryo that has just started to develop soon after conception becomes heavily reliant on essential nutrients to support its growth [14, 15]. Babies that are born to mothers that are undernourished or overweight during pregnancy may be at risk of low or high birth weight, which can further place them at risk of chronic diseases such as type 2 diabetes, obesity, and heart disease [15–18]. In fact, more than 20 million children in the world are born with low birth weight, especially in low-income countries [18].

One major indicator of maternal malnutrition is anemia, a condition that involves the depletion of iron levels in the body and that is often attributed to heavy bleeding during menstruation, the underconsumption of iron as an important nutrient, or a general poor ability of the body to absorb iron [1]. Research has shown that more than 20% of maternal deaths are related to iron deficiency [19]. Another significant indicator of maternal malnutrition is iodine deficiency, which can not only lead to miscarriage and stillbirth but also cause serious brain developmental consequences for the child [1, 9]. A poor maternal diet during pregnancy coupled with a lack of breastfeeding can lead to nutrient deficiencies for both the mom and baby that specifically affects the gut microbiota and affects many other pathways, such as epigenetic controls, the transcription of genes involved in metabolism, and others that may increase the likelihood of acquiring noncommunicable diseases later in life [17, 20, 21]. Maternal diet during pregnancy also influences the gut microbiome and the development of organ systems in the newborn [13]. Because pregnancy is known to be a dynamic process through which pregnant people experience both external and internal changes to their body, it is important to understand the role of the remodeling of the gut microbiota throughout the progression of pregnancy where maternal diet as an external and environmental factor facilitates positive gut microbial changes [13]. Research has shown that pregnancy-related changes to the gut microbiome are more vulnerable to maternal diet, even more so than obesity status or weight-gain trajectory throughout pregnancy [13, 22]. Also, a number of studies have pinpointed a relationship between maternal diet, the gut microbiome, and fetal development, especially to highlight that maternal diet further shapes and educates the fetal immune system, which assists in the development of gut microbiota early in life for the infant [13]. Because of these outcomes, nutrients play vital roles in a healthy pregnancy for both the mother and the baby.

Nutrient Requirements for Pregnant People

The key nutrients that are most important for maternal and child health outcomes include folic acid, iron, calcium, protein, other B vitamins, iodine, choline [1, 10, 23–26], and omega-3 fatty acids [10]. Eating healthy foods that contain these ingredients along with a daily prenatal vitamin often helps meet nutrient needs [10, 27]. Micronutrient deficiencies are still quite common in many countries around the world, such as among women and children in sub-Saharan Africa, where the intake of fatty acids, in particular, is low among many pregnant people [28]. One strategy that has been recommended to improve the intake of these essential nutrients is to prepare enriching foods at home that contain lipid-based nutrient supplements; these supplements have the potential to offer both essential fatty acids and can be a good source of protein for both women and children [28]. One study aimed to examine the impact of this strategy and found that prenatal lipid-based nutrient consumption reduced the prevalence of low gestational weight in Ghana and overall was found to contribute to improved child growth in sub-Saharan Africa [28].

Although pregnant people should take necessary steps to ensure that these nutrients are incorporated into their diet, they should do so with caution by recognizing that too much of certain vitamins or supplements can have counterproductive and harmful effects on the body and for the baby, and it can lead to serious birth defects [10, 26]. These nutrients are described in detail in this section, but individuals should always consult with their medical provider to make a fully informed decision about their pregnancy diet.

Folic Acid

Folic acid is part of the family of B vitamins and serves to prevent neural tube defects among pregnant people [10, 26, 27, 29], which specifically can help to prevent major fetal defects that affect the brain and spinal cord [10, 27, 29, 30]. People who are planning to become pregnant should begin taking folic acid 1 month before getting pregnant. In addition, folic acid is recommended to be taken consistently throughout the entire duration of the pregnancy [26, 31]. Before pregnancy, they are recommended to take 400 micrograms of folic acid per day, and this dosing should be increased to 600 micrograms per day during pregnancy. This is considered a high dose, which can often be difficult to obtain from food alone, so pregnant people are recommended to work with their medical provider to determine whether a prenatal vitamin that contains at least 400 mcg/day is indicated [10]. Moreover, some foods that contain folic acid include green leafy vegetables, berries, nuts, beans, and citrus fruits [10, 27, 30].

Other B Vitamins

Vitamins B_6 and B_{12} are important during pregnancy because they both help in the formation of red blood cells; B_6 also helps the body use protein, fat, and carbohydrates, and B_{12} helps maintain the nervous system [10]. Pregnant people are recommended to take 1.9 milligrams of B_6 and 2.6 micrograms of B_{12} daily during pregnancy [10]. Examples of foods that contain B_6 include beef, liver, pork, ham, whole-grain bread, and bananas [10]. Examples of foods that contain B_{12} include meat, poultry, and milk. Pregnant people who adhere to a vegetarian diet may consider taking supplements [10].

Iron

Iron is important to ensure optimal levels of red blood cell production in the body, for both the mother and the baby, since during pregnancy the amount of blood in the body is expected to increase [26, 29]. For the baby, iron as an essential nutrient will promote the baby's overall growth and development [31], making it essential for the development of red blood cells that supply oxygen to the fetus [10, 26]. Recent data have shown that at least 10% of all pregnant people have an iron deficiency [29]. The recommended dose of iron per day is 27 milligrams [10, 26, 27], which can be found in most prenatal vitamins; however, a medical provider may recommend an iron supplement on a case-by-case basis. Examples of iron-rich foods include lean red meat, poultry, and dried beans, and peas [10, 27]. Iron is commonly taken with vitamin C, whether that is through a vitamin C supplement or by consuming foods that are high in vitamin C, because it plays a strong role in increasing iron absorption in the body. Examples of vitamin C–rich foods include citrus fruits, broccoli, tomatoes, and strawberries [10].

Calcium

Calcium is another essential vitamin that is crucial in supporting the formation of bones and teeth in the developing fetus [27]. Taking calcium can also reduce a pregnant person's risk of pre-eclampsia, which is a serious medical condition that can cause a sudden rise in blood pressure [26]. Pregnant adults are recommended to take 1000 milligrams of calcium per day. For pregnant teenagers, the recommended dose increases to 1300 milligrams of calcium per day [26]. Examples of calcium-rich foods include milk, cheese, yogurt, and green leafy vegetables [10, 27]. Taking calcium along with vitamin D, whether that is through a vitamin D supplement or by consuming foods that are high in vitamin D, can help improve calcium absorption in the body [26]. Pregnant people are recommended to incorporate 600 international units of vitamin D per day [27]. Examples of vitamin D-rich foods include fortified milk and fatty fish such as salmon [10, 27]; vitamin D can also be obtained from natural sunlight [10].

Protein

Protein intake is important, and pregnant people are encouraged to consume about 60 grams of protein per day to support the fetal tissue. A few options for protein-rich foods include beans, peas, eggs, lean meats, and unsalted nuts and seeds [26, 30].

Iodine

Iodine is an essential nutrient that supports healthy brain development [10, 29]. Pregnant people are recommended to take 27 milligrams of iodine daily during pregnancy. Importantly, many prenatal supplements do not contain iodine, so foods that contain iodine should be incorporated into the diet [29]. Examples of iodine-rich foods include iodized table salt, dairy products, seafood, meat, and eggs [10].

Choline

Choline is an essential nutrient that is important for the development of the fetal brain and spinal cord [10, 29]. Pregnant people are recommended to take 450 milligrams of choline per day during pregnancy. More than 90–95% of all pregnant people do not meet this recommendation [29]. Examples of choline-rich foods include milk, eggs, peanuts, and soy products [10].

Omega-3 Fatty Acids

Omega-3 fatty acids are natural fats found in fish and have shown to have positive effects for the fetus, especially for brain development before and after birth [10, 29]. To consume the recommended amount of omega-3 fatty acids, pregnant people should aim to have two or three servings of fish or shellfish per week, where one serving is measured as 4 ounces [10]. Pregnant people should take caution to ensure that fish they consume does not contain high levels of mercury because that can lead to birth defects; fish with high mercury levels are typically caught from local waters and include shark, swordfish, and tilefish [10]. Examples of food products that contain omega-3 fatty acids and are safe to eat include flaxseed, broccoli, cantaloupe, kidney beans, spinach, cauliflower, and walnuts [10].

Dietary Guidelines During Pregnancy

Weight Gain During Pregnancy

Weight gain should be expected for every pregnant person. Although people commonly say that a pregnant person should "eat for two" while pregnant [10], the actual amount of weight gain that is recommended depends on several factors, such as how much the individual weighed before pregnancy, their overall body mass index, and physical activity level [26], and should not be assumed as the amount needed to "eat for two." Rather, pregnant people should think of it as eating twice as *healthy* during pregnancy because of the need to maintain both their and their baby's health [10]. For individuals that were at a healthy weight before pregnancy, they should expect to gain an additional 25–35 pounds during pregnancy [26]. For individuals that were underweight during pregnancy, they should expect to gain between 28–40 pounds during pregnancy; for individuals that were overweight before pregnancy, they should expect to gain between 15 and 25 pounds; and for individuals that were obese before pregnancy, they should expect to gain about 11–20 pounds [10]. This weight gain can be further broken down depending on how far along a pregnant person is during their pregnancy. During the first trimester, the total weight gain should be between 1 and 4 pounds. During the second and third trimesters, an extra 1 pound per week is expected to be gained. Ultimately, regular appointments during pregnancy with a medical provider can ensure continued weight monitoring throughout [26, 32]. Box 11.1 highlights these general weight-gain expectations.

Box 11.1 Expected Weight Gain During Pregnancy

Weight before pregnancy	Expected overall weight gain for a single fetus (pounds)
Underweight	28–40
Healthy Weight	25–35
Overweight	15–25
Obese	11–20

Calorie Intake

The overall recommended calorie intake during pregnancy depends on individual weight-gain goals [26]. Although a medical provider can work with pregnant people on an individual basis to identify those goals, the general recommendation is that pregnant people should not increase their calorie intake from baseline during the first trimester of pregnancy [26]. During the second trimester, pregnant people are recommended to increase their calorie consumption by 340 calories/day. In the third trimester, pregnant people are recommended to consume an additional 450 calories per day [26]. These guidelines are provided for pregnant people who are expecting to have one child; those expecting twins should consume about 600 extra calories per day, and those expecting triplets should eat 900 extra calories per day [10].

Recommended Intakes of Foods and Drinks

Pregnant people can safely consume a range of foods during pregnancy, especially those that are high in essential nutrients such as folic acid, vitamin D, and calcium. Options for vegetables include carrots, cooked greens, pumpkin, spinach, and sweet potatoes; fruits include bananas, honeydew, mango, and tomatoes; dairy includes skim or 1% milk and soymilk; and proteins include beans and peas, lean beef, nuts and seeds, and poultry [30]. Figure 11.1 shows these recommended food options and the nutrients that they provide.

Fluid intake is incredibly important during pregnancy [30]. Pregnant people are recommended to consume between 2–3 liters of fluids, which can include water or other beverages; however, beverages high in sugar content like juice and soda should be avoided. For water specifically, pregnant people should aim to drink about 8–12 cups of water per day [10].

The following food and drinks should be avoided during pregnancy because they can adversely affect the health of the mother and baby, which could have long-term implications, especially for child development. First, no amount of alcohol is recommended during pregnancy, so it should never be consumed [26, 30]. Second, foods with high levels of mercury (mostly fish or seafood) should be avoided. For white tuna specifically, or albacore, no more than 6 ounces per week should be consumed [26]. The following seafood should never be consumed, even in small amounts: tilefish, shark, swordfish, marlin, orange roughy, or king mackerel [26].

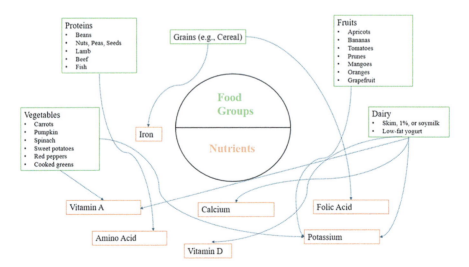

Fig. 11.1 Recommended food options and their nutrients

Acquiring any kind of disease during pregnancy can lead to complications; efforts to prevent foodborne diseases in particular should be implemented, so pregnant people should avoid eating foods that may contain germs, foods such as refrigerated meat spreads, unpasteurized juices, raw milk, or cheeses or unwashed fruits and vegetables [26, 30]. Finally, pregnant people should avoid consuming more than 200 milligrams of caffeine per day, which usually equates to about three glasses of a caffeinated beverage.

Special Requirements for High-Risk Pregnancies

Pregnant people should incorporate several additional nutritional considerations into their diet if they have a high-risk pregnancy. Box 11.2 describes some of the common conditions that may increase the chances for a high-risk pregnancy.

Box 11.2 Common Conditions Related to High-Risk Pregnancies
Anemia

Pregnant people who have anemia, which is a condition that does not enable to body to produce enough red blood cells in the body, may be at increased risk for maternal mortality and morbidity; anemia may also diminish a pregnant person's productivity because that may lead to less red blood cell support for oxygen to be transported to the body's tissues [1].

Overweight or obesity

Being overweight or obese, or having excess weight, during pregnancy can place pregnant people at greater risk for several pregnancy and childbirth-related complications, such as high blood pressure, pre-eclampsia, preterm birth, and gestational diabetes [10, 13, 33]. Obesity, specifically, can further increase pregnant people's risk of birth injury, cesarean birth, or birth defects [10]. Infants that are born to obese mothers may further have an increased risk of chronic conditions such as obesity [34, 35], diabetes [36], asthma [34], cardiovascular disease [37], and altered brain development [38]. Recent data have suggested that over 300 million reproductive-age women are obese due to factors such as access to energy-dense and nutrient-poor foods, and sedentary lifestyles [13, 39, 40]. Those who are overweight or obese should develop both a nutrition plan and an exercise plan, in consultation with their medical provider, for prevention of these conditions during their pregnancy [2, 10]. Physical activity is particularly important both before and during pregnancy for maintaining a healthy body mass index and in achieving positive pregnancy outcomes, which include a decreased risk of preterm birth and reduced chances of having children with low birth weight [2].

(continued)

Gestational diabetes

Gestational diabetes is a condition where glucose tolerance is impaired in a pregnant person; this condition increases the risk of complications such as microsomes, which make the infant larger than normal, or hypoglycemia. Pregnant people have to closely monitor their blood glucose levels, follow a controlled carbohydrate diet, and possibly take insulin if prescribed. One study found that a higher intake of sugary beverages during pregnancy was associated with higher glycemic results on the test for glucose tolerance [41].

Nutrition Therapy During Breastfeeding and Lactation

After childbirth, a mother enters into a lactation period during which time their body produces milk that can be fed to their child through breastfeeding. Mothers who choose to breastfeed should continue to maintain a healthy and nutrient-rich diet during this lactation period so that those nutrients can be passed on to the child as a continued effort to ensure child development [42]. When mothers are breastfeeding, those nutrients promote growth and overall health for their baby [43].

Calorie Intake

That mothers continue to consume more calories than they did before pregnancy—about 330 to 400 more calories per day—is normal for their body to produce enough milk to feed their baby [43]. The Mayo Clinic recommends that these calories be obtained from nutrient-rich food options such as whole-grain bread with one tablespoon of peanut butter (16 g), a medium apple or banana, and 8 ounces of yogurt (2022). The actual amount of additional calories that are needed during the breastfeeding period will also depend on other factors, such as the mother's age, body mass index, and physical activity level [44].

Suggested Food and Nutrient Options While Breastfeeding

The main goal when selecting nutrient-rich options during lactation is to consume foods that are high in energy in order to fuel milk production and to consume a variety of foods so that the flavor of breast milk will change accordingly [43]. This will not only expose the baby to different types of flavors, but will also help ensure that the baby can more easily adapt to eating solid foods later in their development. Recommended foods include those that are rich in protein, such as meat, beans, lentils, and eggs. Although seafood can be added to this list, the seafood product must continue to be low in mercury [43, 44]. Additionally, mothers who are breast-feeding can also eat a variety of whole-grain foods such as bread, fruits, and vegetables. Finally, mothers should ensure they are continuing to take their vitamin and mineral supplements but only with medical provider consultation [43], to avoid toxicity from exceeding the amount of iron or folic acid that is needed for a mother who is no longer pregnant but is breastfeeding [44].

The Centers for Disease Control and Prevention (CDC) states that mothers need an increased amount of iodine and chlorine during lactation [44], especially because breast milk is the only source from which the newborn will be able to consume these nutrients [29]. Specifically, mothers are recommended to take 290 micrograms of iodine and 550 milligrams of chlorine daily for the entire first year after giving birth [44]. Some of the foods mentioned above will support mothers during lactation to meet these nutrient goals, such as consuming eggs and seafood; however, iodine and chlorine can also be found in dairy products, iodine can be found in iodized table salt, and chlorine in specific can be found in meats, beans, peas, and lentils [44].

Recommended Fluid Intake

Mothers who are breastfeeding are encouraged to self-monitor their urine color to determine whether they need to increase fluid intake. Generally, more fluids should be consumed if the color of the urine appears dark yellow [43]. Also, mothers are recommended to drink at least one additional glass of water or some other beverage after every breastfeeding session with their baby [43]. Although mothers are generally free to select any beverage besides water that they want to consume after breast-feeding, they should be wary of beverages with high sugar content because sugar can contribute not only to weight gain [43] but also to the onset of other chronic conditions, such as diabetes. Lastly, mothers should be conscientious about their daily caffeine intake and limit themselves to three glasses of a caffeinated beverage a day to avoid agitating their baby or interfering with their sleep schedule [43, 44]. Common caffeinated beverages include coffee, soda, energy drinks, and tea [44].

Food and Drinks to Avoid

Mothers should continue to avoid alcohol during the lactation period if they are breastfeeding [43]. However, some levels of alcohol can be consumed with caution as alcohol typically takes about 3 h to clear out of breast milk for a typical 12 oz glass of beer, wine, or other liquor. This will also depend largely on the mother's weight, so consulting with a medical provider continues to be important to ensure that alcohol is not passing through breast milk to the baby [43]. One strategy to avoid any risk of alcohol transmission to the baby is to pump milk before consuming alcohol and store it away for feeding [43]. As discussed before, no more than three glasses of a caffeinated beverage should be consumed while breastfeeding, to avoid agitating the baby or interfering with their sleep pattern [43, 44]. Finally, even though seafood can have a number of essential nutrients such as omega-3 fatty acids, mothers should take caution to minimize their consumptions of seafood high in mercury [43, 44] to avoid potential brain and nervous system problems for both themselves and their baby. Throughout the breastfeeding period, overall, mothers should monitor their baby to look for signs of any agitations, allergic reactions, or other adverse effects, such as diarrhea, rash, or wheezing, after feeding [43]. Even if the mother maintains a nutrient-rich and recommended diet during lactation, the baby could be allergic to some ingredients, or the nutrients may not otherwise suit their gut microbiome [43].

Special Guidelines for Mothers Following Vegan or Vegetarian Diets

Generally, individuals that maintain a vegan or vegetarian diet may be at risk for becoming nutrient deficient, especially in vitamin B_{12} and iron. Mothers should take steps to ensure that they select foods high in iron such as cereal, peas, dry fruit, and raisins [43]. As discussed previously, pairing these foods with other foods that are high in vitamin C, such as lemons and tangerines, can facilitate iron absorption [43]. Low levels of vitamin B_{12} for both breastfeeding women and their child can be harmful to their health; for the infant in particular, it can place them at a greater risk of neurological damage [44]. For this reason, mothers should consult their medical provider to determine whether nutrient supplements for iron, vitamin B_{12}, and other nutrients may be recommended for them [43, 44].

Contraindications to Breastfeeding

Even though all mothers will be in a lactation period after childbirth, breastfeeding their child may not always be advisable for them, and they should therefore make sure to have open communication with their medical provider on the best feeding option for their newborn. In general, a mother should not breastfeed their baby if the baby is diagnosed with a rare genetic metabolic disorder that can affect feeding, if the baby has galactosemia, if the mother has HIV and is either currently not on treatment or has not been taking treatment long enough to suppress the virus, if the mother is taking any illicit drug or are consuming alcohol, or if the mother is suspected to have Ebola virus disease [44]. There may also be other circumstances for which mothers should not breastfeed, such as temporarily acquiring an infection like chickenpox, mpox, or herpes virus with sores visible on the breast; if they are taking certain medications; or if they have untreated, active tuberculosis [44]. Finally, even though much research indicates that breastfeeding alone can be sufficient as an infant's only food source during their first 6 months of life [45], if breastfeeding mothers are not consuming the appropriate nutrients during this period or if they have an infant who is at risk of osteopenia, then they should consider taking additional supplements to augment their breastfeeding diet as an approach to prevention [46].

Barriers and Challenges to Healthy Nutrition During Pregnancy

From a public health perspective, pregnant people may face barriers and challenges to healthy nutrition during pregnancy, many of which will be unique to social determinants that surround them. Research has found that in the United States, almost 11% of all households were food insecure and disparities exist in how healthy food is distributed across society [47]; *food insecurity* is defined as having limited or uncertain access to adequate food [48]. Low-income, racial and ethnic minorities, and single-parent homes are more likely to experience food insecurity than their counterparts are [48]. Geographically, certain regions, such as rural areas and deserts, may have a reduced availability of healthy food options where individuals can readily access healthier options [48]. Identifying these barriers and implementing public health interventions are important for promoting consistency and the maintenance of a nutrient-rich diet among mothers in order to achieve positive maternal health outcomes.

The United Nations Children's Fund (UNICEF) releases their strategic plan for nutrition every 10 years; this plan includes their Conceptual Framework on the Determinants of Maternal and Child Nutrition [49]. Their most recent framework uses a systems thinking model to recommend that experts should first identify enabling determinants for maternal and child nutrition, which may include governing factors such as political, financial, social, and public actions that influence outcomes. These enabling factors also include resources, such as having access to environmental, financial, and human resources, and norms, such as positive actions that facilitate positive nutritional outcomes. After these enabling factors have been identified, the underlying determinants need to be understood, determinants such as food, practices, and services, which comprise a combination of the availability of nutrient-rich food, adherence to recommended dietary practices, and support services that work together to facilitate positive maternal and child nutritional outcomes. Collectively, these factors can address barriers to healthy nutrition, facilitate the development and implementation of interventions that foster healthy diets, and promote an overall self-care system that can be integrated into one's routine and daily lifestyle.

Educational Initiatives and Strategies for Future Directions

Research suggests that many women do not have sufficient knowledge of healthy nutrition during pregnancy [50], where some may even have formed their beliefs on the basis of popular practices [45]. Abdalla and colleagues conducted a study among

468 pregnant people in Egypt, where they administered a questionnaire to test their nutritional knowledge. The results suggested that even though a majority of participants were able to correctly identify breast milk as the only food that a baby requires during the first 6 months of its life, only 20% were aware of the harmful effects of caffeine during pregnancy, especially its role in provoking premature birth [45]. The commonly reported knowledge sources among participants included friends and family (60%) and doctors or previous educational institutions (45%) [45]. When stratifying according to family income levels, women with more higher income levels had higher knowledge scores compared to those with lower income levels. Alehegn and colleagues (2021) also found similar results in their qualitative study, where participants stated not receiving adequate maternal nutrition despite recognizing the importance of receiving counseling provided by nutritionists [50], a finding consistent with other studies [51, 52].

Among healthcare practitioners, the major identified barrier to providing adequate nutritional counseling among their patients was a shortage of clinic time. Staying up to date on the most current nutritional information and preparing their educational content ahead of time were contributing factors that led to inadequate counseling provided during the time of the visit between the mother and nutrition experts [50]. Other gaps included specifically providing counseling on expected weight gain during pregnancy and offering different platforms for counseling in general [52]. However, even receiving nutritional information through counseling sessions can be perceived as overwhelming among some women [53], where there may be more of a preference to conduct an online search for information on a case-by-case basis when needed and to rely on their intuition when making dietary decisions as opposed to being attentive when this information is provided more comprehensively during a visit with their healthcare provider [53].

Personal and cultural beliefs are also important factors in determining whether women have the correct nutritional knowledge or whether their knowledge may be informed by misbeliefs, such as through the practice of food taboos [54, 55]. Food taboos are recognized as one of the major factors contributing to maternal undernutrition during pregnancy [54, 55]. In a community-based study, Acire and colleagues (2023) found that cultural dictates, individual characteristics, and societal norms were major reasons why many food taboos and misconceptions were being followed [54]. During pregnancy, there was also the common belief that women are not to engage in certain behaviors such as shaving their hair, having sex, or touching needles [54]. These findings demonstrate a need to ensure that educational campaigns are tailored to address misconceptions, misinformation, and taboos that may be rooted in cultural traditions [55]. Another factor is maternal literacy [18], where research findings that represented more than 500 pregnant people demonstrate that low birth weight is associated with maternal illiteracy and low income.

Education is important to promote maternal nutrition both during pregnancy and after delivery during the breastfeeding period in order to ensure that the newborn child(ren) receive(s) proper nutrition for their development. Admasu and colleagues (2022) conducted a study to understand the impact of maternal nutrition education on the early initiation of breastfeeding among 310 pregnant people in Hawaii [56]. Their findings indicated that breastfeeding practice was significantly higher among pregnant people that received education compared to those that did not. This indicates that providing sustained education to pregnant people could lead to optimal breastfeeding outcomes among new mothers [56]. In all phases of pregnancy, tailoring educational initiatives to meet the unique needs of pregnant people becomes crucial, where, especially in underdeveloped regions and among low-income populations, offering unconditional cash incentives can facilitate the uptake of recommended nutritional behaviors during pregnancy [57].

Several approaches are available to increase healthy nutrient consumption during pregnancy, such as making dietary modifications, taking supplements like prenatal vitamins, meal planning, and reinforcing the importance of consuming healthy foods [1]. Several organizations have recommended educational strategies to reinforce the importance of these approaches to promote maternal health. These recommendations take into consideration past successful programs such as the Women, Infants, and Children (WIC) special supplemental nutrition program in the United States, which has been known to be associated with a lower risk of stillbirth among pregnant people that participate [58]. The following subsections describe some of these approaches.

Building Community Health Worker Capacity

Community health workers (CHWs) work to establish relationships with underserved or priority populations, provide education and resources, and facilitate access to and the uptake of healthy behaviors. In the context of maternal nutrition, these relationships can play instrumental roles in educating and counseling mothers to promote behavior change as a way to be more proactive about consuming recommended nutrients and supplements during pregnancy, recognizing and treating comorbid conditions, engaging in conversations about family planning, and maintaining a stable connection with their medical provider during all stages of pregnancy [1]. CHWs can also collaborate with other organizations, especially those involved in policymaking, to advocate for policies and strategies that address structural reasons for poor maternal nutrition [1]. Enhancing community health worker activities through the use of mobile or other technological devices can improve reproductive, maternal, newborn, and child health and nutrition services, especially in under-resourced or difficult-to-reach settings [59].

Engaging the Entire Household, Including the Partners of Pregnant People

Any one person is fully responsible for their health because of the relationship between underlying factors that may play a role in influencing their decisions, including social and environmental factors like culture, beliefs, values, religion, community norms, and gender-based policies. For this reason, educational initiatives should also consider engaging the immediate family members of pregnant people, especially their partners, to normalize and encourage discussions around sexuality, family planning, and nutritional practices in the entire household [1]. In one study, a questionnaire was administered among 84 households to solicit data on maternal diet and breastfeeding practices, and the researchers found that partners were left out of breastfeeding and dietary decision-making; however, contrary to these practices, paternal inclusion was recommended in this decision-making process to improve maternal and child health outcomes [60].

Creating Support Groups

Even within mothers' support systems, such as their immediate household or with their partners, mothers may not always feel comfortable discussing sensitive topics such as body changes during pregnancy, physical or mental pain, challenges that they may be experiencing, psychological changes that influence their confidence and self-esteem, and changes in their sexual needs and desires during pregnancy [1]. Therefore, the creation of mothers-only support groups can be empowering for mothers because they can be part of a community that encourages the uptake of optimal health choices during pregnancy [1, 61]. For these groups to be effective, however, the facilitators and barriers to utilization must be understood, especially because data show that only 27% of reproductive-age women participate in such groups [62]. Acharya and colleagues performed a mixed-methods study among 1000 women and their family members, who participated in in-depth interviews and focus group discussions to understand the reasons for participating in groups for mothers, and they found that highest level of educational attainment was strongly associated with participation [62]. They also found that participation was connected to women's interests in learning something new, women's awareness of the meeting schedule and location, and their level of engagement with staff and workers from healthcare organizations [62]. Further, mentoring relationships that are formed within programs like these among pregnant people are known to yield favorable outcomes for fetal growth and neonatal birth weight; in one study, women that participated in a mentoring program had a significantly higher weight-for-length score for their newborns [2].

Organizing a Nutrition Campaign

Southern Oregon launched a nutrition campaign that brought together community and organizational leaders to implement strategies to improve birth outcomes [11]. This campaign included the development of educational resources and training curricula for CHWs and healthcare providers. This campaign ensures that all resources and materials are tailored to meet the cultural needs of people of childbearing age not only to increase engagement but also to facilitate access to and retention in reproductive care [11]. Strategies like these can also help promote diet diversity during pregnancy [61], which can provide a range of healthy options for mothers from different cultural backgrounds and traditions.

Promoting Meal Planning

Public health and nutrition practitioners can encourage pregnant people to use the tools available for meal planning. One such tool is the MyPlate food-planning guide made available by the United States Department of Agriculture [10, 63]. This tool helps individuals learn how to make healthy food choices for every meal and even offers personalized meal plans to meet each person's unique needs, such as by taking into account their height, prepregnancy weight level, and current physical activity level [10]. The use of technology can also facilitate the personalization of nutritional goals for each individual to ensure a healthy pregnancy, prevent fetal developmental issues, and reduce the chances for noncommunicable diseases later in life [20]. Smartphone apps, in particular, have been commonly used in pregnancy to positively impact lifestyle behaviors [64]. This tool is also an excellent way for individuals to become more informed and knowledgeable about the healthy food options that are available to them.

UNICEF further recommends tangible key action steps for future direction that public health and nutrition practitioners can take to improve maternal nutrition [65]. These include establishing a governance system that comprises of leaders who not only make data-driven recommendations on strengthening policies and programs but also play integral roles in mobilizing institutions and other resources to improve maternal nutrition; establishing policies that protect people from consuming unhealthy foods and beverages and instead institute efforts to improve access to healthy and affordable nutrient-rich foods; using multiple communication strategies to raise awareness about resources that are available to improve maternal nutrition; and eliminating gender norms within communities where girls and women do not currently realize their rights to healthy food [65].

Conclusion

Maternal nutrition is important to ensure the health of both the mother and the baby during all pregnancy stages, including the conception, antenatal, and postnatal periods. Pregnant people are encouraged to consume the essential and recommended nutrients for a healthy pregnancy and fetal growth and development. Pregnant people are recommended to partner with a medical provider who can provide them with guidance throughout their pregnancy and during the 6 month period after giving birth to ensure the health of their newborn. Mothers to be and pregnant people are also encouraged to engage in educational initiatives to stay informed on up-to-date nutritional guidelines and to prevent misinformation, as well as involve their family members in decision-making when appropriate.

Further Practice

1. _____ is an essential nutrient that is responsible for the development of red blood cells that supply oxygen to the fetus.

   a. Iron
   b. Vitamin B$_{12}$
   c. Vitamin D
   d. Folic acid

2. _____ is a vitamin that, when paired with iron, can help increase the absorption of iron.

   a. Calcium
   b. Folic acid
   c. Vitamin B$_{12}$
   d. Vitamin C

3. Which of the following foods or drinks should never be consumed while pregnant?

   a. Seafood
   b. Coffee
   c. Alcohol
   d. Red meat

4. Which of the following conditions increases the risk of maternal mortality and morbidity by resulting in the significant loss of red blood cells?

   a. Hyperemesis
   b. Anemia
   c. Gestational diabetes
   d. Phenylketonuria

5. Why is it important to continue consuming an increased number of calories during the lactation period after delivery?

   a. It is needed for breast milk production.
   b. It is needed to ensure that the body does not experience a drastic change in weight.
   c. It is needed to ensure that the mother does not experience postpartum depression.
   d. All of the above are true.

6. Mothers are recommended to drink one additional glass of water or another beverage immediately after each breastfeeding session to maintain their recommended daily fluid intake.

   a. True
   b. False

7. _____ is a public health intervention that serves as a community forum for current and future mothers to feel empowered to discuss sensitive topics such as body changes during pregnancy and how to increase healthy nutrient consumption.

   a. Support groups
   b. Community health workers
   c. Town halls and listening sessions
   d. Educational campaign with household members

8. Which of the following is true?

   a. Fish caught from local waters typically contain high levels of mercury and are not recommended for consumption during pregnancy.
   b. Omega-3 fatty acids contain healthy fats from certain fish but should not be consumed during pregnancy, because they contain high levels of mercury.
   c. Vitamin C is a vitamin that, when taken with calcium, can improve the body's absorption of calcium.
   d. Folic acid is part of the D vitamin family and can promote healthy brain or spinal cord development for the fetus.

9. When it comes to weight gain during pregnancy, a woman should generally aim to "eat for two" in order to gain enough weight to support both herself and her child.

   a. True
   b. False

10. How many grams of protein is a pregnant person encouraged to consume per day?

    a. 50
    b. 60
    c. 70
    d. 80

11. How much water should a pregnant person consume per day?

    a. 6–8 cups
    b. 7–9 cups
    c. 8–10 cups
    d. 9–11 cups

12. _____ is a condition during which glucose tolerance is impaired in a pregnant person and that may increase the risk of birth-related complications such as developing hypoglycemia.

    a. Gestational diabetes
    b. Anemia
    c. Obesity
    d. Hyperemesis

Critical Thinking Short-Answer Questions

1. One of your close friends recently informed you that they are 3 weeks pregnant, and they are asking you, as someone who has studied maternal nutrition, for advice on what to do to maintain healthy nutrition during pregnancy. What are three suggestions you would give to your friend and why?
2. If you were working with a team on designing an educational campaign to promote nutrition awareness among those of childbearing age, what would your key messages be and why? Please discuss three to five key messages.
3. Think about the community that you are involved in currently—a community can be considered your local neighborhood, city, or county location, your racial or ethnic group, or some other group that shares a similar value or belief as you. What unique challenges do you think pregnant people in your identified community may face in ensuring a healthy pregnancy? Identify three to five challenges and discuss why they are unique to your community and what strategies you would suggest to overcome those challenges.

Practice Test Answer Key

1. a
2. d
3. c
4. b
5. a
6. a
7. a
8. a
9. b
10. b
11. c
12. a

References

1. CARE USA, & DiGirolamo A. Maternal nutrition & maternal and child health [Program brief]. Cooperative for Assistance and Relief Everywhere, Inc. (CARE). 2013. https://www.care.org/wp-content/uploads/2020/06/MH-2013-Maternal-Nutrition-Maternal-and-Child-Health.pdf
2. Apostolopoulou A, Tranidou A, Tsakiridis I, Magriplis E, Dagklis T, Chourdakis M. Effects of nutrition on maternal health, fetal development, and perinatal outcomes. Nutrients. 2024;16(3):375. https://doi.org/10.3390/nu16030375.
3. de Rooij SR, Wouters H, Yonker JE, Painter RC, Roseboom TJ. Prenatal undernutrition and cognitive function in late adulthood. Proc Natl Acad Sci U S A. 2010;107(39):16881–6. https://doi.org/10.1073/pnas.1009459107. Epub 2010 Sep 13. PMID: 20837515; PMCID: PMC2947913
4. Torres N, Bautista CJ, Tovar AR, Ordáz G, Rodríguez-Cruz M, Ortiz V, Granados O, Nathanielsz PW, Larrea F, Zambrano E. Protein restriction during pregnancy affects maternal liver lipid metabolism and fetal brain lipid composition in the rat. Am J Physiol Endocrinol

Metab. 2010;298(2):E270–7. https://doi.org/10.1152/ajpendo.00437.2009. Epub 2009 Nov 17. PMID: 19920218; PMCID: PMC2822484

5. Mathur P, Pillai R. Overnutrition: current scenario & combat strategies. Indian J Med Res. 2019;149(6):695–705. https://doi.org/10.4103/ijmr.IJMR_1703_18. PMID: 31496522; PMCID: PMC6755771

6. Godfrey KM, Reynolds RM, Prescott SL, Nyirenda M, Jaddoe VW, Eriksson JG, Broekman BF. Influence of maternal obesity on the long-term health of offspring. Lancet Diabetes Endocrinol. 2017;5(1):53–64. https://doi.org/10.1016/S2213-8587(16)30107-3. Epub 2016 Oct 12. PMID: 27743978; PMCID: PMC5245733

7. Antony AC, Vora RM, Karmarkar SJ. The silent tragic reality of hidden hunger, anaemia, and neural-tube defects (NTDs) in India. Lancet Reg Health-Southeast Asia. 2022;6:100071.

8. Hsu CN, Tain YL. The first thousand days: kidney health and beyond. Healthcare (Basel). 2021;9(10):1332. https://doi.org/10.3390/healthcare9101332. PMID: 34683012; PMCID: PMC8544398

9. Cortés-Albornoz MC, García-Guáqueta DP, Velez-Van-Meerbeke A, Talero-Gutiérrez C. Maternal nutrition and neurodevelopment: a scoping review. Nutrients. 2021;13(10):3530. https://doi.org/10.3390/nu13103530.

10. Nutrition during pregnancy. ACOG. 2024. https://www.acog.org/womens-health/faqs/nutrition-during-pregnancy

11. Nutrition Before Pregnancy is Critical for Fetal Development and Lifelong Health | OHSU. 2024. https://www.ohsu.edu/school-of-medicine/moore-institute/nutrition-pregnancy-critical-fetal-development-and-lifelong

12. Koletzko B, Godfrey KM, Poston L, Szajewska H, van Goudoever JB, de Waard M, Brands B, Grivell RM, Deussen AR, Dodd JM, Patro-Golab B, Zalewski BM, Early Nutrition Project Systematic Review Group. Nutrition during pregnancy, lactation and early childhood and its implications for maternal and long-term child health: the early nutrition project recommendations. Ann Nutr Metab. 2019;74(2):93–106. https://doi.org/10.1159/000496471. Epub 2019 Jan 23. PMID: 30673669; PMCID: PMC6397768

13. Barrientos G, Ronchi F, Conrad ML. Nutrition during pregnancy: influence on the gut microbiome and fetal development. Am J Reprod Immunol. 2023;91(1):e13802. https://doi.org/10.1111/aji.13802.

14. Hales CN, Barker DJ. Type 2 (non-insulin-dependent) diabetes mellitus: the thrifty phenotype hypothesis. Diabetologia. 1992 Jul;35(7):595–601. https://doi.org/10.1007/BF00400248.

15. Marshall NE, Abrams B, Barbour LA, Catalano P, Christian P, Friedman JE, Hay WW, Hernandez TL, Krebs NF, Oken E, Purnell JQ, Roberts JM, Soltani H, Wallace J, Thornburg KL. The importance of nutrition in pregnancy and lactation: lifelong consequences. Am J Obstet Gynecol. 2022;226(5):607–32. https://doi.org/10.1016/j.ajog.2021.12.035.

16. Stephenson J, Heslehurst N, Hall J, Schoenaker D, Hutchinson J, Cade K, Poston L, Barrett G, Crozier S, Kumaran K, Yanjik C, Barker M, Baird J, Mishra G. Before the beginning: nutrition and lifestyle in the preconception period and its importance for future health. Lancet. 2018;391:1830–41. https://doi.org/10.1016/S0140-6736(18)30311-8.

17. Bazer FW, Spencer TE, Wu G, Cudd TA, Meininger CJ. Maternal nutrition and fetal development. J Nutr. 2004;134(9):2169–72. https://doi.org/10.1093/jn/134.9.2169.

18. Berhe K, Weldegerima L, Gebrearegay F, Kahsay A, Tesfahunegn A, Rejeu M, Gebremariam B. Effect of under-nutrition during pregnancy on low birth weight in Tigray regional state, Ethiopia; a prospective cohort study. BMC Nutr. 2021;7(1):72. https://doi.org/10.1186/s40795-021-00475-7.

19. Black RE, Allen LH, Bhutta ZA, et al. Maternal and child under nutrition study group. Maternal and child under nutrition: global and regional exposures and health consequences. Lancet. 2008;371:243–60.

20. Alabduljabbar S, Zaidan SA, Lakshmanan AP, Terranegra A. Personalized nutrition approach in pregnancy and early life to tackle childhood and adult non-communicable diseases. Life. 2021;11(6):467. https://doi.org/10.3390/life11060467.

21. Bangarusamy DK, Lakshmanan AP, Al-Zaidan S, Alabduljabbar S, Terranegra A. Nutri-epigenetics: the effect of maternal diet and early nutrition on the pathogenesis of autoim-

mune diseases. Minerva Pediatr (Torino). 2021 Apr;73(2):98–110. https://doi.org/10.23736/S2724-5276.20.06166-6.

22. Gohir W, Whelan FJ, Surette MG, Moore C, Schertzer JD, Sloboda DM. Pregnancy-related changes in the maternal gut microbiota are dependent upon the mother's periconceptional diet. Gut Microbes. 2015;6(5):310–20.

23. Kupka R, Mugusi F, Aboud S, et al. Randomized, double-blind, placebo-controlled trial of selenium supplements among HIV-infected pregnant women in Tanzania: effects on maternal and child outcomes. Am J Clin Nutr. 2008;87:1802.

24. de Benoist B. Conclusions of a WHO technical consultation on folate and vitamin B12 deficiencies. Food Nutr Bull. 2008;29(Suppl 2):S238–44.

25. Kovacs CS. Vitamin D in pregnancy and lactation: maternal, fetal, and neonatal outcomes from human and animal studies. Am J Clin Nutr. 2008;88:520S–8S.3.

26. National Library of Medicine. Pregnancy and nutrition. MedlinePlus. 2024. Retrieved on August 2, 2024 from https://medlineplus.gov/pregnancyandnutrition.html

27. Pregnancy diet: Focus on these essential nutrients. Mayo Clinic. 2022, February 18. https://www.mayoclinic.org/healthy-lifestyle/pregnancy-week-by-week/in-depth/pregnancy-nutrition/art-20045082

28. Adu-Afarwuah S. Impact of nutrient supplementation on maternal nutrition and child growth and development in sub-Saharan Africa: the case of small-quantity lipid-based nutrient supplements. Matern Child Nutr. 2020;16(S3):e12960. https://doi.org/10.1111/mcn.12960.

29. Hart TL, Petersen KS, Kris-Etherton PM. Nutrition recommendations for a healthy pregnancy and lactation in women with overweight and obesity – strategies for weight loss before and after pregnancy. Fertil Steril. 2022;118(3):434–46. https://doi.org/10.1016/j.fertnstert.2022.07.027.

30. Nutrition during pregnancy. Johns Hopkins Medicine. 2019, November 19. Retrieved on August 2, 2024 from https://www.hopkinsmedicine.org/health/wellness-and-prevention/nutrition-during-pregnancy

31. Billah SM, Raynes-Greenow C, Ali NB, Karim F, Lotus SU, Azad R, Sari M, Mustaphi P, Maniruzzaman M, Rahman SMM, Dibley MJ, Kelly PJ, El Arifeen S. Iron and folic acid supplementation in pregnancy: findings from the baseline assessment of a maternal nutrition service Programme in Bangladesh. Nutrients. 2022;14(15):3114. https://doi.org/10.3390/nu14153114. PMID: 35956291; PMCID: PMC9370216

32. Aoyama T, Li D, Bay JL. Weight gain and nutrition during pregnancy: an analysis of clinical practice guidelines in the Asia-Pacific region. Nutrients. 2022;14(6):1288. https://doi.org/10.3390/nu14061288. PMID: 35334946; PMCID: PMC8949332

33. Lindsay KL, Milone GF, Grobman WA, Haas DM, Mercer BM, Simhan HN, Saade GR, Silver RM, Chung JH. Periconceptional diet quality is associated with gestational diabetes risk and glucose concentrations among nulliparous gravidas. Front Endocrinol (Lausanne). 2022;13:940870. https://doi.org/10.3389/fendo.2022.940870. PMID: 36133312; PMCID: PMC9483841

34. Liu S, Zhou B, Wang Y, Wang K, Zhang Z, Niu W. Pre-pregnancy maternal weight and gestational weight gain increase the risk for childhood asthma and wheeze: an updated meta-analysis. Front Pediatr. 2020;8:134.

35. Perng W, Oken E, Dabelea D. Developmental overnutrition and obesity and type 2 diabetes in offspring. Diabetologia. 2019;62(10):1779–88.

36. Lecoutre S, Maqdasy S, Breton C. Maternal obesity as a risk factor for developing diabetes in offspring: an epigenetic point of view. World J Diabetes. 2021;12(4):366–82.

37. den Harink T, Roelofs MJM, Limpens J, Painter RC, Roseboom TJ, van Deutekom AW. Maternal obesity in pregnancy and children's cardiac function and structure: a systematic review and meta-analysis of evidence from human studies. PLoS One. 2022;17(11):e0275236.

38. Basak S, Das RK, Banerjee A, Paul S, Pathak S, Duttaroy AK. Maternal obesity and gut microbiota are associated with fetal brain development. Nutrients. 2022;14(21):4515.

39. Gonzalez-Perez G, Hicks AL, Tekieli TM, Radens CM, Williams BL, Lamouse-Smith ES. Maternal antibiotic treatment impacts development of the neonatal intestinal microbiome and antiviral immunity. J Immunol. 2016;196(9):3768–79.

40. Parrettini S, Caroli A, Torlone E. Nutrition and metabolic adaptations in physiological and complicated pregnancy: focus on obesity and gestational diabetes. Front Endocrinol. 2020;11:611929.
41. Ramakrishnan U, Grant F, Goldenberg T, Zongrone A, Martorell R. Effect of women's nutrition before and during early pregnancy on maternal and infant outcomes: a systematic review. Paediatr Perinat Epidemiol. 2012 Jul;26(Suppl 1):285–301. https://doi.org/10.1111/j.1365-30 16.2012.01281.x.
42. National Academies Press (US). Meeting maternal nutrient needs during lactation. Nutrition During Lactation - NCBI Bookshelf; 1991. https://www.ncbi.nlm.nih.gov/books/NBK235579/
43. Breastfeeding nutrition: Tips for moms. Mayo Clinic. 2022. https://www.mayoclinic.org/healthy-lifestyle/infant-and-toddler-health/in-depth/breastfeeding-nutrition/art-20046912
44. Maternal diet and breastfeeding. Breastfeeding Special Circumstances. 2024, February 9. Retrieved on August 2, 2024 from https://www.cdc.gov/breastfeeding-special-circumstances/hcp/diet-micronutrients/maternal-diet.html
45. Abdalla M, Zein MM, Sherif A, Essam B, Mahmoud H. Nutrition and diet myths, knowledge and practice during pregnancy and lactation among a sample of Egyptian pregnant women: a cross-sectional study. BMC Pregnancy Childbirth. 2024;24(1):140. https://doi.org/10.1186/s12884-024-06331-3.
46. Bijari BB, Salmeei S, Niknafs P, Jamali Z, Mousavi H, Sabzevari F, Daee Z, Bagheri MM. Osteopenia of prematurity and its maternal and nutrition-related factors among preterm infants admitted to the NICU Department of Afzalipour Medical Center. Majallah-i Dānishgāh-i ʿUlum-i Pizishkī-i Kirmān. 2023;30(6):339–43. https://doi.org/10.34172/jkmu.2023.57.
47. Herman D, Baer MT, Adams E, Cunningham-Sabo L, Duran N, Johnson D, Yakes E. Life course perspective: evidence for role of nutrition. Matern Child Health J. 2014;18:450–61. https://doi.org/10.1007/s10995-013-1280-3.
48. Hartline-Grafton H, Hassink S. Food insecurity and health: practices and policies to address food insecurity among children. Acad Pediatr. 2021;21(2):205–2010. https://doi.org/10.1016/j.acap.2020.07.006.
49. UNICEF. UNICEF Conceptual Framework on Maternal and Child Nutrition. 2020. Retrieved on August 30, 2024 from https://www.unicef.org/media/113291/file/UNICEF%20Conceptual%20Framework.pdf
50. Alehegn MA, Fanta TK, Ayalew AF. Exploring maternal nutrition counseling provided by health professionals during antenatal care follow-up: a qualitative study in Addis Ababa, Ethiopia-2019. BMC Nutr. 2021;7(1):20. https://doi.org/10.1186/s40795-021-00427-1.
51. Feyisa BR, Mulatu Y, Fentahun F, Biru B, Atlantis E. Nutrition, stress, and healthcare use during pregnancy are associated with low birth weight: evidence from a case–control study in West Ethiopia. Front Public Health. 2023;11:1213291. https://doi.org/10.3389/fpubh.2023.1213291.
52. Kavle JA. Strengthening maternal nutrition counselling during routine health services: a gap analysis to guide country programmes. Public Health Nutr. 2022;26:363. https://doi.org/10.1017/S1368980022002129. Epub ahead of print
53. Daigle Millan K, Poccia S, Fung TT. Information seeking behaviors, attitudes, and beliefs about pregnancy-related nutrition and supplementation: a qualitative study among US women. Nutr Health. 2022;28(4):563–9. https://doi.org/10.1177/02601060211038842. Epub 2021 Dec 21
54. Acire PV, Bagonza A, Opiri N. The misbeliefs and food taboos during pregnancy and early infancy: a pitfall to attaining adequate maternal and child nutrition outcomes among the rural Acholi communities in northern Uganda. BMC Nutr. 2023;9(1):126. https://doi.org/10.1186/s40795-023-00789-8.
55. Bhanbhro S, Kamal T, Diyo RW, Lipoeto NI, Soltani H. Factors affecting maternal nutrition and health: a qualitative study in a matrilineal community in Indonesia. PLoS One. 2020;15(6):e0234545. https://doi.org/10.1371/journal.pone.0234545.
56. Admasu J, Egata G, Bassore DG, Feleke FW. Effect of maternal nutrition education on early initiation and exclusive breast-feeding practices in South Ethiopia: a cluster randomised control trial. J Nutr Sci. 2022;11:e37. https://doi.org/10.1017/jns.2022.36.

57. Huda TM, Alam A, Tahsina T, Hasan MM, Khan J, Rahman MM, Siddique AB, Arifeen SE, Dibley MJ. Mobile-based nutrition counseling and unconditional cash transfers for improving maternal and child nutrition in Bangladesh: pilot study. JMIR Mhealth Uhealth. 2018;6(7):e156. https://doi.org/10.2196/mhealth.8832. PMID: 30021707; PMCID: PMC6070725

58. Angley M, Thorsten VR, Drews-Botsch C, Dudley DJ, Goldenberg RL, Silver RM, Stoll BJ, Pinar H, Hogue CJR. Association of participation in a supplemental nutrition program with stillbirth by race, ethnicity, and maternal characteristics. BMC Pregnancy Childbirth. 2018;18(1):306. https://doi.org/10.1186/s12884-018-1920-0.

59. Carmichael SL, Mehta K, Srikantiah S, Mahapatra T, Chaudhuri I, Balakrishnan R, Chaturvedi S, Raheel H, Borkum E, Trehan S, Weng Y, Kaimal R, Sivasankaran A, Sridharan S, Rotz D, Tarigopula UK, Bhattacharya D, Atmavilas Y, Pepper KT, Rangarajan A, Darmstadt GL, Ananya Study Group*. Use of mobile technology by frontline health workers to promote reproductive, maternal, newborn and child health and nutrition: a cluster randomized controlled trial in Bihar, India. J Glob Health. 2019;9(2):0204249. https://doi.org/10.7189/jogh.09.020424. PMID: 31788233; PMCID: PMC6875677

60. Chakona G. Social circumstances and cultural beliefs influence maternal nutrition, breastfeeding and child feeding practices in South Africa. Nutr J. 2020;19(1):47. https://doi.org/10.1186/s12937-020-00566-4.

61. Canada LG. Influence of Nutrition Knowledge on the Association between Maternal Nutrition and Birth Outcomes. 2023. www.academia.edu. https://www.academia.edu/102941154/Influence_of_Nutrition_Knowledge_on_the_Association_between_Maternal_Nutrition_and_Birth_Outcomes

62. Acharya A, Chang C, Chen M, Weissman A. Facilitators and barriers to participation in health mothers' groups in improving maternal and child health and nutrition in Nepal : a mixed-methods study. BMC Public Health. 2022;22(1):1660. https://doi.org/10.1186/s12889-022-13859-6.

63. MyPlate | U.S. Department of Agriculture. n.d.. https://www.myplate.gov/

64. Brown HM, Bucher T, Collins CE, Rollo ME. A review of pregnancy iPhone apps assessing their quality, inclusion of behaviour change techniques, and nutrition information. Matern Child Nutr. 2019;15(3):e12768. https://doi.org/10.1111/mcn.12768. Epub 2019 Feb 6. PMID: 30569549; PMCID: PMC7650606

65. UNICEF. Maternal nutrition: Preventing malnutrition in pregnant and breastfeeding women. 2010. Retrieved on August 2, 2024 from https://www.unicef.org/nutrition/maternal

Exploring Food Label Characteristics, Accessibility, and Regulation in an Era of Technological Advancements and Shifting Consumer Needs

12

Harit Agroia (ORCID)

Learning Objectives

After completion of this chapter, students will be able to

1. Understand the concept of food labeling and its relevance for consumer informed dietary decision-making
2. Identify major policies that serve to regulate food labels, including policy implementation, enforcement, and challenges to implementation
3. Apply a systems framework to understand the public health impact of the corporate role in transparent food labeling
4. Understand the triadic relationship between consumers' personal, cognitive, social, environmental, and behavioral factors that play roles in facilitating consumer food-purchasing behavior
5. Become familiar with educational initiatives, including technology-based interventions, which are designed to improve consumer accessibility to food label information

---

Introduction

A substantial intersection exists between food labeling, nutrition, and public health sciences. Although diet-related diseases such as diabetes, hypertension, and obesity can affect anyone, notable disparities in disease morbidity and mortality have been observed among vulnerable populations, such as those with lower socioeconomic

H. Agroia (✉)
San Jose State University, San Jose, CA, USA

© The Author(s), under exclusive license to Springer Nature
Switzerland AG 2025
A. K. Mitra, D. Vanoh (eds.), *Essentials of Clinical and Public Health Nutrition*,
Nutrition and Health, https://doi.org/10.1007/978-3-031-95373-6_12

status, who may face limited food options, face food insecurity, or have lower rates of health literacy. Those who seldom monitor their nutrition and dietary patterns and can easily access a vast number of options available for the same food product may be less likely to refer to food labels. An adequate understanding of food labels and their characteristics can help improve consumer dietary decision-making. This includes an understanding of the current landscape of food label policy regulations and the responsibility of corporations in promoting transparency in food labeling. Moreover, consumer preferences in receiving food label information, especially food-processing information such as organic or gluten-free foods, or foods that contain clear allergen information, are evolving with time. These factors and shifts collectively present opportunities to identify current gaps in food-labeling policies and strategies that can inform future directions. In a new age of technology, the use of smartphone applications and other digital forms of information-sharing about food labels can raise awareness and increase knowledge and accessibility to food label information among consumers.

The Concept and Relevance of Food Labeling

Food labels are commonly found on the back, front, or side of food packaging; their purpose is to provide the consumer with a snapshot of the main ingredients that can be found in the food product. These ingredients can include basic nutritional information such as the number or amount of carbohydrates, calories, sugar, sodium, fiber, protein, and vitamins included in the product [1]. Research shows that although most people refer to food labels when grocery shopping, the nutritional information that they seek on the label varies greatly [2]. For example, if a consumer is interested in purchasing a box of cereal, they may consider how much sugar, fiber, or vitamin content was added to the cereal to decide whether to purchase it. Depending on individual dietary preferences or health needs, consumers may place greater value on certain ingredients when deciding to purchase a particular food item. A person who is looking to increase their fiber intake for health reasons may select a cereal that is high in fiber; a person who is looking to reduce their sugar intake for health reasons may select the cereal with the lowest amount of added sugar. A questionnaire administered through Facebook between January and March 2016 revealed that people in younger age groups who are in the process of obtaining or have obtained higher education are more likely to refer to food labels when shopping for weekly groceries [2]; however, these individuals may place greater importance on the overall quality of the item according to customer reviews of the food product instead of the nutritional ingredients within it when deciding which product to purchase. Among those consumers that read food labels, research shows that 60% of them refer to its sugar content to assess the product's level of healthiness [3]. Overall, women, older adults, educated individuals, and obese individuals are found to more commonly refer to food labels [4]. The primary reason why some individuals do not refer to food labels ingredients is because of their limited understanding of food labels [2, 5].

Food Labeling, Public Health, and the Prevention of Diet-Related Diseases

Food labeling can play a significant role in preventing diet-related diseases, many of which are driven by the consumption of food products that are high in salt, sodium, fat, and overall calories. Approximately 75% of Americans do not consume the Federal Food Drug Administration (FDA)'s recommended levels of fruits, vegetables, or dairy; 63% exceed the recommended level of added sugar, and 77% exceed the limits for saturated fat [6]. The consumption of sodium is of particular importance given that 90% of Americans exceed the chronic disease reduction limits of sodium intake [6]. These dietary patterns place many Americans at a heightened risk of chronic diseases, which may further impact their quality of life. Cardiovascular diseases, in particular, can be prevented by choosing heart-healthy foods such as fruits and vegetables and by avoiding foods that contain added sugars and saturated fats [7]. To prevent hypertension, a consumer may select foods that are lower in sodium and cholesterol [7]. In a study conducted in university dining facilities, sales data on prepackaged food were analyzed to compare foods that were categorized as high calorie, low calorie, high fat, or low fat. The results showed that nutrition labels can significantly reduce the purchase of high-calorie and high-fat foods [8]. Among children and adolescents in particular, rates of chronic disease, especially diabetes and childhood obesity, are rising. Educating mothers through the use of food labels can be a key determinant in decreasing these rates and improving overall health among children and adolescents.

Characteristics of Food Labels for Clear and Comprehensive Interpretation

Being able to accurately understand food labels requires an understanding of nutritional information, including the nutrition facts label, front-of-pack (FOP) labels, and label claims.

Nutrition Facts Label

On most food packages, important nutritional information is displayed on the nutrition facts label [9] (Fig. 12.1). These nutrition facts, which are often found on the back of the package, are designed to provide consumers with easy-to-interpret nutritional information that can facilitate informed decision-making. Table 12.1 provides the key nutritional information that is found on most nutrition facts labels [9].

Front-of-Pack Labels

Front-of-pack (FOP) labels are placed on the front of the food package and are designed to quickly grab consumers' attention while shopping for food [11]; most

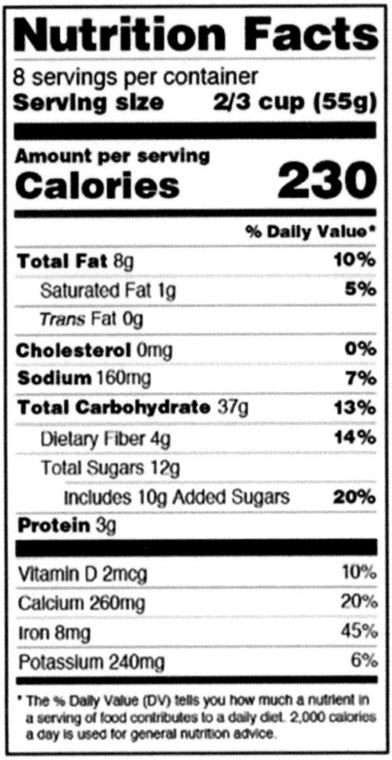

Nutrition Facts

8 servings per container

Serving size   2/3 cup (55g)

Amount per serving

Calories   230

	% Daily Value*
Total Fat 8g	**10%**
Saturated Fat 1g	**5%**
Trans Fat 0g	
Cholesterol 0mg	**0%**
Sodium 160mg	**7%**
Total Carbohydrate 37g	**13%**
Dietary Fiber 4g	**14%**
Total Sugars 12g	
Includes 10g Added Sugars	**20%**
Protein 3g	
Vitamin D 2mcg	10%
Calcium 260mg	20%
Iron 8mg	45%
Potassium 240mg	6%

* The % Daily Value (DV) tells you how much a nutrient in a serving of food contributes to a daily diet. 2,000 calories a day is used for general nutrition advice.

Fig. 12.1 Nutrition facts label [10]

consumers spend no less than a few seconds reviewing food product nutrition information prior to making a purchasing decision [12]. FOP labels are placed as complementary material on food packages to help consumers, especially those who may have less knowledge or awareness of nutritional guidelines, and are placed for consumers to identify healthy foods that can easily be incorporated into their regular eating plan; however, FOP labels should not be the only source of nutritional information on food packages [11]. In the United States, the FDA has conducted extensive research into understanding whether FOP labels would be effective prior to implementing them on food products across the nation [11]. In one study, the authors found evidence that FOP labels are noticed more often and earlier in the food-purchasing process compared to nutrition facts labels [13]. Globally, similar research has informed the implementation of FOP labels. However, significant debate remains about which FOP label designs are most effective among consumers [14]. In an 18-country analysis of the effectiveness of FOP labels, the results showed that the use of attractive color schemes on food labels increased consumer likelihood for navigating toward healthier food options and that FOP labels can be a good tool to guide the general consumer population toward food products that will benefit their health [15]. These findings are supported by other studies [15–20]. FOP labels

Table 12.1 Nutrition facts label components and their definitions

Label components	Label component definition
Serving size	The serving size is considered a reference point for consumers to understand the portion that most individuals consume of the food product; this is not a recommendation for how much of the product one should eat. This serving size is calculated by taking the average of how much of the product most people generally consume in one serving.
Serving size per container	The serving size per container provides an estimation of the number of servings, or portions, that are available in one container of the food product.
Calories (Amount per serving)	Calories refer to the amount of food energy that a consumer may get from one serving of the food product [10]. The number of calories displayed is for one serving of the food product. If a consumer has more than one serving of the product, then the number of calories that is consumed multiplies according to the number of servings that the consumer has had. The general nutrition recommendation is for adults to consume up to 2000 calories per day [9]; however, individual calorie needs per day may vary depending on several factors, such as physical activity level, age, height, and weight [10].
Calories from fat	The total calories from fat denote how many of the total calories come from fat; most of the time, the amount of total fat that is displayed on the food label is broken down into either saturated fats or trans fats. Saturated and trans fats are generally considered as unhealthy fats and can cause health issues like obesity or heart disease if consumed at high levels or beyond recommended amounts.
Cholesterol	Although cholesterol has health benefits and is a necessary component of the human diet, consuming too much of it can increase the risk of developing health issues such as heart disease or obesity. Cholesterol is included on the nutrition food label for individual consumer-monitoring purposes.
Sodium	Sodium refers to the amount of salt that was used to prepare the food product. Regularly eating foods that are high in sodium may increase consumers' risk of hypertension, kidney disease, or stroke.
Total carbohydrates	The total carbohydrates listed on the nutrition label comprise a range of healthy or unhealthy ingredients [9], which is why the nutrition label should be closely reviewed to understand the specific ingredients that comprise the total carbohydrates. Foods that contain healthy carbohydrates consist of anything that has been *unprocessed*, such as whole grains, vegetables, or beans. Foods that contain unhealthy carbohydrates consist of more *processed* ingredients, such as white bread or pastries.
Protein	Protein is important because it provides the body with energy and strength, especially the muscles, tissues, and bones [9]. These days, many consumers track their protein intake and aim to eat protein-rich foods to maintain their daily calorie targets. Eating foods with high protein can also reduce the urge to keep eating or eat a higher quantity of food throughout the day because protein can keep a person feeling full for a long period of time; however, other elements of the nutrition label should still be reviewed for sugar, total calories, carbohydrates, and other aspects to gauge how healthy the protein-rich food really is overall [9].
Vitamins and minerals	Vitamins are generally listed on nutrition labels given their ability to dissolve in the body, either through fat or water, which can be beneficial for health. Currently, food labels are required to display the levels of vitamin D, calcium, iron, and potassium due to deficiency in these vitamins among most Americans [9]. Other vitamins, such as A and C, were historically reported under FDA requirements but are only voluntarily reported now given that most Americans are maintaining minimum amounts of these nutrients in their body [10].

can also promote online purchasing behaviors among consumers who want to make healthy food choices but may not invest a large amount of time into reviewing the detailed nutrition facts [21]. In the United States, placing FOP labels on food products is completely voluntary and is therefore not closely regulated by the FDA [9]. Food corporations display FOP labels on food products in two common ways: (1) nutrient-specific labeling and (2) summary labels.

Nutrient-Specific Labels

In nutrient-specific labels, the goal is to highlight the total calorie content and the amount of select nutritional ingredients that were included in the food product, such as total fat, sugar, and sodium [19]. Nutrient-specific labels ensure that the consumer can clearly identify unhealthy ingredients in a food product. Two main types of nutrient-specific labels are used on FOP labels: (1) guideline daily amounts (GDAs) and (2) warning labels.

Guideline Daily Amounts

Guideline daily amount (GDA) labels show how much of the food product may be consumed to maintain a balanced diet [19]. The guideline ingredient amounts are usually displayed as the total per unit and/or as a percentage of the individual reference intake. For example, most adults are provided a guideline to consume a maximum of 2000 calories per day.

Warning Labels

The purpose of warning labels is to alert the consumer to ingredients that may be found in a food product that may adversely affect their health, most commonly high levels of sodium or sugar [19]. Traffic lights (TLs) or multiple traffic lights (MTLs) are two design approaches that are used to display warning labels. These two design approaches are similar to those seen on the GDA food label [19]; however, on these warning labels, color schemes become important factors that serve to draw consumers' attention and communicate the potential harmful impact of the food product that they may be considering purchasing. In Canada, more than 3500 consumers from shopping centers were surveyed, where results showed that FOPs containing warnings were effective in discouraging purchasing behavior and that, in contrast, labels that highlighted the positives of the food product encouraged purchasing behavior [18]. An eye-tracking study conducted among consumers recruited through various supermarkets, Internet platforms, and newsletters found that TL labels are more efficiently processed by consumers given the quick and friendly color-coded

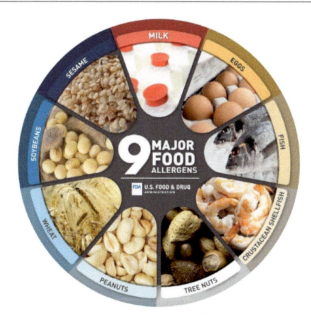

Fig. 12.2 Nine major food allergens [38]

way of communicating nutritional information on the FOP label [22]. Other studies have also shown the high performance of TL labels in influencing consumer purchasing intention [23]. General health warning statements can also be a simpler approach to convey information about other ingredients on a food label, such as allergen information [19]. These statements are usually short in text and lean into the consumers' average attention time in reading food labels when grocery shopping. The United States is among several countries that have adopted warning statements for regular use on FOPs. Nine major food allergens commonly found on these labels are depicted in Fig. 12.2.

Summary Labels

Summary labels use automated processing methods, such as algorithms, to determine whether the food product is overall healthy on the basis of the combination of ingredients used to produce the food product [19]. As a result, in contrast to nutrient-specific labels, summary labels do not focus on displaying specific ingredients that may be harmful to the consumer, because the algorithm is based on an overall assessment of the healthiness of the food product [19]. Across the globe, various methods are used to score food products to classify the products as healthy or unhealthy; Fig. 12.3 provides a summary and comparison of some of these methods.

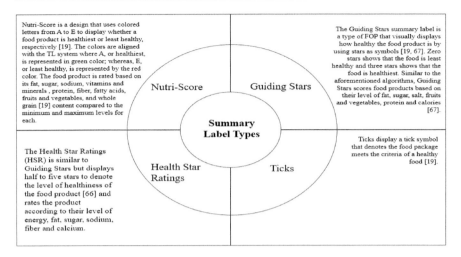

Nutri-Score is a design that uses colored letters from A to E to display whether a food product is healthiest or least healthy, respectively [19]. The colors are aligned with the TL system where A, or healthiest, is represented in green color; whereas, E, or least healthy, is represented by the red color. The food product is rated based on its fat, sugar, sodium, vitamins and minerals , protein, fiber, fatty acids, fruits and vegetables, and whole grain [19] content compared to the minimum and maximum levels for each.

The Guiding Stars summary label is a type of FOP that visually displays how healthy the food product is by using stars as symbols [19, 67]. Zero stars shows that the food is least healthy and three stars shows that the food is healthiest. Similar to the aforementioned algorithms, Guiding Stars scores food products based on their level of fat, sugar, salt, fruits and vegetables, protein and calories [67].

The Health Star Ratings (HSR) is similar to Guiding Stars but displays half to five stars to denote the level of healthiness of the food product [66] and rates the product according to their level of energy, fat, sugar, sodium, fiber and calcium.

Ticks display a tick symbol that denotes the food package meets the criteria of a healthy food [19].

Fig. 12.3 Summary label types, definitions, and examples

Label Claims

The FDA has established three main types of label claims, which include health claims, nutrient content claims, and structure/function claims [24].

> **Box 12.1 The Three Types of Label Claims**
> 1. *Health claims*: Health claims are statements that food corporations make about the food product that suggest that the ingredients can lower the risk of disease or health-related conditions [9]. These statements, based on scientific research, may be reviewed by the FDA under the Nutrition Labeling and Education Act of 1990. For example, a food corporation may make a health claim that their whole wheat bread is high in dietary fibers and can help control diabetes.
> 2. *Nutrient content claims*: Nutrient content claims are regulated by the FDA and are used to display nutritional information pertaining to specific vitamins and minerals in the food product; their overall goal is to communicate the positive attributions of the food product [9]. Examples of nutrient content claims include "high in antioxidants," "high in fiber," and "less sugar" [9].
> 3. *Structure/function claims*: Similar to health and nutrient content claims, the structure/function claims are designed to communicate the positive attributes of the food product by describing how the ingredients can improve the structure or function of the body [24]. The Dietary Supplement Health and Education Act of 1994 established regulatory requirements for the use of structure/function claims [24]. Examples include "fiber improves digestion," "contains vitamin C to build immunity," and "contains vitamin E to improve eye health."

Other Types of Food Labels

Gluten-Free Labels

The FDA estimates that more than three million people in the United States have celiac disease [25], a disease that increases the production of antibodies that attack the small intestine when a person is exposed to foods that contain gluten. The FDA ensures that products that do not contain gluten and meet the definition of *gluten-free* are appropriately labeled as "gluten-free." [25]; examples of foods that contain gluten include beer, cake, and bread.

Plant-Based Milk Alternatives

Plant-based milk alternatives (PBMAs) are options for consumers who are lactose intolerant, who are vegan, or who are not able to or do not prefer to consume regular milk as part of their diet. PBMAs are composed of nuts, such as hazelnuts, coconuts, and almonds, and seeds, such as oats, rice, and soy [26]. PBMA products also have nutrition facts labels; the FDA recommends selecting PBMAs that are high in protein, vitamin D, calcium, and potassium and low in fat and sugars [26]. In 2023, the FDA released recommendations for food corporations on including PBMA statements on products; the goal of this statement was to promote consumer transparency, an increased understanding of what ingredients makeup the PBMA product, and whether PBMA products can be seen as a healthier alternative to milk [26].

Organic Food Labels

The organic food label is widely sought out by many consumers in their commitment to preserve the environment and/or to be more health conscious [27]; this label reflects a rigorous review process conducted by the United States Department of Agriculture (USDA) to ensure that the product adheres to standards that promote ecological balance and conserves biodiversity such as through assessment of soil quality, animal raising practices, and pest and weed control [28]. The USDA strictly requires that products labeled as organic must demonstrate that they have not been produced by the use of synthetic fertilizers, sewage sludge, irradiation, and genetic engineering [28]. Despite these USDA certification and testing processes, however, some entities have questioned the reliability of the organic food label. As such, consumers may consider ensuring that their food products are purchased from reputable grocery stores, farmers markets, or direct from farms.

Clean Labels

Due to concerns for health, allergens, environmental sustainability, or lifestyle, consumers have increasingly become conscientious about selecting healthier food options [29]. This concern has increased in parallel with the development of more-industrialized countries that have overcome the long-standing problems of food insecurity among their populations, where the ability to choose one food option over another was often not feasible for many individuals and households [29]. Research shows that individuals tend to become more conscious about healthier food choices as they grow older in age [29]. Consumers have also become much more aware of technological and manufacturing advancements that may play roles in introducing harmful ingredients into food-processing systems, which can further be detrimental to health in the short or long term [29]. These harmful ingredients may include pesticides, artificial ingredients, additives, or colorants [29]. Given this shift in consumer preferences, a new consumer-driven trend in labeling emerged to differentiate healthier foods from those that are unhealthy; this label is known as the "clean label" [29]. Even though the clean label is not new, the increased use of the label is driven by the aforementioned factors. Although there is no standard definition of the label to provide clear interpretation of its use, most individuals familiar with the label consider it to be associated with a product that contains as few ingredients as possible, often fewer than five ingredients [29]. Other sources indicate that the clean label may also imply that the product is organic, natural [29], and free from additives or preservatives [30]. Overall, the degree of acceptability for a product with a clean label depends on its perceived naturalness [31].

Genetically Engineered Food Labeling

The Food, Drug, and Cosmetic Act mandates additional food labeling if the ingredients have been derived from genetically engineered (or genetically modifiable) sources [32]. In 2016, the National Bioengineered Food Disclosure Law was enacted, which created nationwide standards in the United States for labeling food products that have been genetically modified [32]. To produce genetically engineered ingredients, genetic material from one organism is inserted into the genetic code of another to create the mass production of food items [33]. In the United States, only some crops are grown through genetic modification but of those that are grown, it often constitutes a large percentage. For example, genetically modified soybeans make up 94% of all those soybeans that are planted, and most of the corn grown in the country is genetically modified.

Major Food Label Regulations

In the United States, the FDA regulates most products, except for meat and poultry; meat and poultry are regulated by the USDA Food Safety and Inspection Service [FSIS] [34]. The labels produced by both entities, including the information required on the nutrition labels, align with one another to maintain consistency. The following are major regulatory policies that have been enacted to establish and enforce food-labeling requirements.

Standards of Identity

In 1939, the FDA established its standards of identity (SOI), which aimed to promote transparent and honest dealings with food products [35]. The necessity of SOI originated from marketplace competition among multiple corporations that sold similar products and where each contained significant variations in the ingredients. For example, two companies may sell fruit pie, but the fruit pie of one company may contain significantly less fruit than the other. Establishing an SOI ensures that the same products, even when sold by different companies, maintain the same level of essential characteristics. Examples of products that have established SOIs include milk, bread, peanut butter, and ketchup [35].

Nutrition Labeling and Education Act of 1990

The Nutrition Labeling and Education Act of 1990, or NLEA, was enacted to give the FDA full authority to require nutrition labeling on most food packages [36]. This included the authority to define what specific nutritional ingredients should be reported on these labels and how these ingredients should be calculated. For example, the FDA defined what "serving sizes" should represent which was "an amount customarily consumed, and which is expressed in a common household measure that is appropriate to the food." This act was also the first to require the FDA to establish formal definitions for the different levels of nutrients, such as calories, proteins, and fats, and established FDA authority to approve health claims [36]. The Code of Federal Regulations (CFR) Title 21 provides basic requirements on how nutrition information should be displayed on food packaging, as well as food- and nutrition-labeling requirements [37]. The nutrition label had not changed for decades since NLEA's initial enactment, but in 2016, the FDA issued new requirements to update the label to better align with shifting consumer needs [10, 32]. Since the passing of this initial major law, nutrition-labeling policy has proven to be an evolving process, which makes it important for practitioners to monitor federal activity on the topic.

Food Allergen Labeling and Consumer Protection Act of 2004

The Food Allergen Labeling and Consumer Protection Act of 2004 requires that ingredients that many people are known to be allergic to be listed as a "contains" statement on the ingredients list of the food package [9]. These ingredients include milk, fish, tree nuts, peanuts, shellfish, wheat, eggs, soybeans, and sesame [9]; see Fig. 12.2. Sesame was added as an ingredient as part of the 2021 Food Allergy Safety, Treatment, Education, and Research Act. The FDA requires food corporations to list these ingredients on the food packages; certain foods that may pose increased risk for hypersensitivity reactions may require the implementation of additional labeling requirements [38]. To implement policy provisions, the FDA provides guidance to the food industry, consumers, and stakeholders to ensure that they are properly assessing and managing any allergens that may be present in the food. This guidance is further supplemented with food-sampling inspections to ensure that consumers are not inadvertently exposed to an allergen [38]. The public is notified immediately through product recall notices if any issues are found during this inspection process, and the product may be permanently removed from the market if the issues cannot be corrected [38]. Separately, some corporations may voluntarily include an additional statement on the food label that states that the product "may contain" certain allergens based on their evaluation of food-processing practices; however, this specific statement is voluntary, and consumers should interpret it with caution [38] because "may contain" can sometimes be seen as both an ambiguous and contradictory statement [39].

Menu and Vending Machine Labeling

Consumer social patterns include frequent dining at restaurants and retail food establishments. Although the role of menu labeling on healthier food product purchasing has been a topic of debate for many years, some research shows that it can effectively encourage lower-calorie purchases in dining and retail food establishments [40–42]. In 2010, the Affordable Care Act was enacted into law as part of an overall healthcare reform effort in the United States, and it included food-labeling implications for restaurants and retail food establishments [32]. In 2014, the FDA expanded on this law and published a new rule for menu labeling for menus and vending machines to ensure that nutrient information is provided to consumers that dine in these establishments or that purchase from vending machines [32]. Specifically, chain restaurants that have more than 20 locations are required to display nutrition information similar to what one would expect to find on a regular food product [32].

Corporate Role in Transparent Food Labeling

Although food labeling has shown clear benefits for consumer health and has been a major focus of advocacy among consumers themselves, food corporations and businesses have made every effort to oppose labeling efforts [43–45]. The industry has stated its reasons for opposition as being entirely consumer focused, where consumers may "get confused" or become "overwhelmed" by the information provided on the label [45]. After the passing of NLEA in 1990, food corporations became fearful that labeling would market some food products as healthier than others in a clearer way, such that consumers would be more likely to purchase healthier products, hence driving up profits for corporations that produce those products [45]. In the years and decades since NLEA's passing, the FDA has continued to strengthen its food-labeling policies by using research to pinpoint the types of ingredients that would later be mandated to be included on these labels; for example, due to rising obesity and diabetes rates in the United States, the FDA added a rule requiring food companies to specify the total sugar content on the label and how much of this content is attributable to added sugars [46]. Each time the FDA released draft guidance for these new rules, the agency invited public comments to ensure that feedback was captured for any improvements that needed to be made to the rule; most of these public comments came from food corporations that opposed the rule entirely [43, 46]. These corporations strongly advocated against this rule by arguing that mandating "added sugars" to the food label would not be correctly interpreted, or could be misinterpreted, by consumers [43, 46]. Despite these major oppositions, consumers have maintained consistency in their demand for more information, not less [43]. These demands are fueled by concern for their own health and the health of their dependents, including children, elderly people, and disabled people, among a plethora of other factors [43]. Given this, regulatory efforts that facilitate transparent food labeling can play a major role in fostering consumer trust and well-being, including raising knowledge that enables them to make informed food-purchasing decisions [47] and to align with consumer demands.

Box 12.2 Benefits of Transparent Food Labeling

1. Food labeling *increases awareness among consumers* of public safety by labeling foods that contain allergens or other harmful ingredients. Ensuring food labels clearly label foods that contain these ingredients can reduce health risks and potential future liability to the food corporation [47].

2. Food labeling improves *consumer motivation to make informed and confident food-purchasing decisions* so that they are able to select the food products that are best aligned with their health goals, cultural values, and preferences [47].

3. Food labeling *promotes the availability of important nutritional information*, including the ingredients that can be found in the food product. This can improve consumer knowledge and awareness, particularly so that consumers understand the level of vitamins and minerals, calories, sugars, saturated fats, and sodium found in the food product. This can also help the consumer to easily identify any ingredients in the food product that may pose health risks [47].

4. Food labeling *reduces impacts on the environment*, which improves sustainability.

5. Food labeling *protects against consumer misinformation* and promotes trust among consumers regarding product authenticity [47] and with the brand or food corporation that made the food product available in the market. When a food corporation has transparently labeled the food product, it also shows that the corporation is compliant with the regulations put in place to ensure food safety [47]. Further, consumers can easily identify whether the product is organic, genetically modified, or gluten-free [47].

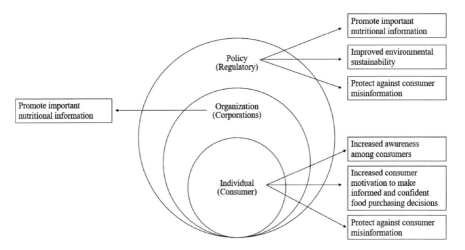

Fig. 12.4 Systems framework for understanding the benefits of transparent food labeling at the individual, organizational, and policy levels

These benefits can impact the individual consumer and food corporations and can guide regulatory policymaking processes toward increased transparency. This relationship is depicted in Fig. 12.4.

Challenges in Implementing and Enforcing Food-Labeling Policies

The World Health Organization (WHO) identified key factors that play roles in being able to successfully implement and enforce food-labeling policies [48]. These factors include cultural values; the resources required to implement and enforce the policy; the policy impact on human rights, health, inequities, and inequalities; the overall acceptability of the policy among stakeholders; and the feasibility of implementation, monitoring, evaluation, and enforcement [48]. In some countries and among communities of different ethnic backgrounds, the perception of body image, body weight, and obesity differ, where some communities may not perceive being overweight to be a significant problem that needs to be addressed [48]. Across genders, women may be more self-conscious about their body image and weight and perceive being overweight to be a serious problem. These differences in values among different communities could hamper enforcment of certain food-labeling policies given how the information could be perceived. Resource implications are also challenges because some countries or organizations may be limited in their capacity to make changes to their food and nutrition labels in order to comply with regulatory requirements [48]; on an individual level, even with the availability of updated nutritional information on food labels, individuals may face difficulty making healthy food purchases due to socioeconomic status even though knowledge and food literacy levels support positive attitudes toward healthy food product purchasing. Also, even if nutritional labels are largely accepted by most people generally, there could be inequalities in being able to access healthier foods or access foods that are considered healthier within certain communities according to their personal values, beliefs [48], cultures, or traditions. From a feasibility standpoint, resource availability as well as other barriers to implementation and enforcement can be seen with competing industry interests or priorities and, in some instances, a lack of media or public campaign support [48].

Finally, even if an organization were completely successful in its implementation and enforcement, the evaluation of such large-scale policies can be challenging because implementation can differ vastly and because not every food label is approved by the FDA, such as FOP labels, which can create confounding effects on consumer purchasing behavior. So, even though these large-scale policies exist, a lack of standardization can hamper comparisons of food corporation performance or different food products with one another for meaningful interpretation. No one standard way but rather many ways are available for designing FOP labels because of the lack of policies that work to institute one informed recommendation. For governmental regulatory agencies, enacting such policies has become incredibly challenging due to opposition from food corporations and their lobbyists [19]. Specifically for food corporations that may receive negative ratings for their food product under a standardized rating system, opposing these policies and instead having the freedom to decide on a FOP label that could better highlight the positive attributes of their food product to ultimately influence the consumer are in their best interest. Labels such as MTL and warning labels can deter a consumer from purchasing their food products [19], which may negatively impact the corporation's revenue and presence in the food business market. To minimize this opposition, countries like the United States have discussed the possibility of excluding certain food corporations from the policy development process [19, 49]; however, a high degree of complexity is involved in being able to do so because the policy development process requires a fair and unbiased evaluation of the food product to classify it as truly healthy or unhealthy.

Shifting Consumer Needs and Evolving Health Priorities

Research shows that consumer food-purchasing intentions can be driven by a range of factors that can be either logical or emotional in nature [50, 51]. For example, from an emotional standpoint, an individual that is going grocery shopping while experiencing hunger cravings may be more inclined to select food products on the basis of their cravings rather than on the basis of the nutritional information provided on the food label. This individual may also be less likely to spend more than a few seconds reviewing a food label, whether it is a nutrition facts label or an FOP label, to make a purchasing decision. The same behavior is likely to occur for a consumer who may be limited in financial resources to purchase certain products even if they are labeled as healthy [50]. In contrast, an emotional response can be more immediately triggered once a consumer sees an FOP label [51]. Consumers may further have varying levels of baseline skills in, knowledge of, or openness to considering new information that can affect their ability to process a nutrition label to therefore be able to act on it in an informed way [50]. In one study, researchers implemented an online questionnaire among 783 participants to understand consumer intentions on using food labeling to make healthier food choices [52]. Their results indicated that a combination of consumer baseline knowledge, food literacy, attitude toward the food, and their social influences, such as opinions or preferences of those in their network circle, was associated with food-purchasing behavior [52]. From a logical standpoint, consumers who have chronic diseases such as obesity or diabetes are more likely to use food label information due to being more aware of nutritional recommendations [53]. Consumers that are motivated to maintain their health or are committed to preserving the environment may benefit from actionable labels that promote the purchase of organic food options [27]. Some research shows that reading nutritional information is also predicted by having higher education, being female, and being older in age [54]. For these reasons, labels should be designed to ensure that the information provided on the label increases knowledge and that this knowledge can then be translated into purchasing behavior [50], such as by creating colorful labels [55].

Although consumer food choices have historically been driven largely by flavor and price, these factors have evolved in developed countries, where a majority of the population is working and has a greater sense of affluence [29]. Today, consumers are more interested in learning how food is produced and whether the ingredients within it are healthy, natural, or organic [29]. Research shows that consumers' priorities have shifted to the following factors, which guide their decision-making in purchasing food products: Situational factors such as time, social and physical surroundings, coping, assimilation, intentionality, and attribution; sociocultural factors such as cultural economical influence, trust in industry, and changing beliefs, norms, habits, and attitudes; extrinsic product characteristics such as risk perception, sustainability, and claims/label packaging; intrinsic product characteristics such as appearance, taste, smell, and texture; biological and physiological factors such as age and gender, physical condition, genetic factors, and physiology; and psychological factors such as cognition, emotion/motivation, decision-making, memory, previous experiences, and personality traits all contribute to an individual's decision to purchase food products [29]. The level of healthiness, taste, cost, and convenience are major drivers of food purchasing [56, 57]. Shifting consumer needs are depicted in Fig. 12.5, where the social cognitive framework is applied to understand the triadic relationship between the various personal, cognitive, social, environmental, and behavioral factors of consumes, which collectively play a role in facilitating consumer food-purchasing behavior. This framework shows that these factors can play a bidirectional role in food-purchasing behavior, which can differ among individuals, communities, and populations as a whole.

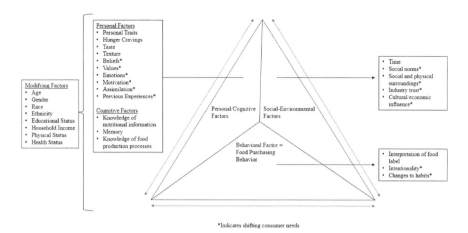

Fig. 12.5 Social cognitive framework of shifting consumer personal and social-environmental factors in food-purchasing behavior

Role of Technology in Enhancing Food Label Information Accessibility

With the growth of new technology, many consumers rely both on the Internet and social media to weigh their food options and opt to shop online for their groceries. Convenience and ease of information access through technological means are key reasons why consumers may obtain information from these sources [50]. Therefore, digital interventions play significant roles in improving consumer knowledge and in facilitating behavior change [50]. For example, food basket feedback or automated food swap recommendations can be incorporated into online grocery shopping platforms [50] to provide real-time feedback on how healthy a purchase is and to share ways that some products can be quickly swapped for healthier alternatives before checkout. Consumers are also increasingly using quick response (QR) barcodes [47] to quickly scan a food product by using their smartphones and retrieve nutritional information during their in-person shopping experience. These electronic methods can supplement or entirely replace hard-copy materials such as brochures and certifications [47] that consumers may now find harder to seek out when searching for nutritional information; the process of locating hard-copy material may become so difficult for some that they may find it altogether inconvenient and ultimately give up on the process . Another technological advancement is smart packaging, which includes sensors on the food product to track how fresh the food product is in real time [47]; smart packaging can help consumers be better informed and be able to realistically plan out their meals to achieve overall health goals and to minimize future waste. For consumers with environmental and sustainability concerns, blockchain technology can easily help identify the origin of a product by backtracking its production within the supply chain [47]. As a more comprehensive approach, augmented reality labeling allows consumers to scan the food label and retrieve full information about the product, from its ingredients to its production to recipe recommendations [47]. Because a large majority of food products come to market from the global supply chain, this technological approach can illuminate the production process more clearly, decrease any worries or concerns about the food, and ensure informed decision-making [58].

Educational Initiatives to Improve Public Awareness

Education is highly important for consumers to be able to identify food products that are transparently labeled and compliant with governmental regulations [47]. Education is also important for consumers to understand what labels were voluntarily indicated on the food product and how to decipher the overall level of healthiness of the product without over-reliance on the front-of-pack voluntary labeling by food corporations.

Box 12.3 "The New Nutrition Facts Label: What's in It for You" Educational Initiative

The *"The New Nutrition Facts Label: What's in It for You"* initiative is an educational initiative launched by the FDA to raise awareness of the changes that were made to the nutrition label in 2016 [59] because most consumers were accustomed to the old label that had been in effect since the early 1990s. Specific changes included making key ingredients easier to find, such as through bolder font, listing nutrients in order of importance, and requiring vitamin D and potassium to be listed on the label [59]. This campaign was designed for many audiences, including healthcare professionals and educators, to share updated information about the nutrition facts label to their patients, clients, or students. A noteworthy component of the campaign was the outreach component, which utilized various methods to increase public awareness of the updated label, such as social media, indoor/outdoor advertising, videos, and downloadable educational materials [59].

In addition to this campaign, the FDA also made an interactive label available on their website that allows consumers to easily place their cursor over any part of the updated label to find a description of what the updated information means [59]. Another set of more-recent initiatives are being implemented by the FDA in alignment with the United States' 2022 National Strategy on Hunger, Nutrition, and Health, which aims to increase healthy eating and physical activity by 2030 to ultimately prevent diet-related diseases such as diabetes and hypertension [60]. The FDA is working to expedite these efforts by supplying consumers with nutrition information, encouraging healthier food purchasing, and discouraging the purchase of foods with high sodium or sugar content [59]. Also, efforts are being made to ensure that consumer misinformation is avoided—for example, food corporations that put health claims on food packaging stating that the product will prevent disease without any scientific evidence [9]. Using technological devices and providing financial incentives [50] may engage the public in these important initiatives.

Future Directions and Conclusion

Given the strong opposition from food corporations on back-of-pack labeling, the food industry has increasingly shifted toward the use of FOP labels that have yet to be more closely regulated for information accuracy. Food corporations may utilize FOP labels to make claims that would serve their profit-driven interests and ones they believe would attract more customers or put them at a greater advantage over their competition in the food market [58]. These types of claims can be misleading and potentially have harmful effects on people's long-term health if these foods are, in fact, not healthy to eat [58]. Although the United States Federal Food, Drug, and Cosmetic Act and the Federal Trade Commission has made policy statements on deception and their guide for using environmental marketing claims (e.g., a product is "environmentally friendly") [58, 62], research has only recently led to stronger governmental regulatory action on promoting transparency on FOP labels. These actions include the United States National Strategy on Hunger, Nutrition, and Health, where the first FOP labeling system was proposed [63]. This also includes the FDA's recent 2023 plans to launch a rigorous study to examine FOP labels for the purposes of issuing a future final rule [63]. In 2023, the Transparency, Readability, Understandability, Truth, and Helpfulness (TRUTH) in Labeling Act was introduced by the United States Senate to establish mandatory FOP labels for both food and beverages [63]. To strengthen food-labeling policies and to improve implementation and enforcement, mandating FOP labels could pave the way to restricting the sale or marketing of foods that contain ingredients harmful to health—for example, banning foods with warning labels from future sales [61].

One point of consumer misinformation is what is meant for a food product to be truly considered "healthy." The current use of the term *healthy* requires updating given that its definition was initially established by the FDA in 1994 [6]. In September 2022, the FDA proposed an updated definition to better align with recent guidelines to ensure that food marked as healthy is truly healthy for the general population. In this definition, the FDA aimed to build on its past definition by encouraging the consumer to build sustainable diets consistent with recommended dietary guidelines [6, 64]. This means that the food product must contain food from at least one of the following food groups: proteins, dairy, vegetables, fruits, or grains. Because the corporate use of healthy labels is not currently required by the FDA, in this recent evaluation, the FDA has recognized that the label is used quite frequently; therefore, the entity will propose a universal symbol that consumers can easily use to identify food products that meet the definition of healthy [6].

These proposed steps by the FDA appear to be promising to encourage informed healthy dietary decision-making and to prevent diet-related chronic conditions among consumers. How these plans will inform the enactment of future policies and whether they can be implemented and enforced to achieve desired nutritional changes among consumers remain to be seen.

Further Practice

1. Which of the following is not a food label regulatory entity?

    a. US Federal Food and Drug Administration
    b. US Department of Meat and Poultry Products
    c. US Department of Agriculture
    d. US Food and Safety Inspection Service

2. Which of the following are major drivers of food purchasing among consumers?

    a. Taste, the presence of microplastics, cost, and convenience
    b. The level of healthiness, taste, cost, and convenience
    c. The level of healthiness, artificial coloring, cost, and convenience
    d. Taste, cost, genetic engineering, and convenience

3. Which government regulation made the placement of the nutrition facts label mandatory on food packages?

    a. Food Allergen Labeling and Consumer Protection Act of 2004
    b. Nutrition Labeling and Education Act of 1990
    c. Affordable Care Act of 2010
    d. All of the above

4. What is one reason why some consumers may not read food labels?

    a. Consumers rely on the government to ensure all food products are safe to eat.
    b. A majority of consumers are at least of average or above average health and may therefore not have the need to read food labels.
    c. Consumers may not have knowledge of food labels or may not consider themselves as at risk for diet-related diseases.
    d. Food labels should be read only by people who have a diet-related disease.

5. What diet-related disease could be prevented by consuming foods low in sodium content?

    a. Hypertension
    b. Stroke
    c. Both A and B
    d. None of the above

6. The serving size provides an accurate recommendation on how much of the food product one should eat.

   a. True
   b. False

7. A healthy food product requires that foods provide at least _____ of the daily value for one or more of the following nutrients: vitamin A, vitamin C, calcium, iron, protein, or fiber.

   a. 5%
   b. 10%
   c. 15%
   d. 20%

8. What kind of food label alerts the consumer of any ingredients in a food product that may potentially be harmful to their health?

   a. Nutrition label
   b. Nutrient label
   c. Organic label
   d. Warning label

9. For a food product to be labeled organic, what food production process must it not have gone through?

   a. Synthetic fertilizers
   b. Irradiation
   c. Genetic engineering
   d. All of the above

10. Which government regulation requires that the ingredients to which many people are known to be allergic be listed as a "contains" statement in the ingredients list of the food package?

    a. Food Allergen Labeling and Consumer Protection Act of 2004
    b. Nutrition Labeling and Education Act of 1990
    c. Affordable Care Act of 2010
    d. National Strategy on Hunger, Nutrition, and Health of 2022

11. Approximately _____ or more of processed foods in the market contain genetically engineered ingredients.

    a. 15%
    b. 18%
    c. 70%
    d. 63%

12. Which educational initiative was launched by the FDA to raise awareness of the changes that were made to the nutrition label in 2016?

    a. National Strategy on Hunger, Nutrition, and Health of 2022
    b. The Updated Nutrition Facts Label: Food Choices through Empowerment
    c. The New Nutrition Facts Label: What's in It for You
    d. National Strategy on Nutrition, Food Labels, and Health of 2023

Critical Thinking Short-Answer Questions

1. How would you, as a consumer, say your dietary needs have shifted over the past 5–10 years, and how have these shifts affected your food-purchasing behaviors?
2. In your opinion, what strategies can be employed to reduce opposition from food corporations to promote transparent front-of-pack food labeling? Why do you believe these strategies are likely to be successful?
3. What types of digital interventions can promote informed purchasing behaviors among consumers who shop at in-person grocery stores?

Answer Key

1. b
2. b
3. b
4. c
5. c
6. b
7. b
8. d
9. d
10. a
11. c
12. c

References

1. Food labels. Centers for Disease Control and Prevention. 2022, September 20. https://www.cdc.gov/diabetes/managing/eat-well/food-labels.html#:~:text=The%20label%20breaks%20down%20the,information%20can%20differ%20a%20lot.
2. Viola GCV, Bianchi F, Croce E, Ceretti E. Are food labels effective as a means of health prevention? Deleted J. 2016;5(3):jphr.2016.768. https://doi.org/10.4081/jphr.2016.768.
3. Todd JE, Variyam JN. The decline in consumer use of food Nutrition labels, 1995–2006. Economic Research Report; 2008. https://ideas.repec.org/p/ags/uersrr/56466.html

4. Satia JA, Galanko JA, Neuhouser ML. Food nutrition label use is associated with demographic, behavioral, and psychosocial factors and dietary intake among African Americans in North Carolina. J Am Diet Assoc. 2005;105(3):392–402. https://doi.org/10.1016/j.jada.2004.12.006.
5. Ollberding NJ, Wolf RL, Contento IR. Food label use and its relation to dietary intake among US adults. J Am Diet Assoc. 2010;110(8):1233–7. https://doi.org/10.1016/j.jada.2010.05.007.
6. Nutrition, C. F. F. S. a. A. Use of the term healthy on food labeling. U.S. Food and Drug Administration. 2024.
7. Choose Heart-Healthy Foods | NHLBI, NIH. 2022, March 24. NHLBI, NIH. https://www.nhlbi.nih.gov/health/heart-healthy-living/healthy-foods.
8. Cioffi CE, Levitsky DA, Pacanowski CR, Bertz F. A nudge in a healthy direction. The effect of nutrition labels on food purchasing behaviors in university dining facilities. Appetite. 2015;92:7–14. https://doi.org/10.1016/j.appet.2015.04.053.
9. Understanding food labels. The Nutrition Source. 2023, February 2. https://www.hsph.harvard.edu/nutritionsource/food-label-guide/
10. Nutrition, C. F. F. S. a. A. Changes to the Nutrition Facts label. U.S. Food and Drug Administration. 2024, March 28.
11. Nutrition, C. F. F. S. a. A. Front-of-Package nutrition labeling. U.S. Food And Drug Administration. 2024, March 28. https://www.fda.gov/food/food-labeling-nutrition/front-package-nutrition-labeling.
12. Sanjari SS, Jahn S, Boztug Y. Dual-process theory and consumer response to front-of-package nutrition label formats. Nutr Rev. 2017;75(11):871–82. https://doi.org/10.1093/nutrit/nux043.
13. Becker MW, Bello NM, Sundar RP, Peltier C, Bix L. Front of pack labels enhance attention to nutrition information in novel and commercial brands. Food Policy. 2015;56:76–86. https://doi.org/10.1016/j.foodpol.2015.08.001.
14. Temple NJ, Fraser J. Food labels: a critical assessment. Nutrition. 2014;30(3):257–60. https://doi.org/10.1016/j.nut.2013.06.012.
15. Pettigrew S, Jongenelis M, Jones A, Herçberg S, Julia C. An 18-country analysis of the effectiveness of five front-of-pack nutrition labels. Food Qual Prefer. 2023;104:104691. https://doi.org/10.1016/j.foodqual.2022.104691.
16. Mazzù MF, Romani S, Marozzo V, Giambarresi A, Baccelloni A. Improving the understanding of key nutritional elements to support healthier and more informed food choices: the effect of front-of-pack label bundles. Nutrition. 2023;105:111849. https://doi.org/10.1016/j.nut.2022.111849.
17. Grummon AH, Musicus AA, Moran AJ, Salvia MG, Rimm EB. Consumer reactions to positive and negative front-of-package food labels. Am J Prev Med. 2023;64(1):86–95. https://doi.org/10.1016/j.amepre.2022.08.014.
18. Acton RB, Kirkpatrick SI, Hammond D. Comparing the effects of four front-of-package Nutrition labels on consumer purchases of five common beverages and snack Foods: results from a randomized trial. J Acad Nutr Diet. 2022;122(1):38–48.e9. https://doi.org/10.1016/j.jand.2021.07.014.
19. Temple NJ. Front-of-package food labels: A narrative review. Appetite. 2020;144:104485. https://doi.org/10.1016/j.appet.2019.104485.
20. Shangguan S, Afshin A, Shulkin M, Ma W, Marsden D, Smith J, Saheb-Kashaf M, Shi P, Micha R, Imamura F, Mozaffarian D. A meta-analysis of food labeling effects on consumer diet behaviors and industry practices. Am J Prev Med. 2019;56(2):300–14. https://doi.org/10.1016/j.amepre.2018.09.024.
21. Santos O, Alarcão V, Feteira-Santos R, Fernandes J, Virgolino A, Sena C, Vieira CP, Gregório MJ, Nogueira P, Graça P, Costa A. Impact of different front-of-pack nutrition labels on online food choices. Appetite. 2020;154:104795. https://doi.org/10.1016/j.appet.2020.104795.
22. Siegrist M, Leins-Hess R, Keller C. Which front-of-pack nutrition label is the most efficient one? The results of an eye-tracker study. Food Qual Prefer. 2015;39:183–90. https://doi.org/10.1016/j.foodqual.2014.07.010.

23. Lima M, Ares G, Deliza R. How do front of pack nutrition labels affect healthfulness perception of foods targeted at children? Insights from Brazilian children and parents. Food Qual Prefer. 2018;64:111–9. https://doi.org/10.1016/j.foodqual.2017.10.003.

24. Nutrition, C. F. F. S. a. A. Label claims for conventional foods and dietary supplements. U.S. Food and Drug Administration. 2024, March 28. https://www.fda.gov/food/food-labeling-nutrition/label-claims-conventional-foods-and-dietary-supplements

25. Nutrition, C. F. F. S. a. A. Gluten-Free labeling of foods. U.S. Food And Drug Administration. 2022, March 7.

26. Nutrition, C. F. F. S. a. A. Plant-Based Milk Alternatives (PBMA). U.S. Food and Drug Administration. 2023, February 22.

27. Aitken R, Watkins L, Williams J, Kean A. The positive role of labelling on consumers' perceived behavioural control and intention to purchase organic food. J Clean Prod. 2020;255:120334. https://doi.org/10.1016/j.jclepro.2020.120334.

28. Understanding the USDA organic label. USDA. 2016, July 22. https://www.usda.gov/media/blog/2016/07/22/understanding-usda-organic-label.

29. Asioli D, Aschemann-Witzel J, Caputo V, Vecchio R, Annunziata A, Næs T, Varela P. Making sense of the "clean label" trends: A review of consumer food choice behavior and discussion of industry implications. Food Res Int. 2017;99:58–71. https://doi.org/10.1016/j.foodres.2017.07.022.

30. Ingredion. The clean label guide to Europe. 2014.

31. Maruyama S, Streletskaya NA, Lim J. Clean label: why this ingredient but not that one? Food Qual Prefer. 2021;87:104062. https://doi.org/10.1016/j.foodqual.2020.104062.

32. Mayne ST, Spungen J. The US Food and Drug Administration's role in improving nutrition: labeling and other authorities. J Food Compos Anal. 2017;64:5–9. https://doi.org/10.1016/j.jfca.2017.07.015.

33. Center for Food Safety | about GE Foods | About Genetically Engineered foods. Center for Food Safety. n.d.. https://www.centerforfoodsafety.org/issues/311/ge-foods/about-ge-foods

34. Food labeling. UC Food Safety. 2024, January 18. https://ucfoodsafety.ucdavis.edu/processing-distribution/regulations-processing-food/food-labeling

35. Nutrition, C. F. F. S. a. A. Standards of identity for food. U.S. Food and Drug Administration. 2024, March 14. https://www.fda.gov/food/food-labeling-nutrition/standards-identity-food.

36. Wartella EA, Lichtenstein AH, Boon CS. History of nutrition labeling. Front-of-package nutrition rating systems and symbols - NCBI Bookshelf. 2010. https://www.ncbi.nlm.nih.gov/books/NBK209859/.

37. 21 CFR Part 101 – Food labeling. n.d. https://www.ecfr.gov/current/title-21/chapter-I/subchapter-B/part-101?toc=1

38. Nutrition, C. F. F. S. a. A. Food allergies. U.S. Food and Drug Administration. 2024, April 12. https://www.fda.gov/food/food-labeling-nutrition/food-allergies.

39. Soon JM. Food allergen labelling: "may contain" evidence from Malaysia. Food Res Int. 2018;108:455–64. https://doi.org/10.1016/j.foodres.2018.03.068.

40. Finkelstein EA, Strombotne KL, Chan N, Krieger J. Mandatory menu labeling in one fast-food chain in King County, Washington. Am J Prev Med. 2011;40(2):122–7. https://doi.org/10.1016/j.amepre.2010.10.019.

41. Elbel B, Kersh R, Brescoll VL, Dixon LB. Calorie labeling and food choices: A first look at the effects on low-income people in New York City. Health Aff. 2009;28(Supplement 1):w1110–21. https://doi.org/10.1377/hlthaff.28.6.w1110.

42. Bassett MT, Dumanovsky T, Huang C, Silver L, Young C, Nonas C, Matte T, Chideya S, Frieden T. Purchasing behavior and calorie information at fast-food chains in New York City, 2007. Am J Public Health. 2008;98(8):1457–9. https://doi.org/10.2105/ajph.2008.135020.

43. Transparency in food labeling. Union of Concerned Scientists. 2016, July 19. https://www.ucsusa.org/resources/transparency-food-labeling.

44. Kyle TK, Thomas DM. Consumers believe nutrition facts labeling for added sugar will be more helpful than confusing. PubMed. 2014;22(12):2481–4. https://doi.org/10.1002/oby.20887.

45. Nestle M. Food politics: how the food industry influences nutrition and health. Berkeley and Los Angeles: University of California Press; 2002.
46. Food Marketing Institute (FMI). Comments on food labeling: revision of the Nutrition and supplement facts labels. Docket No. FDA-2012-N-1210. Comment ID No. FDA-2012-N-1210-0802. 2015 October 13. Washington, DC: US Food and Drug Administration.
47. Admin. Role of transparent food labeling in ensuring food safety for consumers. KENAFF. 2023, October 19; https://kenaff.org/wp/2023/10/12/role-of-transparent-food-labeling-in-ensuring-food-safety-for-con-sumers/#:~:text=Accurate%20and%20transparent%20labeling%20helps,their%20trust%20in%20the%20industry
48. Engelhardt K, Erichsen D, Allen T, World Health Organization. Implementing nutrition label-ling policies: a review of contextual factors (Biotext Pty Ltd, Ed.) [Review]. World Health Organization; 2021. https://iris.who.int/bitstream/handle/10665/345119/9789240035089-eng.pdf?sequence=1
49. Moodie R, Stuckler D, Monteiro CA, Sheron N, Neal B, Thamarangsi T, Lincoln P, Casswell S. Profits and pandemics: prevention of harmful effects of tobacco, alcohol, and ultra-pro-cessed food and drink industries. Lancet. 2013;381(9867):670–9. https://doi.org/10.1016/s0140-6736(12)62089-3.
50. Schruff-Lim E, Van Loo EJ, Van Kleef E, Van Trijp J. Turning FOP nutrition labels into action: A systematic review of label+ interventions. Food Policy. 2023;120:102479. https://doi.org/10.1016/j.foodpol.2023.102479.
51. David IA, Da Silva Gomes F, Silva LAA, Coutinho GMS, Pacheco LB, Figueira JSB, Pereira MG, Oliveira L, Souza GGL, Mota BEF, Stariolo JB, Lemos TC, Lobo I, Campagnoli RR. Use of event-related potentials to measure the impact of front-of-package labels on food-evoked emotion. Food Qual Prefer. 2023;111:104995. https://doi.org/10.1016/j.foodqual.2023.104995.
52. Sousa I, Mucinhato RMD, Prates CB, Zanin LM, Da Cunha DT, Capriles VD, De Rosso VV, Stedefeldt E. Do Brazilian consumers intend to use food labels to make healthy food choices? An assessment before the front-of-package labelling policy. Food Res Int. 2023;172:113107. https://doi.org/10.1016/j.foodres.2023.113107.
53. Lewis JE, Arheart KL, LeBlanc WG, Fleming LE, Lee DJ, Davila EP, Cabán-Martinez AJ, Dietz NA, McCollister KE, Bandiera FC, Clark JD. Food label use and awareness of nutri-tional information and recommendations among persons with chronic disease. Am J Clin Nutr. 2009;90(5):1351–7. https://doi.org/10.3945/ajcn.2009.27684.
54. Mehanna A, Ashour A, Mohamed DT. Public awareness, attitude, and practice regard-ing food labeling, Alexandria, Egypt. BMC Nutr. 2024;10(1):15. https://doi.org/10.1186/s40795-023-00770-5.
55. Bandara B, De Silva D, Maduwanthi B, Warunasinghe W. Impact of food labeling information on consumer purchasing decision: with special reference to Faculty of Agricultural Sciences. Procedia Food Sci. 2016;6:309–13. https://doi.org/10.1016/j.profoo.2016.02.061.
56. Jo J, Lusk JL. If it's healthy, it's tasty and expensive: effects of nutritional labels on price and taste expectations. Food Qual Prefer. 2018;68:332–41. https://doi.org/10.1016/j.foodqual.2018.04.002.
57. U.S.: Factors impacting consumers food purchasing decisions 2021 | Statista. Statista. 2022, February 24. https://www.statista.com/statistics/1289086/impacts-on-consumers-food-purchasing-decisions-in-the-us/
58. Admin. Process labeling: the challenges of transparency. Food and Drug Law Institute (FDLI); 2017. https://www.fdli.org/2017/08/process-labeling-challenges-transparency/
59. Nutrition, C. F. F. S. a. A. The nutrition facts label. U.S. Food and Drug Administration. 2024, March 5. https://www.fda.gov/food/nutrition-education-resources-materials/nutrition-facts-label.
60. Nutrition, C. F. F. S. a. A. FDA's nutrition initiatives. U.S. Food and Drug Administration. 2023, October 19. https://www.fda.gov/food/food-labeling-nutrition/fdas-nutrition-initiatives.

61. Ares G, Antúnez L, Curutchet MR, Giménez A. Warning labels as a policy tool to encourage healthier eating habits. Curr Opin Food Sci. 2023;51:101011. https://doi.org/10.1016/j.cofs.2023.101011.

62. Dingell JD, & Committee on Energy and Commerce, U.S. House of Representatives. FTC Policy Statement on Deception. In Cliffdale Associates, Inc. 1983. pp. 103–174. https://www.ftc.gov/system/files/documents/public_statements/410531/831014deceptionstmt.pdf

63. Bolas M. The struggle to put health concerns in food labels – Penn LDI. Penn LDI. 2024, February 13. https://ldi.upenn.edu/our-work/research-updates/the-struggle-to-put-health-concerns-in-front-of-package-food-labeling/

64. Dietary Guidelines for Americans, 2020–2025 and Online materials | Dietary Guidelines for Americans. n.d.. https://www.dietaryguidelines.gov/resources/2020-2025-dietary-guidelines-online-materials

Understanding the Impact of School Meal Programs on Children's Nutrition and Health

13

Jody L. Vogelzang ⓘ

Learning Objectives

After completing this chapter, you will be able to

- Describe the evolution of school meals in the US
- Summarize the changes in school meals since the Healthy Hunger-Free Kids Act (HHFKA) of 2010
- Discuss common characteristics of smart snacks
- Summarize contributors to food waste in schools
- Compare the US and foreign school lunch programs

History of School Lunches in the United States

School meals in the United States (US) began in the late nineteenth century. Meals were unpredictable and usually undertaken by private organizations interested in children and education. In the 1800s, families were larger than today, jobs were scarce, and wages were low. These social determinants of health contributed to children's arriving at school hungry and unfocused and having difficulty learning. In the early twentieth century, women-driven charities began initiating school meals in large cities across the United States; some schools cooked their meals, and others were prepared in women's homes and carried to schools. A lack of space and equipment challenged rural schools to provide or even reheat school meals. Partnerships between parents and school employees produced innovative ways of using donated food to feed rural students [1].

J. L. Vogelzang (✉)
Grand Valley State University, Allendale, MI, USA
e-mail: vogelzjo@gvsu.edu

A. K. Mitra, D. Vanoh (eds.), *Essentials of Clinical and Public Health Nutrition*,
Nutrition and Health, https://doi.org/10.1007/978-3-031-95373-6_13

295

The 1930s began the federal involvement in school meals by providing food commodities. During this time, the number of schools offering school meals increased, as did the number of students who took advantage of these meals. The United States' entry into World War II depleted the availability of food commodities, and much of what was sent to schools was instead being used to feed the troops. Consequently, the number of schools serving meals declined significantly. However, the government was able to assist with cash payments instead of commodities, thereby rescuing school meals. In 1946, the National School Lunch Act was passed by US Congress, which permanently established the school lunch program and nutritional standards [1]. Since the 1940s, nutritional standards have been modified following changes in the nation's dietary guidelines (Table 13.1).

Source: Adapted from Gunderson, G (2003) The National School Lunch Program Background and Development Nova Science Publishing.

The twenty-first century includes several significant changes in school meals. In 2010, the Healthy Hunger-Free Kids Act (HHFKA) was passed on the federal level, making it the first nutritional change to school meals in almost 20 years. The objective was to increase the availability of fruits, vegetables, whole grains, and fat-free milk; reduce sodium and saturated fat and trans-fat levels; and meet the nutrition needs of school children within calorie requirements [2]. Significant meal changes focused on reducing added sugars and sodium and increasing whole grains [3]. In 2018, the US Department of Agriculture (USDA) issued waivers to schools that wanted more-flexible options for their meal programs in terms of sodium content, fewer whole grains, and adding flavored milk. During the COVID-19 pandemic, additional flexibility to the dietary requirements was allowed to accommodate an unstable food delivery system.

In 2023, the secretary of agriculture proposed remodeling the nutrition standards by introducing "common-sense" and "practical" changes to added sugars and sodium that would be implemented over a multiyear period. These changes to school meal choices would better align with the most recent edition of the Dietary Guidelines for Americans [3, 4].

Table 13.1 Significant school lunch changes

Year	Changes enacted
1952	Equalized funding to Hawaii, Alaska, Puerto Rico, Guam, and the Virgin Islands to match the lowest-income states in the continental United States, which established a pilot of extra allotments for "needy schools."
1962	The act modified the funding model for states on the basis of state participation and need rate.
1966	The act established a 2-year pilot program for school breakfast and allowed applications for funding for nonfood needs such as kitchen equipment and increased staffing. The Child Nutrition Act moved all responsibility for school meals to the secretary of agriculture. A school milk program was added to the school lunch.
1968	The amendment broadened the scope of school meals to include public and nonprofit daycare centers.
1970	States were asked to match funds for their school meal programs.

School Meal Perceptions and Consumption

The new HHFKA regulations were enacted for the 2012/2013 school year. Although health and nutrition professionals widely supported the changes outlined in the 2010 HHFKA enactment, others could have been more enthusiastic. The HHFKA became a hotly discussed topic in political circles, in the food industry, and among school food service employees. Opponents of the meal changes expressed concerns about increased spending on more-nutritious meals and more plate waste related to the increase in poorly accepted foods, such as fruits and vegetables. Others were against the federal government's involvement in stemming child obesity by changing lunch choices (eliminating fried foods, adding whole grain entrées, and increasing fruit/vegetables).

Early consumption data taken in the second year of the new school lunch regulations showed that vegetable and entrée consumption significantly increased, whereas fruit and milk intake remained steady [5]. With the full implementation of school lunches following the Dietary Guidelines for Americans, added sugars and sodium will be reduced, and whole grains should be increased. Lifelong health improvements may occur if these dietary changes made in childhood are sustained as students enter adulthood (Table 13.2) [6].

Because of the governmental reimbursement system for school meals, the focus of school meal programs lies heavily on assessing meal participation. For example, the Food Research and Action Center (FRAC) recently reported school meal participation in the 2021–2022 school year by citing the number of meals increased over the prior school year (1.5 billion more meals served in 2021–2022: https://frac.org/news/schoolmeals2023). Also of note was an increase of 1.4 million children participating in school lunch compared to numbers before the COVID-19 pandemic (2018–2019). To prevent our being misled into thinking this increase was directly related to an increase in food quality, note that during the COVID-19 pandemic, free school meals were available and continue to be free of charge in several states; see Fig. 13.1.

Assessing the true success of school meals requires more than looking at just one variable. Counting meal participation does indicate how many students received a nutritious meal; however, this does not indicate meal consumption, satisfaction, or improved health parameters. To support the multifactor success of school meals, we turn to research that has examined consumption, parental perceptions, changes in body mass index (BMI), student satisfaction, and sustained dietary changes at home

Table 13.2 Dietary improvements with full implementation of school lunch adherence to Dietary Guidelines for Americans

Nutrient	Elementary school	Middle school	High school
Added sugar decrease	3.9%	3.8%	1.9%
Sodium decrease	5.6%	5.6%	2.7%
Whole grain increase	22.4%	26.7%	27.7%

Source: Wang (2023) Evaluation of health and economic effects of United States school meal standards consistent with the 2020–2025 Dietary Guidelines for Americans.

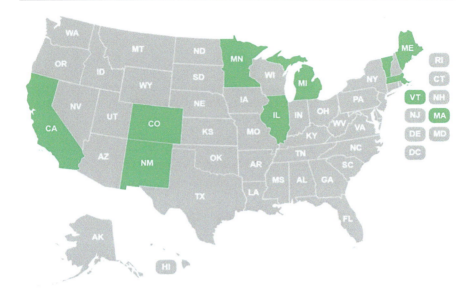

Map created at www.fla-shop.com

Fig. 13.1 US states with universal free lunch (green) 2023–2024

and in the community. Research on these factors is relatively recent and still emerging.

Foods that students consumed (not only selected) during lunch had lower nutritional value, and sugar consumption remained high. If students selected chocolate milk as a popular choice, it was unconsumed 55% of the time. White milk consumption was even lower among the students who selected it: It went utterly unconsumed 85% of the time [7].

Research on the impact of the HHFKA demonstrated a decrease in child obesity for low-income 10–17-year-olds [8]. The research from middle school student interviews supports many nutrition changes after the HHFKA; however, they voiced concern over food waste and food refusal [9].

Engaging Students in Healthy Eating

Achieving school meal buy-in requires the support of parents and the community. Although students consume the meals, parents shape children's initial food patterns often on the basis of community ethnicity, norms, and widely available foods. With the introduction of the HHFKA, some parents had negative perceptions, primarily related to the changes made to school meals since they were children.

If parents were students in the 1990s, then their schools could partner with fast food chains for school lunches, and favorites included French fries, square pizzas, ice cream cups, and cinnamon rolls. Today, school lunches strive to meet emerging nutrition guidelines by offering kid-friendly kale salad, vegetable nuggets with dipping sauces, brown rice, steamed or roasted broccoli, and chicken dumplings. Parents should know the purpose of school meals and actively support nutrition guidelines at home [10]. Understanding the impact of school nutrition changes on the significant problem of childhood obesity and lifelong health equips parents to be health advocates who support healthy eating habits and the connection between healthy, nutrient-dense foods and better focus in the classroom, as depicted in Fig. 13.2. Parental support is imperative during the middle school years, when students develop eating patterns that will persist into adulthood [9, 10].

US Department of Agriculture and US Department of Health and Human Services. Dietary Guidelines for Americans, 2020–2025. 9th Edition. December 2020. Available at DietaryGuidelines.gov.

Preparing foods that meet nutrition guidelines is a primary step toward improved health; however, making these foods tasty and attractive should not be overlooked. Parents, school staff administrators, and other community interested parties must consider the trade-offs between ensuring that more students eat school meals and that the meals appeal to the tastes of all students [2]. The sights and smells of food items can make the difference between food getting into the mouth or the garbage bin [11].

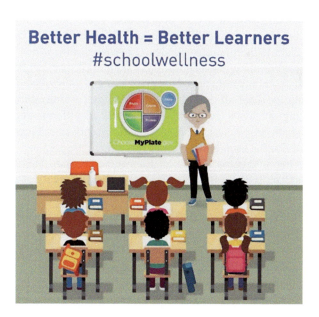

Fig. 13.2 Advantages of HHFKA meals

Table 13.3 Federal reimbursement for school meals, 2020–2021

Reimbursement	Breakfast	Lunch
Free meal reimbursement	$1.89	$3.60
Reduced meal reimbursement	$1.59	$3.20
Student fully paid meal reimbursement	$0.32	$0.42

Source: Taken from FRAC, available at https://frac.org/wp-content/uploads/SchoolMealsReport2022.pdf

In addition to adherence to nutrition guidelines, school nutrition professionals must also stay within cost guidelines. During the 2020–2021 school year, schools received reimbursements at the rates reported in Table 13.3.

Methods to increase the acceptance of school meals must also address student consumption behaviors. School nutrition professionals often employ innovative methods to encourage students to choose healthier food. These techniques, known as "nudges," are highly effective in making healthy choices the easiest and most motivating behavior change. For instance, preslicing fruits and pairing them with contrasting colors, such as halved strawberries with banana slices, can nudge students toward increased fruit intake.

Other schools have increased the available menu choices by adding salad bars, deli sandwich bars, and soup bars. Although evidence suggests that using these strategies may improve meal participation, uncertainty about whether the strategies make a lifelong change in eating behaviors persists [12].

There may be a better answer than removing familiar foods from school meals and replacing them with unfamiliar foods to improve health, which leads to a discussion on the impact of nutrition education in student classrooms. Food-based curricula are found in schools from preschool to high school. School gardens are widely used as teaching tools for all ages. In addition, many customizations of food and nutrition cooking curricula are targeted at schools in different settings and age groups [13]. School-based programs impact students and school health most when consistently provided at each grade level [14].

Introducing the Integrative Nutrition Education Program (INEP) curriculum appears to depend on school culture and has greater school uptake and a more holistic approach to teaching. Program content and lesson formats must be simple and adaptable, allowing for alignment with existing curricula and time constraints (Table 13.4) [15].

Table 13.4 Best practices for the integration of nutrition in an educational program

Best practice	School examples
Early nutrition intervention	Starting with preschool
Well-trained and motivated teachers	Teachers willing to be role models by eating with students
Partnership between teachers, nutrition educators, and stakeholders	Bringing individuals and the community together to support a common vision
Longer program durations (10–15 h total to show improvement; 50 h to show behavior change)	A supportive environment (school administrators and parents)

Source: Adapted from Large, A., Morgan, R., Kalas, S., Appleton, K., & Giglia, R. (2023). Determining best practice for school-based nutrition and cooking education programs: A scoping review. *Issues in Educational Research*, *33*(3), 1047–1065.

School Breakfast and Competitive Foods

School Breakfast

A 2-year school breakfast pilot program started in 1965 and served about 80,000 nutritionally challenged students. US Congress permanently established school breakfast in 1975. During the 2022–2023 school year, approximately 14.3 million children participated in school breakfast, with 79% receiving a free or reduced-price breakfast [16]. Schools that choose to serve breakfast have creatively addressed how to get more children to eat first thing in the morning. Some offer school breakfast, usually consisting of a piece of fruit, a cereal bar, and a drink of either milk or juice in the cafeteria. However, most cafeterias are far from lockers and classrooms, so morning meals are rushed or avoided.

Other schools have committed to a program called Breakfast after the Bell (BATB). In these schools, the students can grab breakfast from a conveniently located cart or kiosk and bring it into the classroom for consumption. Documented improvements in school breakfast participation, diet quality, and student behavior were seen by using this approach to breakfast. However, the effect of Breakfast in the Classroom (BIC) on BMI, weight status, academic achievement, and attendance was mixed [17].

Innovative schools provide breakfast for students who arrive late for their first class. These schools offer a grab-and-go breakfast in the administrative offices, where students check in for a tardy class pass. The goal of this approach is not to reward tardiness but rather to help reset the chaotic start to the day, potentially increasing school attendance [18]. On average, children in schools using breakfast carts in the classroom are in lower grades, and those using the grab-and-go breakfast are in higher grades [16, 19].

A second-chance breakfast is yet another creative approach to school breakfast. In this model, students are offered another opportunity to eat breakfast after the school day has started. Many middle and high school students are not hungry first thing in the morning but are ready to eat breakfast after their first class, helping them focus on their classes until lunchtime [16].

Smart Snacks

As schools complied with the HHFKA in the 2012/2013 school year on school lunch and breakfast, another application of these standards, this time for competitive foods, was positioned for implementation in the 2014/2015 school year [20]. The Smart Snacks in School regulation focuses on food sold à la carte in the school store, vending machines, and other venues where food is sold to students. The infographic in Fig. 13.2 compares snacks in schools before and after the standards had been implemented.

As with school lunch, the implementation of these changes caused some consternation. Across the United States, schools commonly raised funds through the sale of food items and had to reconsider a shift to food items that met HHFKA smart snack guidelines, or nonfood sales, to recast their income stream. Under the 2014 standards, snack bars, food in vending machines, food sold to students during fundraisers, or food sold anytime during the school day needed to meet the requirements of "smart snacks." However, states were allowed to apply for an exemption for infrequent deviation from the Smart Snacks in School guidelines [22]. The law requires that the state agency set an upper limit on the number of fundraisers that would be allowed. If the agency decides not to establish an upper limit, it will elect to prohibit any exempt fundraisers from being held in schools. The ability of 50 states to determine their exemptions has created diversity in the application of Smart Snacks in School legislation [22].

According to the US Department of Agriculture (USDA), a snack must meet the following nutrition standards: It must be a grain product that has whole grain as the first ingredient or have fruit, a vegetable, a dairy food, or a protein food as a first ingredient, or it must be a combination food that contains at least ¼ cup of fruit and vegetable (e.g., ¼ cup of raisins with enriched pretzels); in addition the food must meet the nutrient standards for calories, sodium, fats, and total sugars. Food companies have reformulated many snack favorites to meet these requirements. These ingredient-modified snacks are often marketed in similar packaging to that of the original, hampering student's ability to discern which are "smart" and which are not [23]. Foods that compete with school breakfast, lunch, and snacks are "competitive foods." In one research study on 72 schools from kindergarten to twelfth grade (K–12), 80% provided access to competitive foods, and 75% of these foods were compliant with Smart Snacks in School guidelines (Fig. 13.3). Competitive food was more available in schools that did not provide free breakfast or lunch [24].

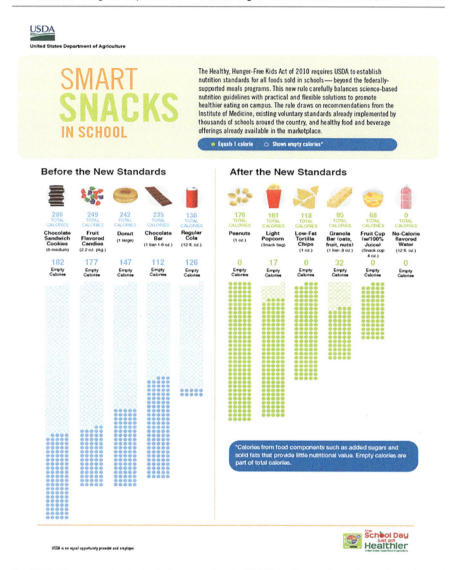

Fig. 13.3 Empty snack calories before and after the HHFKA. (*Source*: https://www.fns.usda.gov/tn/guide-smart-snacks-school)

Earlier in this chapter, the carryover of food behavior learned in grades K–12 to adulthood was discussed. Regarding how smart snacks emerged on college campuses, the carryover was disappointing. In a research study, a university campus reviewed the nutrition quality of snack items in 25 vending machines in public access locations (academic buildings, sports venues, and libraries). The results showed that less than 2% of the 890 items evaluated complied with Smart Snacks in School criteria [20]. Additional research is needed on lifelong changes in food behavior related to improved nutrition standards in K–12.

School Meal Safety and Sustainability

Food safety and food sustainability are vital to all food establishments. Food service in schools must meet federal, state, and county regulations, like other dining establishments must. Kitchens are regularly inspected, and inspection outcomes are available to the public. Commonly noted school food service citations may be related to personnel who lack training. The USDA mandates 6 hours of professional education for full-time employees and 4 h for part-time employees. Key critical violation and serious violation trends (terms used to delineate the severity of the violation) were a lack of food safety knowledge and temperature controls from start to finish in the food preparation process [21]. Specifically, the most common critical violations in descending order of occurrence were management and employee food safety knowledge, facilities that maintain proper storage, potentially hazardous food temperatures during preparation, and adequate handwashing sinks (Reynolds 1).

A study sponsored by the USDA investigated food safety concerns in the school meal environment (USDA). As more schools look to include made-from-scratch (instead of using highly processed preprepared) meals and sourcing more fresh fruit and vegetables, food safety knowledge is more important than ever. Culinary skills are also critical to the creation of palatable made-from-scratch meals. A shortage of formally trained food service personnel limits the implementation of creative, healthy meals, as noted in Fig. 13.4.

In addition to a lack of skills and training, cooking from scratch requires adequate preparation time and kitchen equipment, such as steamers and convection ovens. Space is often an issue in school kitchens, so attention must be paid to adequate shelving and counter space so that raw meats are prepared separately from a green salad to prevent cross-contamination. An inviting serving line contributes to the attractiveness of fresh and colorful fruits and vegetables.

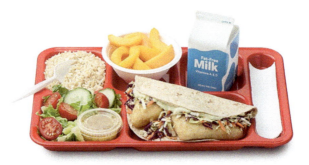

Fig. 13.4 An example of an HHFKA school lunch: brown rice, sliced peaches, green salad, fish tacos with avocado crema coleslaw, and milk. (*Source*: https://www.fns.usda.gov/tn/school-meals-trays-many-ways)

Food Waste

Controlling and eliminating school meal food waste is a challenge. Although no benchmark existed for food waste before the implementation of the HHFKA, after the implementation of the HHFKA, food waste was estimated in middle schoolers to be about 50% of the food served. Plant-based entrées were the most likely food item partially or entirely thrown out after mealtime [25]. There are many reasons for food waste: unfamiliar food items, food items not presented attractively, negative attitudes of school teachers and staff, and poor parent support. Enhanced school nutrition education may positively impact acceptance and decrease food waste, particularly if food tasting occurs before the new food item becomes part of the menu rotation.

Another way to prevent food waste is to stop before it hits the cafeteria line. Doubling down on meal forecasting, accurate food ordering, uniform portion sizes, and strict adherence to recipe instructions can stop food waste. Unserved meal entrées can be recovered and used for snacks. Student "share tables" are used to voluntarily return uneaten food (within food safety guidelines) to a common table so that those who are still hungry can have an extra portion or so that the food can be used for a snack or donated to a food charity.

Box 13.1 Ways to Increase Food Intake and Decrease Food Waste
- Food must be attractive and healthy.
- Schedule recess before lunch.
- Carve out adequate time for students to eat lunch.
- Schedule lunch later on (around noon) so that students eat more.
- Provide grab-and-go lunches for high schoolers who use the lunch period for catch-up.
- Keep lunch lines short to maximize eating time.

Source: Adapted from What You Can Do to Help Prevent Wasted Food. USDA FNS-553-2020.

Food waste occurs in school meals and when students bring lunches prepared at home. In a study completed with third graders, students with meals from home consumed about 67.3% of their meals. Students who consumed a school-provided lunch consumed close to 70% of a school lunch [26]. This indicates that a personalized lunch taken from home is not consumed more than an HHFKA meal prepared at school.

The most accurate method of tracking food waste is by weighing trash after a meal and analyzing the composition and weight of the discarded food [27]. This method is time-consuming but provides accurate information that can be used for behavior change. For example, the results of bin waste for meals consumed in the classroom can be compared between grades and can instigate friendly competition to work toward reduction. When mixed classes consume meals in a cafeteria, differentiating waste on the basis of class level is more challenging. However, the information gained from a bin audit can help food service personnel address general waste generators.

Effective School Nutrition Worldwide

Countries around the globe offer school meals. As expected, countries differ in how food is sourced, food items are served, and who has access to school meals. In 2022, the Global Child Nutrition Foundation (GCNF) published survey data on global school meals. The data indicate that the children who most benefited from school meals were less likely to be served one. Although approximately 330.3 million children globally received food through school meal programs in the school year that began in 2020, this only scratched the surface of need. Just over 25% of all children in higher and lower grades participated in school meals. Funding for school meals predominantly came from government sources, where some countries fund 100% of the meal cost and other countries shoulder closer to 70% of the cost [28].

School meals likely contain universal grain, oil, and legume staples worldwide. In more-affluent areas, the meals included meat, fruits, and staple foods. Food procurement was most likely to come from domestic markets and reflect cultural and heritage foods. The diversity of school meal programs in the continents of Asia, Oceania, Europe, and North America are further examined (Table 13.5).

Oceana

In 2020, Australia and New Zealand introduced changes in school meals. The first pilot school lunch in Australia was introduced in Tasmania, an island state with the smallest income per capita. The evaluation of the 20-day pilot program indicated that much of the island community favored free school meals, recognizing the

Table 13.5 Global school meal reach

Global area	Percentage benefiting from school meals
Middle East/North Africa	8%
Sub-Saharan Africa	16%
South Asia/East Asia/Pacific	26%
Europe/Central Asia/North America	47%
Latin America/Caribbean	55%

Source: Global Child Nutrition Foundation (GCNF). 2022. School meal programs around the world: results from the 2021 Global Survey of School Meal Programs. Accessed at survey.gcnf. org/2021-global-survey

importance of healthy meals during school hours. Others voiced concerns about the meal's healthiness and the difficulty of affording school lunch if it was not universally free. Hiring registered dietitians to create menus was recommended to ensure that children receive meals that align with the Australian Guide to Healthy Eating. This guide is found in Fig. 13.5.

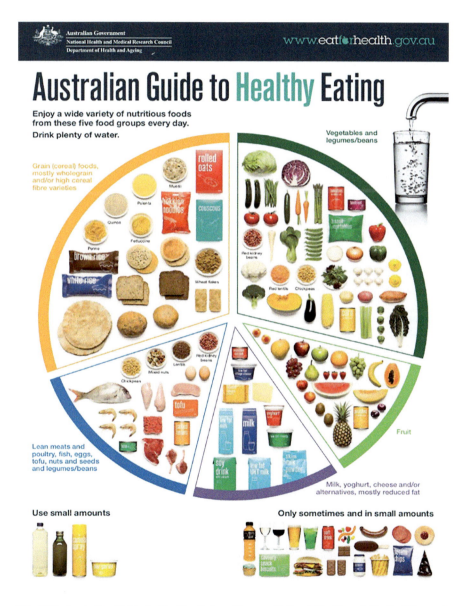

Fig. 13.5 Australian Guide to Healthy Eating. (*Source*: National Health and Medical Research Council https://www.eatforhealth.gov.au/guidelines/australian-guide-healthy-eating)

In the Australian states, school-provided meals are anomalies, where about 90% of students eat meals from home. Culture reinforced that parents were responsible for feeding their children, even away from home. National conversations are addressing the pros and cons of school-provided meals [29].

In 2020, the New Zealand government introduced free lunches for around 200,000 students attending low-income schools (about 27% of the total student body in New Zealand). Free school meals had many advantages, from less stress in the morning to less stigma at mealtime. Parents appreciated the financial aspects of free school meals for their children. Students missed the presence of competitive foods. They perceived that the school meals were of poor quality, particularly in schools that did not prepare meals in-house, leading to surplus food and food waste [30]. Administrative school staff believed that free school lunches required a transition period but made their schools more equitable. They agreed that student and parent buy-in is needed to see the meals as more than "free food" and embrace the meal as a proper and acceptable lunch [30].

Asia

In Korea, students are rarely seen bringing lunch boxes from home. In schools that offer school lunch, 99.9% of the students take it. Most students receiving school lunches were in primary school, whereas most students not taking school lunches were in high school. Eating school lunch (SL) was not dependent on the family's socioeconomic status. From a nutrition viewpoint, school lunches provided more calories than the no-school lunch (NSL) and skipping lunch (SKL) groups did (100 more than NSL and 300 more than SKL). However, those calories were well allocated because SLs provided significantly more protein than did NSLs and SKLs [31].

Most school lunch programs in Korea are prepared in-house and not outsourced to a contract vendor or catered to the school. Like the United States, Korea continues researching the association between school lunches and health outcomes such as childhood obesity. It actively evaluates the possibility of universal school lunches nationwide, as introduced in Seoul in 2021.

European Union (EU)

Europe pioneered school meals in the eighteenth century. Today, school meals are offered in 35 EU countries. Portugal, Finland, Monaco, Iceland, and Luxemburg all had 93% or above coverage for school meals.

Finland, the first country in the world to provide universal free lunch, also has rigorous nutrition guidelines. This country does not allow students to bring lunch from home, perhaps contributing to its high school lunch coverage. Vegetables comprise about 50% of the school lunch tray, followed by grain (25%), a hearty soup (25%), and the national cracker-like Crispbread. Most other EU countries offering school lunches offer targeted or subsidized free lunches, with two countries offering universal free lunches (Finland and Sweden) and two offering no free lunches (Denmark and the Netherlands).

School meals in the European Union reflect the cultural foods of each country, such as sausages, liverwurst, borscht, soft cheeses, and unfamiliar fruits. In France, school meals include culinary classics to preserve French heritage [32]. In the United Kingdom, the impact of school meals on nutritional intake was positively noted in the early grades with above minimum intake of vegetables, protein, and fiber. However, nutritional quality eroded as the school children progressed into upper grades, where more processed foods were commonly consumed [33].

North America

The beginning of this chapter outlined the history of school lunch in the United States, and one may mistakenly believe that the same process and timeline occurred for our northern neighbor, Canada. However, while the United States established school meals in the 1930s and 1940s, Canada chose not to build meals into the school day. In 2017, UNICEF flagged Canada for neglecting child nutrition because it ranked 37 out of the 41 wealthiest countries for its lack of attention to child nutrition [34].

In April 2024, Canada announced that it would implement a national school food program to provide an additional 400,000 school meals yearly for the next 5 years. This five-billion-dollar program will translate into ensuring that two million additional children will receive school meals. The prime minister cited many compelling reasons for providing free school meals, many of which have been covered in this chapter, such as the long-term impact on children's health and improved academic performance [34].

Conclusions

Internationally, school meals are debated, scrutinized, and researched not only from a nutritional standpoint but also as an investment in the health and learning of their youth. Over the past decade, US changes in meal standards have generated interest in child obesity, increased knowledge uptake and test scores, better school attendance, and long-lasting food behavior changes. These emerging outcomes will provide data for future nutritional changes in school meals.

Further Practice

1. What two countries in the European Union provide universal free meals?

   a. Norway and Sweden
   b. Germany and Denmark
   c. Sweden and Finland
   d. The United Kingdom and Luxemburg

2. Which foods are most likely to be a smart snack?

   a. Donut
   b. Peanuts
   c. Fruit-flavored jelly beans
   d. Orange flavored soda

3. Food waste can be lessened or prevented by all the following except

   a. Scheduling recess after lunch
   b. Scheduling lunch close to noon
   c. Presenting foods in an attractive manner
   d. Increasing the time to eat

4. In what year did the United States establish a pilot of extra allotments for "needy schools"?

   a. 1942
   b. 1952
   c. 1962
   d. 1972

5. In the early twentieth century, what charities began initiating school meals in large cities across the United States?

   a. Wealthy corporation foundations
   b. Men's service organizations
   c. The US Senate
   d. Women-driven charities.

6. How did the United States' entry into World War II impact school meals?

   a. Increased the nutritional content
   b. Depleted commodity options
   c. Increased the commodity options
   d. Stopped the government's support of school meals

7. In which of the following countries do 90% of students bring meals from home to school?

   a. Finland
   b. Korea
   c. Australia
   d. New Zealand

8. What is the most common critical food violation in schools?

   a. Adequate handwashing sinks
   b. Management and employee food safety knowledge
   c. Facilities that maintain proper storage
   d. Potentially hazardous food temperatures during preparation

9. A second-chance breakfast occurs _____.

   a. When breakfast is served for lunch
   b. When leftovers from school breakfast can be eaten after school
   c. When a mother drops off a breakfast meal for their child after school starts
   d. When breakfast is served after the first period class

10. Which of the following states does not provide a universal free lunch?

    a. Florida
    b. Colorado
    c. Michigan
    d. Minnesota

11. Which global area has the largest population that receives school meals?

    a. Europe
    b. Sub-Saharan Africa
    c. Latin America
    d. The Middle East

12. Which of the following changes will increase school meal consumption?

    a. Making food more attractive
    b. Scheduling recess after lunch
    c. Shortening the time during which meals are served
    d. Skipping lunch and sending the meal home with students after the last bell

13. Which entrée would be the most likely food item to be partially or entirely thrown out after mealtime?

    a. Spaghetti
    b. Pizza
    c. Beef stew
    d. Lentil meat loaf

14. With the full implementation of school lunches following the Dietary Guidelines for Americans, all of the following should occur except which one?

    a. Increased whole grains
    b. Reduced sugar
    c. Reduced cholesterol
    d. Reduced sodium

15. In what year was the Healthy Hunger-Free Kids Act passed at the federal level?

    a. 2019
    b. 2020
    c. 2021
    d. 2022

Answer Keys

1. c
2. b
3. a
4. b
5. d
6. b
7. c
8. b
9. d
10. a
11. c
12. a
13. d
14. c
15. b

References

1. Gunderson G. The national school lunch program background and development. Nova Science Publishers; 2003. ISBN 1-59033-639-9
2. Moreland-Russell S, Jabbari J, Farah Saliba L, Ferris D, Jost E, Frank T, Chun Y. Implementation of flexibilities to the National School Lunch and breakfast programs and their impact on schools in Missouri. Nutrients. 2023;15(3):720. https://doi-org.ezproxy.gvsu.edu/10.3390/nu15030720
3. Vilsack TJ. Healthy school meals for all: the role of food law and policy. J Food L Pol'y. 2023;19(1):8–20.
4. Gearan EC, Fox MK. Updated nutrition standards have significantly improved the nutritional quality of school lunches and breakfasts. J Acad Nutr Diet. 2020;120(3):363–70. https://doi.org/10.1016/j.jand.2019.10.022.
5. Schwartz MB, Henderson KE, Read M, Danna N, Ickovics JR. New school meal regulations increase fruit consumption and do not increase total plate waste. Child Obes. 2015;11(3):242–7. https://doi-org.ezproxy.gvsu.edu/10.1089/chi.2015.0019
6. Wang L, Cohen JFW, Maroney M, Cudhea F, Hill A, Schwartz C, Lurie P, Mozaffarian D. Evaluation of health and economic effects of United States school meal standards consistent with the 2020-2025 dietary guidelines for Americans. Am J Clin Nutr. 2023;118(3):605–13. https://doi-org.ezproxy.gvsu.edu/10.1016/j.ajcnut.2023.05.03
7. Kaiser R, Hamlin D. The National School Lunch Program and healthy eating: an analysis of food selection and consumption in an urban title I middle school. Educ Urban Soc. 2024;56(2):143–63. https://doi.org/10.1177/00131245221110552.
8. Kenney EL, Barrett JL, Bleich SN, Ward ZJ, Cradock AL, Gortmaker SL. Impact of the healthy, hunger-free kids act on obesity trends. Health Aff. 2020;39:1122–9.
9. Evans RR, Orihuela C, Mrug S. Middle school stakeholder perceptions of school nutrition reform since the healthy, hunger-free kids act of 2010. Am J Health Educ. 2021;52(5):276–87. https://doi-org.ezproxy.gvsu.edu/10.1080/19325037.2021.1955226
10. Meier CL, Brady P, Askelson N, Ryan G, Delger P, Scheidel C. What do parents think about school meals? An exploratory study of rural middle school parents' perceptions. J Sch Nurs. 2022;38(3):226–32. https://doi.org/10.1177/1059840520924718.

11. Rosa PJ, Madeira A, Oliveira J, Palrão T. How much is a chef's touch worth? Affective, emotional and behavioural responses to food images: a multimodal study. PLoS One. 2023;18(10):1–20. https://doi.org/10.1371/journal.pone.0293204.

12. Merlo C, Smarsh BL, Xiao X. School nutrition environment and services: policies and practices that promote healthy eating among K-12 students. J Sch Health. 2023;93(9):762–77. https://doi.org/10.1111/josh.13365.

13. Large A, Morgan R, Kalas S, Appleton K, Giglia R. Determining best practice for school-based nutrition and cooking education programs: a scoping review. Issues Educ Res. 2023;33(3):1047–65.

14. St. Pierre C, Sokalsky A, Sacheck JM. Participant perspectives on the impact of a school-based experiential food education program across childhood, adolescence, and young adulthood. J Nutr Educ Behav. 2024;56(11):4–15.

15. Bergling E, Pendleton D, Owen H, Shore E, Risendal B, Harpin S, Whitesell N, Puma J. Understanding the experience of the implementer: teachers' perspectives on implementing a classroom-based nutrition education program. Health Educ Res. 2021;36(5):568–80. https://doi.org/10.1093/her/cyab027.

16. FitzSimons C, Hayes C. The reach of school breakfast and lunch during the 2022–2023 school year. 2024. https://frac.org/wp-content/uploads/Reach-Report-2024.pdf.

17. Olarte DA, Tsai MM, Chapman L, Hager ER, Cohen JFW. Alternative school breakfast service models and associations with breakfast participation, diet quality, body mass index, attendance, behavior, and academic performance: a systematic review. Nutrients. 2023;15(13):2951. https://doi.org/10.3390/nu15132951.

18. Chandrasekhar A, Xie L, Mathew MS, Fletcher JG, Craker K, Parayil M, Messiah SE. Academic and attendance outcomes after participation in a school breakfast program. J Sch Health. 2023;93(6):508–14. https://doi.org/10.1111/josh.13320.

19. Cuadros MA, Thomsen MR, Nayga RM. School breakfast and student behavior. Am J Agric Econ. 2023;105(1):99–121. https://doi.org/10.1111/ajae.12312.

20. Lambert L, Mann G, Knight S, Partacz M, Jurss MA, Eady M. Impact of smart snacks intervention on college students' vending selections. J Am Coll Health. 2023;71(3):952–8. https://doi-org.ezproxy.gvsu.edu/10.1080/07448481.2021.1909048

21. Reynolds J, Jeong H, Nom CS . School food service directors'national trainig practices. 2022;42(6). https://doi.org/10.1111/jfs.13010

22. Piekarz-Porter E, Lin W, Smart CJF. Snacks fundraiser exemption policies: are states supporting the spirit of smart snacks? J Sch Health. 2019;89:692–7.

23. Harris JL, Hyary M, Schwartz MB. Effects of offering look-alike products as smart snacks in schools. Child Obes. 2016;12(6):432–9. https://doi-org.ezproxy.gvsu.edu/10.1089/chi.2016.0080

24. Cohen JFW, Kesack A, Daly TP, Elnakib SA, Hager E, Hahn S, Hamlin D, Hill A, Lehmann A, Lurie P, Maroney M, Means J, Mueller MP, Olarte DA, Polacsek M, Schwartz MB, Sonneville KR, Spruance LA, Woodward AR, Chapman LE. Competitive foods' nutritional quality and compliance with smart snacks standards: an analysis of a National Sample of U.S. middle and high schools. Nutrients. 2024;16(2):275. https://doi.org/10.3390/nu16020275.

25. Lindke AR, Smith TA, Cotwright CJ, Morris D, Cox GO. Plate waste evaluation of plant-based protein entrees in National School Lunch Program. J Nutr Educ Behav. 2022;54(1):12–9. https://doi.org/10.1016/j.jneb.2021.06.002.

26. Thomas JR, Hanson D, Chinnan-Pothen A, Freaney C, Silverman J. Packed school lunch food consumption: A childhood plate waste nutrient analysis. Nutrients. 2023;15(5):1116. https://doi-org.ezproxy.gvsu.edu/10.3390/nu15051116

27. Cropley M, Sprajcer M, Dawson D. Wastogram: validation of a new tool to measure household food waste. J Environ Psychol. 2022;84. https://doi-rg.ezproxy.gvsu.edu/10.1016/j.jenvp.2022.101896:101896.

28. Global Child Nutrition Foundation (GCNF). School meal programs around the world: results from the 2021 Global Survey of School Meal Programs. 2022. ©.survey.gcnf.org/2021-global-survey
29. Johnson B, Manson A, Gallegos D, Golley R. Australian schools are starting to provide food, but we need to think carefully before we 'ditch the lunchbox'. The Conversation. 2022; https://theconversation.com/australian-schools-are-starting-to-provide-food-but-we-need-to-think-carefully-before-we-ditch-the-lunchbox-193536
30. McKelvie-Sebileau P, Swinburn B, Glassey R, Tipene-Leach D, Gerritsen S. Health, Well-being and nutritional impacts after two years of free school meals in New Zealand. Health Promot Int. 2023;38(4):1–13. https://doi.org/10.1093/heapro/daad093.
31. Kim Y, Son K, Kim J, Lee M, Park KH, Lim H. Associations between school lunch and obesity in Korean children and adolescents based on the Korea National Health and nutrition examination survey 2017-2019 data: A cross-sectional study. Nutrients. 2023;15(3):698. https://doi-org.ezproxy.gvsu.edu/10.3390/nu15030698
32. Maxwell R. Everyone deserves quiche: French school lunch programmes and national culture in a globalized world. Br J Sociol. 2019;70(4):1424–47. https://doi.org/10.1111/1468-4446.12643.
33. Haney E, Parnham JC, Chang K, Laverty AA, von Hinke S, Pearson-Stuttard J, et al. Dietary quality of school meals and packed lunches: a national study of primary and secondary schoolchildren in the U.K. Public Health Nutr. 2023;26(2):425–36. https://doi.org/10.1017/S1368980022001355.
34. Ruetz AT, Martin A, Ng E. A national school food program for all: towards a social policy legacy for Canada. Our Schools/Our Selves; 2022. p. 35–7.

Integrating Food Security and Health for Sustainable Well-being

14

Elizabeth Wall-Bassett (ID)

Learning Objectives

After completing this chapter, you will be able to

- Define food security and hunger, and summarize the scope of food security worldwide
- Investigate the populations most vulnerable to food insecurity and some of the risk factors for food insecurity
- Differentiate the effects of food insecurity on malnutrition
- Explain the strategies and initiatives that address food insecurity

Introduction

Defining Food Insecurity

Food security is defined as households that have consistent, dependable access at all times to enough food for an active, healthy life [1]. In contrast, a household is food insecure when any of its members does not have the resources needed to get adequate amounts of nutritious food [1]. The concept of food insecurity includes components of quantity, quality, suitability, and the psychological and social realms [2, 3]. Food insecurity can be an indicator of trade-offs between paying for basic needs—such as housing, utilities, healthcare, and so on—and using funds for food [4, 5]. In essence, food security is a measure of financial security and public health.

E. Wall-Bassett (✉)
Western Carolina University, School of Health Science, Nutrition and Dietetics Program, Cullowhee, NC, USA
e-mail: ewbassett@wcu.edu

© The Author(s), under exclusive license to Springer Nature Switzerland AG 2025
A. K. Mitra, D. Vanoh (eds.), *Essentials of Clinical and Public Health Nutrition*, Nutrition and Health, https://doi.org/10.1007/978-3-031-95373-6_14

The COVID-19 pandemic also affected food insecurity, which led to increased hunger rates, disrupted food supply chains, and reduced incomes in almost every country around the world [6]. Hunger is a physiological condition that is a consequence of food insecurity; occurs from a prolonged, involuntary lack of food; and results in discomfort, illness, weakness, or pain.

Measuring Food Security

Since 1995, the US Department of Agriculture (USDA) has tracked food security in the United States through an annual survey conducted as a supplement to the US Census Bureau's Current Population Survey [1]. This survey evaluates how households manage their food purchases and intake to save money, sometimes resulting in some members eating less. Food security status is determined by responses to the household food security survey module. This survey includes three general questions for all households, seven questions specifically for adults, and an additional eight questions for households with children. These questions assess conditions over the past year. On the basis of the answers, a scale categorizes households as either food secure (high or marginal food security) or food insecure (low or very low food security).

Box 14.1

High food security is defined by having no reported indication of food access problems or limitations. Marginal food security is defined by one or two reported indications (e.g. anxiety over food insufficiency or a shortage of food in the residence), with no indication of changes in diets or food intake. Low food security is defined by reports of reduced food quality, variety, or desirability in the diet, with little or no indication of reduced food intake. Very low food security is defined by reports of multiple indications of disrupted eating patterns and reduced food intake.

The USDA does not directly measure hunger or the number of hungry people. In contrast, the Food and Agriculture Organization of the United Nations (FAO) has reported on global hunger since 1974, using the term *hunger* interchangeably with the word *undernourishment* [3]. The FAO currently uses the prevalence of undernourishment (PoU) metric to estimate food availability, food consumption, and dietary energy needs annually. Although this measure effectively monitors national and regional trends representative of the entire population, it does not identify specific individuals who are undernourished or their locations.

Integrating Food Security and Health for Sustainable Well-being

Global and National Goals

In 2015, the international community established 17 Sustainable Development Goals (SDGs), with a target for 2023 agenda for sustainable development for peace and prosperity for people, and to address global challenges, including food security and nutrition [7] [Fig. 14.1]. Notably, SDG 2.1.1 uses the prevalence of undernourishment (PoU) to monitor progress toward eliminating hunger, and SDG 2.1.2 measures moderate-to-severe food insecurity to ensure access to safe, nutritious, and sufficient food year-round. The SDGs offer a holistic framework recognizing the interconnected social, economic, and environmental factors affecting food security and nutrition, promoting integrated efforts to achieve sustainable food production and consumption.

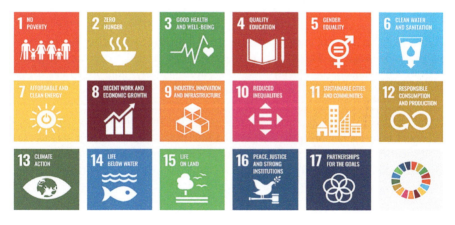

Fig. 14.1 Sustainable development goals

Box 14.2 The SDGs Relevant to Food Security and Nutrition
- *Goal 1: End Poverty* targets economic empowerment, social protection, and inclusive growth to reduce poverty and enhance food security.
- *Goal 2: Zero Hunger* aims to end hunger, improve nutrition, and promote sustainable agriculture, with targets to reduce child stunting and boost small-scale food producers' productivity.
- *Goal 3: Good Health and Well-being* focuses on ensuring healthy lives and nutrition, reducing child mortality, and providing universal health-care access.
- *Goal 12: Responsible Consumption and Production* seeks sustainable food systems, halving food waste, and promoting sustainable agricultural practices.
- *Goal 13: Climate Action* urges action against climate change to protect food security, enhancing resilience to climate hazards and promoting climate education.
- *Goal 15: Life on Land* promotes sustainable land use, halting deforestation, restoring land, and enhancing sustainable land management practices.

The US Department of Health and Human Services (HHS) launched the Healthy People program in 1980, updating it every 10 years to set national health objectives and monitor progress. This program addresses the social determinants of health (SDOHs) by considering factors like economic stability, education, healthcare access, neighborhood conditions, and social context. Informed by past accomplishments and challenges, Healthy People 2030 aims to reduce food insecurity in US households with a focus on upstream actions and health equity [8]. Combining the efforts of both frameworks, the USDA and international bodies strive to increase food security and improve nutrition through comprehensive and integrated strategies that consider various influencing factors and aim for sustainable development and health equity.

Who Is Food Insecure?

Food insecurity is a global, systemic issue affecting diverse individuals and households, transcending demographic and geographic boundaries. It can be temporary or long term and is closely linked to unemployment and economic hardship, primarily driven by poverty. In 2022, 29.6% of the global population (2.4 billion people) experienced moderate or severe food insecurity, with nearly half in Asia, 10.5% in Latin America and the Caribbean, and about 4% in North America and Europe [9]. These populations struggle to consistently meet their dietary needs. Food insecurity disparities exist between poor and wealthy nations and within countries like the United States due to financial and structural barriers. Factors such as affordable housing, social isolation, location, and chronic health issues intersect with social determinants of health, exacerbating food insecurity and health inequities.

Vulnerable groups include women, households with children, single-mother-led households, marginalized communities, racial and ethnic minorities, LGBTQ+ individuals, people with disabilities, and college students [1, 10, 11]. Historical and structural racism and discrimination in economic opportunities, employment, education, housing, and lending often drive these inequities [10, 11].

Food insecurity is particularly severe in rural areas due to persistent challenges in accessing healthy food, with rural women and their families facing unique difficulties in meeting basic needs [12–15]. Rural areas are food deserts, lacking retailers that provide fresh, nutritious, and affordable food. Additionally, both rural and urban areas can be food swamps, where stores predominantly sell unhealthy, calorie-dense junk foods. These conditions complicate efforts to ensure equitable access to healthy food. Tools like the Food Access Research Atlas [16] and Food Environment Atlas [16] help understand and address these challenges by providing insights into food access indicators and factors influencing food choices and health outcomes in rural environments.

The Challenge of Food Security

Addressing the Social Determinants of Health (SDOHs)

Despite surpassing global food production needs, food insecurity persists. The intricate challenge of food insecurity is closely intertwined with the five place-based domains of the SDOHs (economic stability, education access and quality, healthcare access and quality, neighborhoods and built environments, and social and community contexts), reflecting the broader societal and environmental factors influencing

Fig. 14.2 Social determinants of health

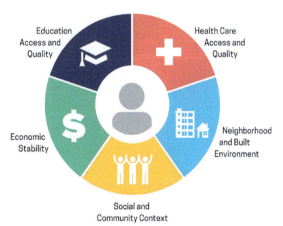

individual well-being (Fig. 14.2). An increasing number of individuals and their families worldwide grapple with unequal access to affordable, nutritious food, heightening the risk of food insecurity and poorer health outcomes. Recognizing and addressing the socioeconomic inequalities that contribute to food insecurity is key to devising effective solutions to this pervasive issue.

Economic Stability

Income is a fundamental driver of food insecurity, impacting not only low-income households but also those above the poverty line, including the "working poor" who struggle to afford necessities despite being employed [Fig. 14.3]. Insufficient wages and benefits, along with unstable employment and a high cost of living, force

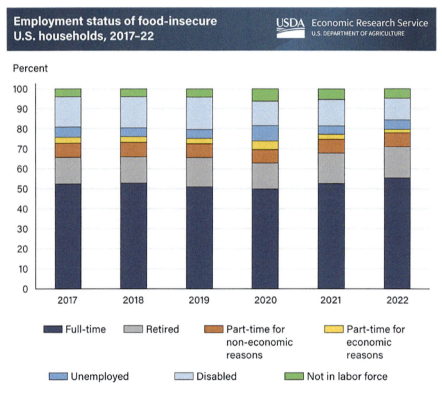

Note: **Food insecure** includes low and very low food security. **Full time** = adult(s) employed full time. **Retired** = adult(s) out of the labor force because of retirement; no adults employed full time. **Part-time for noneconomic reasons** = adult(s) employed part-time by choice; no adults employed full time or retired. **Part-time for economic reasons** = adult(s) employed part time because that was the only job available; no adults employed full time or retired. **Unemployed** = adult(s) unemployed looking for work; no adults employed or retired. **Disabled** = adult(s) out of the labor force because of disability; no one employed, retired, or unemployed. **Not in labor force** = no adults employed, retired, unemployed, or not working because of disability.

Source: USDA, Economic Research Service calculations using data from U.S. Department of Commerce, Bureau of the Census, Current Population Survey Food Security Supplements.

Fig. 14.3 Employment status of US food-insecure households, 2017–2022

individuals to make trade-offs that exacerbate food insecurity. Rising inflation has further strained economically vulnerable people, who often cut food expenses first during financial hardship.

Affordable housing is crucial in mitigating food insecurity because high housing costs directly affect the ability to afford nutritious food. Many households, especially renters, spend a significant portion of their income on housing, leaving less for food and other essentials. This results in housing instability and frequent relocations, further compounding financial difficulties and food insecurity.

Neighborhood and Built Environments

Food insecurity is not solely an issue of individual access to food but also deeply linked to the broader neighborhood and built environments where communities reside. Economic factors like contracts, pricing, and marketing strategies in the food supply chain significantly influence the availability and affordability of nutritious foods. Consolidation within the food system by large corporations limits competition and consumer influence, leading to limited choices and higher costs for nutritious foods, especially in underserved communities. Unhealthy food marketing exacerbates diet-related diseases. Environmental health is critical, with industrial agricultural practices contributing to environmental degradation and impacting the long-term sustainability of food production. Pesticide use poses risks to water, soil, and air quality, affecting both food systems and community health, especially among farmworkers. Safe and affordable transportation, along with accessible routes to healthy food, are vital for addressing food insecurity, particularly for vulnerable populations with limited access to grocery stores and fresh produce. Improving transportation infrastructure and increasing access to healthy food options are essential steps in combating food insecurity and promoting community health and safety.

Healthcare Access and Quality

The intersection between affordable healthcare, medical expenses, insurance coverage, and effective health communication presents a significant challenge to both food security and overall health outcomes. Health issues often escalate medical costs for individuals who struggle with food insecurity, destabilizing household finances and diverting funds away from essential needs like food. The lack of affordable health coverage and rising out-of-pocket expenses push individuals to forgo essential care, exacerbating vulnerabilities to food insecurity and perpetuating a cycle of financial strain and heightened health risks.

Globally, over half of the population lacks access to essential health services, with catastrophic health spending rising and affecting over a billion individuals worldwide [17]. When healthcare costs are burdensome, households face unpaid medical bills and agonizing choices between medical expenses and food. Limited access to affordable healthcare can hinder timely treatment and exacerbate health disparities, leading to increased expenses and further financial strain. Food insecurity contributes to mental health issues, chronic diseases, and developmental impairments in children, impacting long-term economic prospects. Addressing the interplay between healthcare access, food security, and health outcomes is crucial for fostering resilience and well-being within communities.

Social and Community Contexts

People's relationships and interactions with family, friends, coworkers, and community members are critical for shaping their health, well-being, and access to food security. However, various societal challenges can profoundly impact these connections, presenting formidable obstacles to maintaining adequate nutrition and stability. Political instability, unrest, and sanctions disrupt food supply chains, leading to shortages and price fluctuations that affect individuals' ability to access nutritious food. Conflict-affected regions experience disruptions in agricultural production and distribution, exacerbating food shortages and price spikes. Sanctions imposed on countries restrict access to essential resources, impeding trade relationships and hampering individuals' ability to afford food. Food imports and global trade dynamics play crucial roles, especially for countries heavily reliant on imported goods. Fluctuations in commodity prices and trade policies lead to unpredictable food costs, hampering the ability of individuals, particularly those with limited financial means, to afford essential dietary needs. Disruptions in global trade increase food shortages and prices, further compromising food security for vulnerable populations. Discrimination and inequality among vulnerable populations pose significant challenges to food security, perpetuating poverty and marginalization worldwide. Socioeconomic disparities, compounded by factors like race, gender, and ethnicity, result in unequal access to resources and opportunities, including nutritious food, employment, and education. Addressing these systemic barriers is crucial for achieving equitable food security and promoting the well-being of all individuals, regardless of their socioeconomic background or identity.

Education Access and Quality

Access to education empowers individuals to acquire the knowledge and skills essential for decision-making and working efficiency, thereby enhancing food security. Education enables students to utilize techniques and technologies to increase economic opportunities and improve nutritional attainment. However, hungry individuals may struggle to actively engage in learning due to motivational and physiological barriers, potentially hindering educational progress.

For farmers, education plays a vital role in implementing effective farming methods, efficiently managing resources, and adapting to technological innovations. Educated farmers can enhance food production, stimulate economic development, and improve living standards within farming communities. Limited financial resources often hinder farmers' ability to invest in education and adopt new practices, perpetuating food insecurity.

Conversely, a lack of education can exacerbate food insecurity, especially among marginalized populations. Food insecurity can impede educational attainment, particularly among vulnerable populations like women, children, and farmworkers. Families facing economic hardship may prioritize immediate needs over education, causing children to drop out of school and face risks like early marriages and pregnancies. Additionally, food insecurity negatively impacts children's school readiness, hindering their academic success and overall development.

Food Insecurity and Public Health

The Effects of Food Insecurity

Food insecurity has profound effects on health and well-being, contributing to developmental, behavioral, and physical problems and to reduced community cohesion and increased healthcare costs. Poor diet quality can lead to conditions like wasting, stunting, and overweight/obesity. Globally, around one-third of the population experiences malnutrition in various forms, including undernutrition and micronutrient deficiencies [18]. The 2020 UNICEF Conceptual Framework on Maternal and Child Nutrition [19, 20] highlights the connection between malnutrition, diets, and care. Malnutrition exacerbates chronic conditions such as heart disease, stroke, cancer, and diabetes and is a significant social determinant of health [21] (Fig. 14.4).

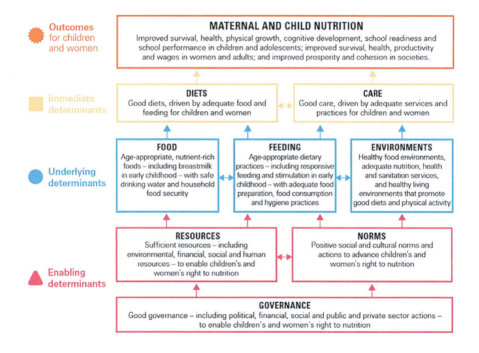

UNICEF Conceptual Framework on the Determinants of Maternal and Child Nutrition, 2020.
A framework for the prevention of malnutrition in all its forms.

Fig. 14.4 UNICEF conceptual framework on the determinants of maternal and child nutrition, 2020

Food insecurity is closely linked to a wide range of physical and psychological challenges, especially in children [22, 23]. Beyond immediate hunger, it affects development and behavioral health, with children in food-insecure households showing increased susceptibility to anxiety, irritability, and depression. This often leads to withdrawn behavior and a greater need for mental health services [24–28]. Physically, these children experience poor health status, more hospitalizations, and more doctor visits. They also face academic challenges, with higher risks of under-achievement, decreased attentiveness, more aggression, more absences, and higher suspension rates [29, 30]. Moreover, food insecurity affects higher education, hindering college students' nutrition, health outcomes, academic progress, and graduation prospects due to associated basic-needs insecurities [31–34].

Undernutrition and Micronutrient Deficiencies

Food insecurity affects a significant portion of the global population, where around 815 million people suffer from undernutrition, resulting in three million child deaths annually [7]. Micronutrient deficiencies, including those in vitamin A, iron, iodine, and zinc, are prevalent worldwide, especially in low- and middle-income countries [35]. Vitamin A deficiency can lead to blindness and increased mortality among children, and iron deficiency causes anemia and maternal mortality. Iodine deficiency affects thyroid hormone synthesis, impacting mental development and reproductive functions. Zinc deficiency compromises immune function, growth, and wound healing, posing risks to pregnant individuals and infants. Adequate intakes of these micronutrients are crucial for overall health and well-being, highlighting the importance of addressing food insecurity and micronutrient deficiencies globally.

Protein-Energy Malnutrition

Protein-energy malnutrition (PEM) is a prevalent global issue, affecting approximately one in nine people [36]. It results from the inadequate intake of both energy (calories) and protein, leading to the depletion of energy stores and tissue proteins. This deficiency often manifests as wasting, with three main types: kwashiorkor, marasmus, and marasmic kwashiorkor. Kwashiorkor is characterized by protein malnutrition; marasmus is primarily an energy deficiency; and marasmic kwashiorkor involves severe shortages of both calories and protein. Acute malnutrition is common in temporary or cyclical settings like emergencies and highly infectious environments. Classic symptoms include edema in kwashiorkor and a frail appearance in marasmus. Complications can include encephalopathy, heart failure, increased infections, and mortality. Treatment involves a comprehensive approach addressing dehydration, nutrient imbalances, and tissue depletion with a gradual restoration of protein and calories [37].

Chronic Malnutrition

Chronic malnutrition occurs when an individual consistently fails to acquire sufficient dietary energy to meet their daily needs, leading to long-term physical and cognitive developmental delays [38, 39]. Stunting, or reduced growth in height, is the most common indicator of chronic malnutrition, but it is only one aspect of the condition. A chronically malnourished child, compared to peers with optimal growth conditions, will likely be shorter [40], have impaired cognitive abilities [41], and face a higher risk of poor health outcomes throughout life. No standardized procedures for treating chronic malnutrition are available, because the causes and consequences of it are multifaceted, encompassing both short-term and long-term impacts on health and development.

Overnutrition and Chronic Conditions

Overnutrition, characterized by excessive calorie intake and insufficient physical activity, is a significant global issue, affecting 2.5 billion adults and 41 million children under five, with one in eight people experiencing obesity [42]. Obesity increases the risk of chronic diseases like high blood pressure, heart disease, cancer, and type 2 diabetes, accounting for a significant portion of global deaths. Obesity results from a complex interplay of genetic, metabolic, behavioral, and environmental factors, but it is largely preventable and manageable. Modifiable risk factors include individual behaviors and environmental influences. Treatment involves assessment and management, with a client-centered approach recommended for improving health outcomes and quality of life [43].

Innovative Approaches to Food Security

Multilevel Strategies

Many resilience approaches help with addressing the complex and interconnected challenges of food insecurity and hunger. The socioecological model examines multiple levels of influence, including individual, interpersonal, community, organizational, and societal factors. It highlights the significance of addressing factors like personal characteristics, social relationships, community environments, organizational structures, and systemic policies to improve food security. SDG 1.5 aims to build resilience among vulnerable populations and reduce their exposure to various shocks and disasters [7]. Proactive health promotion efforts, equity-focused strategies, sustainable agricultural practices, and the integration of nutrition objectives into development policies are highlighted as urgent needs for increasing resilience and capacity building [44].

Focus on Equity

When implementing comprehensive solutions to address food insecurity, particularly in marginalized communities, an equity lens that is culturally appropriate, inclusive, and equitable must be employed. This involves understanding and respecting the cultural backgrounds of the community, considering risks such as occupational hazards and safety in housing and transportation, and addressing barriers to nutritious food, education, and healthcare. Building trust through community engagement and appropriate communication is essential. By engaging community leaders and members, services can be tailored to meet specific needs and overcome barriers. Strong links to culturally appropriate services, facilitated through trusted community figures and translated materials, are essential to making these services accessible and effective.

Strengthening health systems to identify, prevent, treat, and manage malnutrition and diet-related noncommunicable diseases is vital for addressing food insecurity in marginalized communities. For instance, building on and integrating into broader standardized data collection protocols and sharing across all programs serving vulnerable populations help monitor disease progress and trends as well as guide policy and priorities that are targeted and effective. Regular health screenings can help assess and identify individuals at risk of malnutrition or diet-related noncommunicable diseases such as diabetes or cardiovascular conditions. Access to specialized care, including nutritionists and dietitians, is essential for effective, evidence-based, and client-centered diagnoses and treatments of these conditions and for monitoring them, such as providing nutrition counseling and meal planning services that can empower individuals to make healthier food choices and effectively manage their conditions. Community-based nutrition education programs can be implemented to encourage healthy eating habits and prevent malnutrition, especially among vulnerable groups.

Fostering collaboration among federal, state, and local governments, alongside private and nonprofit sectors, is crucial for establishing a resilient food provision infrastructure. Through these partnerships and equitable employment strategies, communities can address systemic issues contributing to food insecurity and overall well-being. Advocating for fair wages and workers' rights, alongside policies supporting paid leave and benefits, aims to ensure access to nutritious food and healthcare services. Additionally, investments in safe housing, quality childcare, and education support family stability and indirectly improve nutrition and health outcomes. These collaborations should incentivize cooperation across sectors to enhance the delivery of food and nutrition benefits, addressing challenges like food deserts and transportation barriers. Initiatives to optimize transportation networks and adjust zoning regulations facilitate access to healthy food, particularly in underserved areas. Connecting federal food programs with local producers supports local economies and reduces food deserts, bolstering community resilience.

Strengthening Food and Nutrition Infrastructure

Strengthening community-based food systems offers a promising pathway toward sustainability and resilience by implementing multifaceted intervention strategies, programs, and policies to address various aspects of nutrition and food access. Initiatives such as biofortification, reformulation, and fortification aim to improve the quality of nourishing foods and enhance diet quality across the lifespan. Supporting smallholder farmers in diversifying their production and fortifying staple foods at the point of manufacture or use are essential strategies. Additionally, fortification mandates ensure that staple foods are enriched with vital nutrients, benefiting broader populations, especially in urban areas. The reformulation of processed foods can lead to products with a healthier profile, reducing the consumption of unhealthy components like excessive sugar and sodium.

The USDA oversees a multitude of hunger and nutrition programs tailored to meet the diverse needs of underserved groups [Table 14.1]. Programs such as the

Table 14.1 Federal food and nutrition assistance in the United States

Program	Purpose	Eligibility criteria
Supplemental Nutrition Assistance Program (SNAP)	To improve the diets of low-income households by increasing access to food and food purchasing	Income, household size, assets, housing costs, work requirements, and other factors More information: www.fns.usda.gov/snap
Commodity Supplemental Food Program (CSFP)	To improve the health and nutrition of low-income older adults at least 60 years of age by supplementing diets with nutritious USDA commodity foods	Age, income, and nutritional risk More information: www.fns.usda.gov/csfp
Food Distribution Program on Indian Reservations (FDPIR)	To provide commodity foods and nutrition education for improving diet quality of low-income households, including older adults, living on Indigenous reservations and of Native American families residing in designated areas near reservations	At least one person who is a member of a federally recognized tribe, income and resource criteria, residence on a reservation or in approved areas near a reservation or in Oklahoma May not participate in FDPIR and SNAP in the same month More information: www.fns.usda.gov/fdpir
The Emergency Food Assistance Program (TEFAP)	To supplement the diets of low-income individuals, including older adults, by providing emergency food and nutrition assistance	Income and employment More information: www.fns.usda.gov/tefap
National School Lunch Program (NSLP); National School Breakfast Program (NSBP)	To assist states in providing free or reduced-price lunches or breakfasts to eligible children	Income of student households attending public or nonprofit private schools of high school grade or under and public or nonprofit residential childcare institutions More information: www.fns.usda.gov/nslp or www.fns.usda.gov/nsbp
Afterschool Snack Program	To assist school-based after-school educational or enrichment programs with providing healthful snacks to children up to age 18	The same income eligibility as that for NSLP and NSBP More information: www.fns.usda.gov/afterschool-snacks
Summer Food Service Program (SFSP)	To ensure that children and teens in lower-income areas continue to receive nutritious meals during long school vacations, when they do not have access to school lunch or breakfast	Meals for all children 18 years of age and younger who come to an approved open site or to an eligible enrolled site in communities, where eligibility is based on income data More information: www.fns.usda.gov/cn

(continued)

Table 14.1 (continued)

Program	Purpose	Eligibility criteria
Child and Adult Care Food Program (CACFP)	To improve the quality and affordability of daycare for low-income families by providing nutritious meals and snacks to children and to adults who receive care in nonresidential daycare centers, meals to children in homeless shelters, and snacks and dinners to youth in eligible after-school care programs	Varies by population served and type of facility More information: www.fns. usda.gov/cn
Special Supplemental Nutrition Program for Women, Infants, and Children (WIC)	To safeguard the health of low-income women, infants, and children up to age five who are at nutritional risk by providing nutritious foods to supplement diets, information on healthy eating, and referrals to healthcare	Pregnant, breastfeeding, and postpartum people, infants up to 1 year of age, and children up to the age of five who are at nutritional risk and if they meet income standards More information: www.fns. usda.gov/wic

Supplemental Nutrition Assistance Program (SNAP), the Special Supplemental Nutrition Program for Women, Infants, and Children (WIC), and child nutrition programs provide access to nutritious foods and alleviate the financial strain of poverty. Investing in safety net nutrition programs further bolsters food security, reaching vulnerable populations in diverse settings. Strategies like incentivizing supermarket development in underserved areas and integrating federal programs with local agriculture initiatives enhance food access while strengthening community resilience. Food literacy also plays a pivotal role in promoting healthier eating habits, with nutrition education programs offering practical guidance on nutrition, meal planning, and cooking skills.

Preventing malnutrition, particularly among vulnerable groups such as children and women, is critical for fostering food security. Investments in the continuum of care for children and adolescents can improve current and future nutrition while breaking the intergenerational cycle of malnutrition [45]. Educational initiatives and support programs aimed at educating mothers and caregivers on proper nutrition during pregnancy and early childhood are vital for healthy development. Supporting appropriate infant and young child feeding practices, policies, and programs that support breastfeeding and ensure access to diverse, nutritious foods are integral to fostering food security [46]. Integrating evidence-based recommendations for breastfeeding and infant nutrition into dietary guidelines underscores the importance of these strategies in bolstering health systems and improving workplace policies.

Sustainability in Agriculture and Food Production

The commitment to Sustainable Development Goals (SDGs) emphasizes eradicating poverty and hunger through sustainable agriculture and food systems. Infrastructure development plays a crucial role in enhancing connectivity between rural and urban areas, promoting responsible land use, and reducing environmental hazards. Optimizing resource use, promoting sustainable pest and weed control, leveraging renewable energy, effectively managing waste, enhancing transportation and storage, and fostering research and education protect both the food system and the environment. Shifting toward sustainable agricultural practices, such as crop rotation and integrated pest management (IPM), ensures long-term viability. Investments in public infrastructure like roads and storage facilities reduce trading costs, incentivizing farmers to cultivate diverse, high-value crops, thus improving food security and diets. Addressing climate change impacts and enhancing market competition are critical for sustainable agriculture and food security. Redirecting domestic agricultural subsidies toward sustainable practices and healthy diets can facilitate transitions to more-resilient and more-equitable food systems, aligning with SDGs and ensuring food security for all.

Incorporating Nutrition and Public Health Objectives into Development Policies

Incorporating nutrition and public health objectives into development policies and programs across the food system can significantly enhance food security by transforming food environments and promoting healthier choices. Strategic policies supporting healthy eating and sustainable agricultural practices can create environments conducive to better health outcomes, reducing chronic disease prevalence and ensuring equitable access to nutritious foods for all. By addressing both supply factors and demand factors, governments can foster environments that make the healthy choice the easy choice, ultimately improving public health.

Creating supportive environments that enable healthier choices is key to preventing chronic diseases. Policies promoting urban planning for walkable cities, incentives for grocery stores in underserved areas, and community-based nutrition education can all contribute to a healthier population. Healthier environments in schools and retail spaces can be achieved through targeted policy interventions like improved nutritional standards in school meals and taxes on unhealthy foods. By making healthy options more accessible, affordable, and attractive, these policies encourage better dietary habits and improve public health outcomes.

Initiatives like the Healthy People framework align grant opportunities and state improvement plans with public health priorities, ensuring that children receive essential nutrients through USDA child nutrition programs and by bolstering breastfeeding support initiatives. Agrifood system policies, such as tariffs and subsidies, can influence the availability and affordability of nutritious foods. Import quotas and tariffs protect domestic agriculture, whereas export bans and taxes ensure that essential foods remain locally available. Subsidies incentivize farmers to grow more-nutritious crops, and land-use regulations and fortification legislation promote agricultural practices that support public health goals, increasing the nutrient content of available foods and promoting balanced diets.

Personal Actions to Help Reduce Food Insecurity

Individuals play a vital role in addressing food insecurity by actively engaging with their communities and advocating for change. One way to make a difference is by informing low-income individuals about available federal and local food-related services and programs. By spreading awareness and providing guidance, individuals can help ensure that those in need are aware of the resources available to them.

Moreover, individuals can work toward increasing the accessibility of existing programs to those who require assistance the most. This may involve collaborating with local organizations to streamline application processes or provide transportation options for those with limited mobility. Additionally, volunteering in these programs allows individuals to directly contribute to their community's well-being while gaining firsthand insights into the challenges faced by those experiencing food insecurity. By monitoring the household food security status of clients and conducting or participating in research to document the effectiveness of food assistance programs, individuals can also contribute valuable data to inform future initiatives and policy decisions. Furthermore, supporting local food production through initiatives not only stimulates food security but also strengthens local economies and fosters community resilience. By joining forces with like-minded individuals and actively participating in the legislative process, individuals can amplify their impact and advocate for systemic changes that address the root causes of food insecurity. Finally, when individuals learn more about food insecurity and document hunger-related needs in their own communities, they can empower themselves to be effective advocates and catalysts for positive change.

Further Practice

1. What is food security?

   a. The ability to produce food within a household
   b. The consistent, dependable access at all times to enough food for an active, healthy life
   c. Having a varied diet with both nutritious and nonnutritious foods
   d. The absence of any anxiety over food insufficiency

2. What does food insecurity indicate about a household?

   a. The household spends too much on nonessential items.
   b. The household has no issues with accessing food.
   c. The household members do not have the resources needed to get adequate amounts of nutritious food.
   d. The household purchases only nutritious food.

3. Which demographic is particularly vulnerable to food insecurity?

    a. Single individuals without children
    b. Households with children, especially single-mother-led households
    c. Wealthy urban communities
    d. Senior citizens living in luxury retirement homes

4. What are some of the primary drivers of food insecurity?

    a. High wages and stable employment
    b. Poverty, unemployment, and economic hardship
    c. Access to affordable housing
    d. The excessive consumption of junk food

5. How does the built environment affect food security?

    a. By providing unlimited access to any type of food
    b. By ensuring all neighborhoods have equal access to fresh, nutritious food
    c. By influencing the availability and affordability of nutritious foods in communities
    d. By making food supply chains immune to economic factors

6. Which of the following best describes the effects of food insecurity on children's mental health?

    a. Improved academic performance and increased attentiveness
    b. Increased susceptibility to anxiety, irritability, and depression
    c. A reduced need for mental health services
    d. Enhanced social skills and community involvement

7. What is a common consequence of chronic malnutrition in children?

    a. Increased height and cognitive abilities compared to peers
    b. Reduced growth in height (stunting) and impaired cognitive abilities
    c. Enhanced immune function and fewer hospitalizations
    d. A lower risk of poor health outcomes throughout life

8. Which of the following micronutrient deficiencies can lead to blindness in and increased mortality among children?

    a. Iron deficiency
    b. Iodine deficiency
    c. Vitamin A deficiency
    d. Zinc deficiency

9. Which Sustainable Development Goal (SDG) specifically monitors progress toward eliminating hunger by using the prevalence of undernourishment (PoU) metric?

    a. SDG 1.5

b. SDG 2.1.1
c. SDG 2.1.2
d. SDG 3.1.1

10. What is the main objective of the Healthy People 2030 program regarding food insecurity in the United States?

    a. To increase global food production
    b. To reduce food insecurity in US households with a focus on upstream actions and health equity
    c. To promote sustainable agricultural practices worldwide
    d. To implement universal basic income policies

11. What does the socioecological model highlight as essential for improving food security?

    a. Individual dietary supplements
    b. Addressing multiple levels of influence, including individual, interpersonal, community, organizational, and societal factors
    c. Increasing agricultural exports
    d. Reducing the number of supermarkets in urban areas

12. Which strategy is crucial for addressing food insecurity in marginalized communities, according to this chapter?

    a. Implementing universal healthcare
    b. Employing an equity lens that is culturally appropriate, inclusive, and equitable
    c. Increasing food imports from high-income countries
    d. Encouraging urban sprawl to reduce population density

13. How can strengthening community-based food systems contribute to food security?

    a. By increasing dependency on imported food
    b. By implementing multifaceted intervention strategies, programs, and policies to address various aspects of nutrition and food access
    c. By reducing the variety of locally grown crops
    d. By promoting the consumption of processed foods

14. Which of the following accurately distinguishes between food insecurity and hunger, according to this chapter?

    a. Food insecurity refers to a lack of access to sufficient, safe, and nutritious food at all times, whereas hunger is a physical sensation that results from not eating enough food.
    b. Food insecurity is a measure of the physical sensation of needing food, whereas hunger is a broader issue involving the inability to regularly access nutritious food.

    c. Food insecurity is a systemic issue involving a lack of consistent access to nutritious food, whereas hunger is a more immediate and personal experience of not having enough to eat.

    d. Food insecurity is a direct consequence of experiencing hunger, whereas hunger is a long-term issue of food access and availability.

15. How do wasting, stunting, and overweight/obesity differ in the context of food insecurity?

    a. Wasting is characterized by inadequate calorie intake, leading to low weight for height; stunting results from chronic undernutrition, leading to reduced height for age; and overweight/obesity is associated with excessive calorie intake and insufficient physical activity.

    b. Wasting refers to reduced height due to prolonged undernutrition; stunting is defined by low weight for height; and overweight/obesity involves both inadequate calorie intake and low nutrient quality.

    c. Wasting and stunting both result from immediate calorie deficiency, whereas overweight/obesity is caused by a lack of access to nutritious food, leading to high body fat accumulation.

    d. Stunting results from acute calorie deficiency; wasting is due to chronic malnutrition; and overweight/obesity occurs from high-quality calorie intake but insufficient physical activity.

Answer Keys

1. b
2. c
3. b
4. b
5. c
6. b
7. b
8. c
9. b
10. b
11. b
12. b
13. b
14. c
15. a

References

1. Rabbitt MP, Hales LJ, Burke MP, Coleman-Jensen A. Household food security in the United States in 2022. (Report No. ERR-325). U.S. Department of Agriculture, Economic Research Service; 2023. https://doi.org/10.32747/2023.8134351.ers.

2. Ballard TJ, Kepple AW, Cafiero C, Schmidhuber J. Better measurement of food insecurity in the context of enhancing nutrition. Ernahr Umsch. 2014;61(2):38–41.
3. Splett PL. Federal food assistance programs: a step to food security for many. Nutr Today. 1994;29(2):6–13.
4. Gundersen C, Engelhard E, Hake M. The determinants of food insecurity among food bank clients in the United States. J Consum Aff. 2017;51:501–18. https://doi.org/10.1111/joca.12157.
5. Calloway EE, Fricke HE, Pinard CA, Smith TM, Yaroch AL. Monthly SNAP benefit duration and its association with food security, hunger-coping, and physiological hunger symptoms among low-income families. J Appl Res Child. 2015;6(2):5.
6. Paslakis G, Dimitropoulos G, Katzman DK. A call to action to address COVID-19-induced global food insecurity to prevent hunger, malnutrition, and eating pathology. Nutr Rev. 2021;79(1):114–6. https://doi.org/10.1093/nutrit/nuaa069.
7. UN. Transforming our world: the 2030 agenda for sustainable development. New York: United Nations, Department of Economic and Social Affairs; 2015.
8. Office of Disease Prevention and Health Promotion. Reduce household food insecurity and hunger – NWS-01. Healthy people 2030. U.S. Department of Health and Human Services. (n.d.). https://health.gov/healthypeople/objectives-and-data/browse-objectives/nutrition-and-healthy-eating/reduce-household-food-insecurity-and-hunger-nws-01
9. FAO, IFAD, UNICEF, WFP and WHO. The state of food security and nutrition in the world 2023. Urbanization, agrifood systems transformation and healthy diets across the rural–urban continuum. Rome, FAO. 2023. https://doi.org/10.4060/cc3017en
10. Food Research & Action Center. The impact of food insecurity on women's health. Available at https://frac.org/blog/impact-food-insecurity-womens-health#:~:text=Research%20from%20the%20U.S.%20Department,14.7%20percent)%20are%20particularly%20high. Last accessed 3/5/24.
11. Coleman-Jensen, A and M Nord. Food insecurity among households with working-age adults with disabilities, ERR-144, U.S. Department of Agriculture, Economic Research Service, January 2013.
12. Sharkey JR, Johnson CM, Dean WR. Relationship of household food insecurity to health-related quality of life in a large sample of rural and urban women. Women Health. 2011;51(5):442–60.
13. Pollin R. Hardship in America: the real story of working families. East Econ J. 2005;31(4):681–3. Retrieved from https://www.proquest.com/scholarly-journals/hardship-america-real-story-working-families/docview/197998537/se-2
14. Berry AA, Katras MJ, Sano Y, Lee J, Bauer JW. Job volatility of rural, low-income mothers: a mixed methods approach. J Fam Econ Iss. 2008;29:5–22. https://doi.org/10.1007/s10834-007-9096-1.
15. Vondracek FW, Coward RT, Davis LA, Gold CH, Smiciklas-Wright H, Thorndyke LE. Introduction. In: Coward RT, Davis LA, Gold CH, Smiciklas-Wright H, Thorndyke LE, Vondracek FW, editors. Rural women's health: mental, behavioral, and physical issues. New York: Springer Publishing Company; 2006. p. 3–5.
16. Economic Research Service (ERS), U.S. Department of Agriculture (USDA). Food Access Research Atlas, https://www.ers.usda.gov/data-products/food-access-research-atlas/
17. World Health Organization; World Bank. Tracking universal health coverage: 2023 global monitoring report. Washington, DC: World Bank; 2023. http://hdl.handle.net/10986/40348
18. UNICEF. UNICEF conceptual framework on maternal and child nutrition. New York, NY: UNICEF Nutrition and Child Development Section, Programme Group; 2020.
19. Bread for the World Institute. 2014 Hunger Report: Ending Hunger in America. Silver Spring: Bread for the World Institute; 2013.
20. World Health Organization. WHO accelerates work on nutrition targets with new commitments [Internet]. 2021. Available from: https://www.who.int/news/item/07-12-2021-who-accelerates-work-onnutrition-targets-with-new-commitments#:~:text=Today%2Cone%20third%20of%20all,8%20million%20deaths%20per%20year
21. WHO. What is malnutrition?. http://www.who.int/features/qa/malnutrition/en/

22. Council on Community Pediatrics, & Committee on Nutrition. Promoting food security for all children. Pediatrics. 2015;136(5):e1431–8. https://doi.org/10.1542/peds.2015-3301.
23. Shankar P, Chung R, Frank DA. Association of Food Insecurity with children's behavioral, emotional, and academic outcomes: a systematic review. J Dev Behav Pediatr: JDBP. 2017;38(2):135–50. https://doi.org/10.1097/DBP.0000000000000383.
24. Alaimo K, Olsen C, Frongillo EA. Food insufficiency and American school-aged children's cognitive, academic, and psychosocial development. Pediatrics. 2001;108:44–51.
25. Ryu JH, Bartfeld JS. Household food insecurity during childhood and subsequent health status: the early childhood longitudinal study–kindergarten cohort. Am J Public Health. 2012;102(11):e50–5. https://doi.org/10.2105/AJPH.2012.300971.
26. Brown JL, Shepard D, Martin T, Orwat L. The economic cost of domestic hunger: estimated annual burden to the United States (Harvard public health study). Sodexo Foundation; 2007. Retrieved from http://us.stop-hunger.org/files/live/sites/stophunger-us/files/HungerPdf/Cost%20of%20Domestic%20Hunger%20Report%20_tcm150-155150.pdf
27. McIntyre L, Williams JV, Lavorato DH, Patten S. Depression and suicide ideation in late adolescence and early adulthood are an outcome of child hunger. J Affect Disord. 2013;150(1):123–9. https://doi.org/10.1016/j.jad.2012.11.029.
28. McLaughlin KA, Green JG, Alegría M, Jane Costello E, Gruber MJ, Sampson NA, Kessler RC. Food insecurity and mental disorders in a national sample of U.S. adolescents. J Am Acad Child Adolesc Psychiatry. 2012;51(12):1293–303. https://doi.org/10.1016/j.jaac.2012.09.009.
29. Howard LL. Does food insecurity at home affect non-cognitive performance at school? A longitudinal analysis of elementary student classroom behavior. Econ Educ Rev. 2011;30(1):157–76. https://doi.org/10.1016/j.econedurev.2010.08.003.
30. Nelson BB, Dudovitz RN, Coker TR, Barnert ES, Biely C, Li N, Szilagyi PG, Larson K, Halfon N, Zimmerman FJ, Chung PJ. Predictors of poor school readiness in children without developmental delay at age 2. Pediatrics. 2016;138(2):e20154477.
31. Olfert MD, Hagedorn-Hatfield RL, Houghtaling B, Esquivel MK, Hood LB, MacNell L, Soldavini J, Berner M, Savoie Roskos MR, Hingle MD, Mann GR, Waity JF, Knol LL, Walsh J, Kern-Lyons V, Paul C, Pearson K, Goetz JR, Spence M, Anderson-Steeves E, Wall-Bassett ED, Lillis JP, Kelly EB, Hege A, Fonenot MC, Coleman P. Struggling with the basics: food and housing insecurity among college students across twenty-two colleges and universities. J Am Coll health. 2023;71(8):2518–29.
32. Broton KM, Mohebali M, Lingo MD. Basic needs insecurity and mental health: community college students' dual challenges and use of social support. Commun Coll Rev. 2022;50:00915521221111460.
33. Gundersen C, Ziliak JP. Food insecurity and health outcomes. Health Aff. 2015;34:1830–9.
34. Richards R, Stokes N, Banna J, Cluskey M, Bergen M, Thomas V, Bushnell M, Christensen R. A comparison of experiences with factors related to food insecurity between college students who are food secure and food insecure: a qualitative study. J Acad Nutr Diet. 2023;123(3):438–453.e2. https://doi.org/10.1016/j.jand.2022.08.001.
35. Victora CG, Christian P, Vidaletti LP, Gatica-Domínguez G, Menon P, Black RE. Revisiting maternal and child undernutrition in low-income and middle-income countries: variable progress towards an unfinished agenda. Lancet (London, England). 2021;397(10282):1388–99. https://doi.org/10.1016/S0140-6736(21)00394-9.
36. Valdés-Sosa PA, Galler JR, Bryce CP, Rabinowitz AG, Bringas-Vega ML, Hernández-Mesa N, Taboada-Crispi A. Seeking biomarkers of early childhood malnutrition's long-term effects. MEDICC Rev. 2018;20(2):43–8. https://doi.org/10.37757/MR2018.V20.N2.10.
37. WHO. Guideline: Updates on the Management of Severe Acute Malnutrition in infants and children. Geneva: World Health Organization; 2013.
38. Bergen DC. Effects of poverty on cognitive function: a hidden neurologic epidemic. Neurology. 2008;71(6):447–51. https://doi.org/10.1212/01.wnl.0000324420.03960.36.
39. Horta BL, Victora CG, de Mola CL, Quevedo L, Pinheiro RT, Gigante DP, Motta JVDS, Barros FC. Associations of linear growth and relative weight gain in early life with human capital at 30 years of age. J Pediatr. 2017;182:85–91.e3. https://doi.org/10.1016/j.jpeds.2016.12.020.

40. Bateson P, Barker D, Clutton-Brock T, Deb D, D'Udine B, Foley RA, Gluckman P, Godfrey K, Kirkwood T, Lahr MM, McNamara J, Metcalfe NB, Monaghan P, Spencer HG, Sultan SE. Developmental plasticity and human health. Nature. 2004;430(6998):419–21. https://doi.org/10.1038/nature02725.

41. Kar BR, Rao SL, Chandramouli BA. Cognitive development in children with chronic protein energy malnutrition. Behav Brain Funct. 2008;4:31. https://doi.org/10.1186/1744-9081-4-31.

42. WHO fact sheet, Obesity and Overweight. 1 March 2024. Accessed May 20, 2024. https://www.who.int/news-room/fact-sheets/detail/obesity-and-overweight

43. Raynor HA, Morgan-Bathke M, Baxter SD, Halliday T, Lynch A, Malik N, Garay JL, Rozga M. Position of the academy of nutrition and dietetics: medical nutrition therapy behavioral interventions provided by dietitians for adults with overweight or obesity, 2024. J Acad Nutr Diet. 2024;124(3):408–15. https://doi.org/10.1016/j.jand.2023.11.013.

44. National Academies of Sciences, Engineering, and Medicine; Health and Medicine Division; Board on Population Health and Public Health Practice; Committee on Informing the Selection of Health Indicators for Healthy People 2030. Leading health indicators 2030: advancing health, equity, and Well-being. National Academies Press; 2020.

45. FAO. Enhancing nutrition in emergency and resilience agriculture responses to prevent child wasting. FAO'S child wasting prevention action plan (2023–2024). Rome; 2022.

46. Indicators for assessing infant and young child feeding practices: definitions and measurement methods. Geneva: World Health Organization and the United Nations Children's Fund (UNICEF), 2021. Licence: CC BY- NC-SA 3.0 IGO; https://creativecommons.org/licenses/by-nc-sa/3.0/igo.

Exploring the Relationship Between Ultra-Processed Foods and Adverse Health Outcomes

15

Fatin Hanani Mazri and Nurul Fatin Malek Rivan

Learning Objectives

After completing this chapter, you will be able to

1. Identify the NOVA food classification system
2. Understand the health implications of ultra-processed foods and their potential mechanism
3. Understand the strategies to reduce ultra-processed food consumption

Introduction

The growth of the food-processing industry in Malaysia has been a key driver of economic progress, providing jobs and boosting the country's gross domestic product (GDP). This sector has made a variety of processed food products easily accessible to consumers through aggressive marketing strategies and distribution networks. Despite this, there is a growing concern that these products often lack essential nutrients and may contain high levels of unhealthy ingredients such as added sugars, fats, and preservatives while containing low levels of dietary fiber, protein, vitamins, and minerals [1]. This has implications for public health in that

F. H. Mazri
Dietetics Programme and Centre for Healthy Ageing and Wellness (H-CARE), Faculty of Health Sciences, Universiti Kebangsaan Malaysia, Jalan Raja Muda Abdul Aziz, Kuala Lumpur, Malaysia
e-mail: fatinhananimazri@ukm.edu.my

N. F. M. Rivan (✉)
Nutritional Sciences Programme and Centre for Healthy Ageing and Wellness (H-CARE), Faculty of Health Sciences, Universiti Kebangsaan Malaysia, Jalan Raja Muda Abdul Aziz, Kuala Lumpur, Malaysia
e-mail: fatinmalek@ukm.edu.my

the increased consumption of these food products could induce eating behaviors linked to various health issues, including cancer, diabetes, and cardiovascular diseases [2]. Thus, making informed choices and balancing processed foods with whole and minimally processed options are important in maintaining a healthy and nutritious diet.

However, a significant shift from consuming whole or minimally processed foods to consuming ultra-processed foods (UPFs) has taken place over the past few decades, driven by several interrelated factors. These include changes in food manufacturing and distribution systems that have increased the marketing of UPFs, lifestyle changes that lead to increased demand for convenience foods, and economic factors that make these foods more affordable and accessible for many people [3]. This shift has made UPFs a significant topic of interest in nutrition and public health. Researchers and health professionals are increasingly concerned about the potential long-term health impacts of a diet high in UPFs. Albeit convenient and often more affordable, these foods are typically energy-dense and nutrient-poor foods, leading to a range of chronic health conditions [4, 5]. Therefore, the rise of the food-processing industry, while economically beneficial, poses a challenge to maintaining a healthy population, highlighting the need for better nutritional guidelines and public awareness campaigns to mitigate the negative health impacts associated with UPF consumption. This chapter delves into the nature of UPFs, their prevalence, and their implications for public health.

Ultra-Processed Foods: Ingredients, Characteristics, and Nutritional Composition

The NOVA food-processing classification system has shifted the focus of nutrition research on processed foods from the previously dominant level of nutrient composition to the level of food products, their ingredients and processing characteristics, and their role in differentiating types of dietary patterns [6]. NOVA classification is one of the superlative techniques recognized by the Food and Agricultural Organization of the United Nations and the Pan American Health Organization as a valid tool to use to observe UPF consumption that can be linked to the nutritional status of an individual [7]. This novel approach categorizes foods into four groups on the basis of the extent and purpose of their processing, providing a comprehensive framework for understanding the impacts of food processing on dietary patterns and health outcomes. Table 15.1 describes foods that are categorized according to the NOVA food-processing classification system and provides examples.

Ultra-processed foods UPFs are industrial formulations made entirely or mostly from substances extracted from foods, derived from food constituents, or synthesized in laboratories. They are highly palatable, habit-forming, characteristically energy-dense foods high in added sugar, salt, oils, saturated fats, and protein

Table 15.1 NOVA food-processing classification system

Group	Degree of processing	Description	Examples
1	Unprocessed or minimally processed foods	These foods undergo minimal processing to remain close to their natural state. Processes include cleaning, trimming, refrigerating, freezing, pasteurizing, and packaging (as long as no additives are included).	Fresh fruits, vegetables, grains, meats, milk, eggs, dried beans, nuts, seeds, fresh fish
2	Processed culinary ingredients	These are substances extracted from whole foods or from nature and used to prepare, season, enhance, and cook Group 1 foods. Although these ingredients are derived from natural foods, they undergo processes, such as pressing, grinding, or refining, that significantly alter their original form to make them suitable for culinary use.	Oils (olive oil, vegetable oil), butter, sugar, salt, honey, starches
3	Processed foods	These foods are created by adding salt, sugar, or oil to Group 1 foods to preserve them or make them palatable. These foods retain the basic identity of their original ingredients but are modified to improve taste, shelf life, or convenience.	Canned vegetables, fruits in syrup, cheeses, freshly baked breads, pickles, smoked meats
4	Ultra-processed foods	These foods are industrial formulations, typically with five or more ingredients. They often contain ingredients not commonly used in home cooking, such as preservatives, emulsifiers, artificial flavors, and colorings.	Packaged snacks, sugary beverages, instant noodles, reconstituted meat products, preprepared meals

Source: Monteiro et al. (2019b) [8]

isolates and often contain artificial additives such as flavors, flavor enhancers, colors, emulsifiers, emulsifying salts, artificial sweeteners, thickeners, and antifoaming, bulking, carbonating, foaming, gelling, and glazing agents. Any example of these classes of additives, as shown on ingredients lists, also qualifies a product as ultra-processed [8, 9]. UPFs are defined as distinct from non-UPFs, not only in terms of their ingredient composition but also in terms of the purpose for which they are processed. These products are designed to be tasteful (often hyperpalatable), convenient (durable, ready to consume), highly profitable (cheap ingredients, value adding), and shelf-stable, often at the expense of nutritional quality, as shown in Table 15.2 [1].

Table 15.2 Nutritional composition of UPFs

Nutritional component	Description
Free or added sugar	High levels of added sugars, including high-fructose corn syrup, glucose, sucrose, and other sweeteners
Saturated and trans fats	High in trans fats and saturated fats, often derived from hydrogenated oils and other industrial processes
Sodium	Elevated levels of sodium, often added for flavor enhancement and preservation
Energy density	High energy density, meaning a high number of calories per serving size, which contributes to excessive calorie intake
Lack of fiber	Generally low in dietary fiber due to the removal of whole food components during processing
Low in essential nutrients	Low in essential vitamins and minerals such as vitamins A, B, C, D, and E; iron; magnesium; and potassium
Protein content	Often contains low-quality protein sources or isolated protein additives rather than whole, high-quality protein from natural sources

---

Box 15.1 Key characteristics of UPFs
- *Multiple processing steps* include extensive processing to alter the food's physical, chemical, and sensory properties.
- *Ingredient complexity* refers to long ingredient lists with many unfamiliar, scientific, or technical names.
- *Additives* are used at high levels to enhance taste, texture, and preservation. Common additives include artificial sweeteners, flavor enhancers, preservatives, and coloring agents.
- *Calorie density and poor nutritional quality* are characteristic of foods high in calories, fats, sugars, and sodium while low in essential nutrients and fiber.
- Aggressive marketing strategies and attractive packaging often feature health claims to promote overconsumption.

The consumption of UPFs is gradually displacing home-prepared meals and the intake of fresh fruits and vegetables in daily diets. This shift is particularly concerning because ultra-processed foods remain fundamentally unhealthy despite being reformulated and marketed as healthier options. Nowadays, many ultra-processed products are labeled as "light" or "diet" or advertised as low in fat or sugar, free from trans fats, and high in fiber, vitamins, and minerals. These modifications can enhance the nutritional profile of the products to some extent, but they do not change the fact that these items are still heavily processed [8]. The inherent issues associated with UPFs, such as the presence of artificial additives, high levels of refined sugars and unhealthy fats, and low levels of essential nutrients, persist despite these changes. Consequently, although these products may appear healthier, they continue to contribute to poor dietary habits and adverse health outcomes [5, 8].

Health Implications of Ultra-Processed Foods and Their Potential Mechanisms

The rapid rise in UPF consumption has paralleled increases in various chronic health conditions, prompting extensive research into the potential health implications of these foods. Although UPFs offer undeniable convenience, their widespread consumption raises critical questions about their impact on public health. Also, although mechanistic research is still in its early stages, emerging evidence indicates that the properties of ultra-processed foods might have synergistic or compounded effects on chronic inflammatory diseases. These effects could operate through recognized or plausible physiological mechanisms, such as alterations to the gut microbiome and increased inflammation [10–12]. Researchers, public health experts, and the public have shown significant interest in ultra-processed dietary patterns, foods, and their components due to their potential role as modifiable risk factors for chronic diseases and mortality. This chapter delves into the evidence linking UPFs to a range of adverse health outcomes, including obesity, metabolic disorders, cardiovascular diseases, cancer, and mental health concerns.

Obesity

One of the significant health implications of consuming ultra-processed foods is obesity. UPFs are typically high in calories but low in nutritional value. They tend to increase the intake of saturated and trans fats, sugars, refined carbohydrates, and sodium while decreasing the intake of fiber, micronutrients, and other beneficial bioactive compounds naturally present in foods [13]. Furthermore, UPFs have been shown to be less satiating and characterized by a greater glycemic response than minimally processed foods [14]. Due to their high energy density, low satiety, and large portion sizes, consuming these products may promote excess energy intake [14]. The ease of preparation associated with UPFs can disrupt normal eating habits, leading to rapid and unconscious food consumption while engaged in routine alternative activities [15, 16]. This can interfere with the neural and digestive signals that regulate hunger and fullness, resulting in overeating [17, 18]. Additionally, the high fat and sugar content of UPFs can affect the brain's reward system in a way that increases food cravings and further promotes overconsumption [19]. Additionally, ultra-processed foods are often designed to be very palatable, leading people to eat more unprocessed or minimally processed foods than they normally would [20].

Research on the health effects of UPFs beyond their nutrient content is still limited. Louzada et al. (2015) [21] discovered that the link between UPF intake and obesity remained significant even after accounting for saturated fat, trans fat, added sugar, and fiber intake. This suggests that nutrient composition alone cannot explain the impact of UPFs on obesity risk. Moreover, associations with obesity and related health outcomes have not been observed for processed foods, which typically do not exhibit the same convenience and palatability as ultra-processed foods. For example, household purchases of processed foods did not correlate with body mass index (BMI) or obesity among Brazilians [15], and processed food intake by preschoolers was not associated with changes in lipid profiles over 4 years [13]. These findings indicate that UPFs may contribute to adverse health outcomes independently of their nutrient content. However, more research is needed to explore hypotheses related to palatability, satiating potential, and convenience to determine whether UPFs have unique characteristics that impact health beyond poor nutrient content.

Cardiometabolic Disorders

Cardiometabolic disorders refer to clusters of interrelated risk factors that increase an individual's chances of developing cardiovascular disease and type 2 diabetes [22]. These risk factors typically include high blood pressure, elevated blood sugar levels (hyperglycemia), abnormal cholesterol levels (dyslipidemia), and excess body fat around the waist (central obesity). The term is often associated with metabolic syndrome, which consists of a specific collection of these risk factors. A strong association exists between consuming ultra-processed foods and cardiometabolic disorders and all-cause mortality [23]. More than 70 long-term prospective epidemiological studies, along with several short-term interventional studies, have consistently found that the consumption of UPFs is associated with weight gain and an increased risk of various diseases, especially cardiometabolic conditions [10, 24].

Excessive energy intake and obesity due to the consumption of UPFs are certainly factors in the development of cardiometabolic risk factors. However, these factors alone do not fully account for the associations observed between UPFs and cardiometabolic risk, as many studies have adjusted for BMI and total energy intake in their models. Numerous UPFs, including condiments, broths, soup powders, and processed meats, contain high levels of salt, which leads to increased sodium intake, a known risk factor for hypertension [25]. UPFs are also a source of trans and saturated fatty acids, which may contribute to an increased risk of dyslipidemia, such as decreasing high-density lipoprotein (HDL) cholesterol [26]. Additionally, UPFs contain numerous chemical additives, synthetic antioxidants, and preservatives, many of which have been linked to an increased risk of obesity, worsened lipid and glucose profiles, and the induction of low-grade inflammation and metabolic syndrome [27, 28]. Finally, those who consume high amounts of UPFs are presumed to consume lower amounts of whole grains, fruits, and vegetables, limiting the intake of micronutrients and bioactive compounds that may reduce cardiometabolic risk [29].

Cancer

Cancer is one of the leading causes of death worldwide. A shred of growing evidence indicates a connection between the level of food processing and higher cancer risk [30]. Recent global data highlight significant shifts in food processing, notably an upsurge in processed food availability, particularly during the historically unprecedented SARS-CoV-2 pandemic lockdown [31]. This surge in processed food availability, in which UPFs contributed to over half of total energy intake, underscores the concerning trend in dietary habits [32]. A recent systematic review revealed that every 10% increase in the proportion of UPFs in the diet was associated with a 4% higher risk of colorectal cancer [33]. Similarly, other systematic reviews have disclosed that diets high in processed foods, such as processed meats, sweets, fried foods, and refined grains, contribute to an elevated risk of cancer [34]. Conversely, Mediterranean-style diets, abundant in fruits, vegetables, extra virgin olive oil, whole grains, and other minimally processed foods, have been associated with a 17% reduction in colorectal cancer risk [35]. Additionally, the authors of a prior meta-analysis incorporating findings from 15 studies observed that individuals with the highest consumption of processed meat exhibited a 9% higher risk of breast cancer compared to those with the lowest intake [36]. These findings suggest that a high intake of ultra-processed foods is linked to an elevated risk of specific cancers affecting particular sites within the body, notably those in the digestive tract and certain hormone-related cancers, such as colorectal and breast cancer.

One potential mechanism by which UPF may contribute to cancer is through the presence of carcinogenic compounds. These compounds, such as heterocyclic amines and polycyclic aromatic hydrocarbons, are formed during the processing and cooking of certain foods, including meats and grilled or smoked foods. In grilled, fried, or roasted meat, the concentrations of these compounds can vary greatly but are generally below levels considered to be carcinogenic [37]. However, if humans have a similar sensitivity to these compounds as animals have, consuming large amounts of meat daily would be necessary to reach carcinogenic levels [38].

Another potential mechanism is the disruption of gut bacteria composition and function unfavorably [39], which, in turn, increases cancer risk through multiple molecular signals, including inhibiting T-cell activity and promoting DNA damage [40]. Furthermore, the high content of additives and preservatives in ultra-processed foods may also contribute to cancer development. These additives and preservatives have been linked to DNA damage and disruption to cellular processes, potentially increasing the risk of cancer. Some contaminants in UPFs have been linked to proinflammation potential [41], endocrine-disrupting effects [42], and dysbiosis [43], which have been proven to promote carcinogenesis in epidemiological, clinical, and experimental studies. For example, the consumption of UPFs was notably associated with an elevated level of inflammatory biomarkers, such as IL-6 concentration, involved in tumor progression at almost every step, including initiation, progression, and metastasis [11]. This evidence sheds light on the broader implications of a processed diet in cancer development, offering a more comprehensive understanding of the potential risks associated with dietary habits.

Mental Health Concerns

UPFs, while convenient and palatable, have been increasingly scrutinized for their negative impact on physical health. However, emerging evidence suggests that UPFs also pose significant risks to mental health. The consumption of ultra-processed foods has been linked to an increased risk of mental health concerns, including depression and anxiety [41]. This link between ultra-processed foods and mental health may be due to several factors. The consumption of these foods can lead to nutritional deficiencies crucial for brain function and mental health. For instance, diets lacking in omega-3 fatty acids, magnesium, zinc, and B vitamins have been linked to higher rates of depression and anxiety. These nutrients are essential for neurotransmitter function and brain health, and their deficiency can disrupt neural communication and mood regulation [44].

Furthermore, emerging but limited evidence indicates that a higher consumption of artificial sweeteners (e.g., aspartame and saccharin) and monosodium glutamate (MSG) may disrupt the synthesis and release of neurotransmitters linked to mood disorders, including dopamine, norepinephrine, and serotonin [45]. Additionally, these substances may affect the hypothalamic-pituitary-adrenal (HPA) axis [46]. The consumption of titanium dioxide nanoparticles, commonly used as food colorants for their whiteness and opacity, has been associated with increased levels of the inflammatory cytokine interleukin-6 in both plasma and the cerebral cortex, leading to neuroinflammation in rats [47]. Inflammation is known to play a role in the development, prevalence, and treatment response of mental disorders, where peripheral inflammation measurements are considered as potential biomarkers for these conditions [48].

On the other hand, the excessive activation of the HPA axis could lead to changes in eating habits by increasing the inclination toward and excessive intake of highly appealing and calorically dense foods, including those categorized as ultra-processed [49]. This is particularly relevant in the context of COVID-19, indicating that individuals may resort to consuming ultra-processed foods as a coping mechanism for stress-induced anxiety stemming from external factors beyond their control [50]. The link between adverse mental health and an increase in the consumption of ultra-processed foods could have repercussions on various metabolic outcomes, as suggested by both experimental (randomized controlled trial) evidence and epidemiological (prospective) evidence, including weight gain or a higher body mass index [3, 24]. Further human studies are needed to discern the specific characteristics of ultra-processed foods that contribute to harm and are needed to determine whether the observed connections between ultra-processed food consumption and mental or related physical health are causal.

Mortality

In recent years, a growing body of evidence has pointed toward the detrimental effects of UPFs on human health, particularly concerning mortality rates. A systematic review reported that a diet with a high intake of UPFs was associated with a higher risk of mortality in a diverse multinational population [51]. Participants with the highest UPF intake ($\geq$ 2 servings/day) exhibited a staggering 28% higher risk of mortality compared to those with minimal or no consumption [52]. This trend was consistent with a large cohort study from France, which showed a 14% higher risk of mortality for each 10% increase in UPF consumption [53], further underlining the grave implications of UPF consumption on mortality rates. Interestingly, the relationship between UPF consumption and mortality appears to be influenced by body weight status and geographical location. Healthy-weight individuals exhibited stronger associations between UPF intake and mortality compared to their overweight and obese counterparts, possibly due to the under-reporting of food intake among the latter group [54]. Moreover, the impact of UPFs on mortality was more pronounced in low- and middle-income countries, aligning with the disproportionate burden of cardiovascular disease in these regions [52].

Several hypotheses have been proposed to elucidate the adverse health outcomes associated with UPF consumption. UPFs are often laden with trans fats, artificial additives, and environmental contaminants, which may contribute to neurotoxicity, carcinogenesis, and inflammatory responses [55, 56]. Furthermore, the energy-dense nature of UPFs, coupled with their low nutritional value, may promote over-consumption and exacerbate the risk of obesity and related comorbidities [57]. Additionally, UPFs could disrupt gut microbiota balance, fostering inflammation and increasing susceptibility to cardiovascular events and mortality [56]. The evidence underscores the urgent need for public health interventions to reduce UPF consumption and promote healthier dietary choices worldwide. By elucidating the intricate link between UPFs and mortality, this research paves the way for targeted strategies to mitigate the global burden of chronic diseases and improve overall population health.

Sleep and Eating Patterns

The modern food landscape has undergone a significant transformation, where the proliferation of UPFs has become increasingly prevalent in our diets. UPFs, characterized by their high energy density, refined carbohydrates, and additives, have been linked to a range of health concerns, including their potential impact on sleep and eating patterns.

Existing research suggests that the consumption of UPFs may have detrimental effects on sleep quality and timing. A study conducted among adults in Brazil discovered that individuals with the highest frequency of UPF consumption and the lowest frequency of minimally processed food consumption had a 144% greater chance of having poor sleep quality compared to individuals with the lowest frequency of UPF consumption and the highest frequency of minimally processed food consumption [58]. Similarly, a large cohort study in France, the NutriNet-Sante Study, demonstrated that UPF consumption was associated with higher odds of chronic insomnia, independent of sociodemographic status, lifestyle, diet quality, and mental health status [59]. Correlatively, a study on adolescents demonstrated similar findings: Higher fresh/minimally processed food consumption is a protective factor for poor sleep quality, whereas higher UPF consumption is a risk factor for poor sleep quality [60]. Aligned with these findings, a recent systematic review and meta-analysis have shown that individuals who consume a greater proportion of UPFs in their diet tend to have poorer sleep quality, shorter sleep duration, and more irregular sleep–wake cycles [61, 62].

The complex interplay between UPF consumption and sleep is further compounded by the circadian rhythm. The circadian rhythm is the daily oscillation of various molecular, physiological, and behavioral process that allow organisms to anticipate and prepare for the changes in body functions throughout the 24-hour day–night cycle [63]. Numerous physiological features exhibit the circadian rhythm, including the sleep–wake cycle, feeding/fasting timing, and the secretion of hormones such as melatonin, cortisol, leptin, and ghrelin [64]. The central circadian clock that generates the circadian rhythm is approximately similar to but slightly different from the 24-hour solar clock, which ranges from 23.5 to 24.9 hours in a healthy adult, thus primarily synchronized to 24-hour time according to sunlight [65].

Other stimuli can also act as time cues or zeitgebers, such as melatonin and eating pattern. Melatonin helps to regulate the sleep–wake cycle by serving as a time cue to the central circadian clock in the suprachiasmatic nucleus (SCN) [66]. Melatonin is associated with decreased sleep latency, increased total sleep time, and improved overall sleep quality [67]. Hence, an alteration in melatonin production could affect sleep and consequently induce misalignment in the circadian rhythm. Melatonin is synthesized from the essential amino acid tryptophan, through the intermediate of serotonin [68]. Protein-rich foods like meat, poultry, fish, eggs, and milk are linked to improved sleep quality due to their high tryptophan content [22]. Besides that, diets rich in fruits, vegetables, legumes, and other sources of dietary tryptophan and melatonin can help regulate the circadian sleep–wake cycle and promote better sleep quality [69]. Nonetheless, highly processed and engineered food contains minimal levels of these nutrients, which may disrupt the circadian rhythm.

The timing of meals may also interact with melatonin in a way that affects the circadian rhythm and metabolism. According to the circadian rhythm, human physiology is naturally aligned for daytime physical activity and eating, whereas nighttime is meant for sleep and fasting [70]. Consuming a meal close to bedtime, when melatonin levels are elevated, has been linked with impaired glucose tolerance because melatonin dampens insulin secretion [71]. Other studies have shown that the consumption of UPFs is linked to late eating. A large-scale cross-sectional study among Italian adults ($n = 8688$) reported that late eaters were associated with a lower intake of minimally processed food but a higher intake of UPFs compared to early eaters [72]. Similarly, a study conducted on university students discovered that UPF consumption was positively correlated with late eating [73]. In summary, late eating patterns often include the consumption of UPFs, which are designed for convenience and easy on-the-go consumption.

Furthermore, the high concentrations of sugar and caffeine frequently present in ultra-processed foods can directly disrupt the circadian sleep–wake cycle [20]. A recent meta-analysis reported that adolescents with a higher intake of fat-rich, sugar-rich foods and higher caffeine intake were associated with poorer sleep characteristics compared to adolescents with a higher consumption of healthy foods [74]. Caffeine consumption can prolong sleep latency, which can potentially reduce both the duration and the quality of sleep by suppressing the production of melatonin, the hormone that regulates the sleep–wake cycle [75]. Thus, excessive caffeine intake, especially later in the day, can disrupt the circadian sleep–wake patterns and lead to poor sleep characteristics, including difficulty falling asleep and reduced sleep duration and quality.

Addressing the impact of UPF consumption on sleep and eating patterns is crucial because these factors are intrinsically linked to overall health and well-being. Research has shown that poor sleep and irregular eating patterns can increase the risk of obesity, type 2 diabetes, and cardiovascular disease [76, 77]. Understanding the multifaceted impact of UPF consumption on sleep and eating patterns emphasizes the need for interventions that promote a shift toward a diet rich in whole, minimally processed foods. By addressing the interconnectedness of diet, sleep, and overall health, individuals can take active steps to improve their well-being and reduce their risk of developing adverse health outcomes that are associated with poor sleep and irregular eating patterns.

Strategies to Reduce UPF Consumption

The rise in UPF consumption in modern diets has become a significant public health concern because these highly engineered and nutrient-poor products have been linked to a range of negative health outcomes, including obesity, chronic diseases, and poor nutritional status. To address this issue, a multifaceted approach that targets individuals, communities, and national and global policies is required (Fig. 15.1).

One key strategy is to increase individual awareness and education about the nature and health impact of UPFs. One study has shown that many consumers are unaware of the distinction between processed foods and ultra-processed foods and exhibit confusion in their perception of the healthiness of these foods [78]. Providing clear and accessible information about the characteristics of UPFs, their nutritional labels, and their connections to health outcomes can empower consumers to make better-informed and healthier choices. Furthermore, establishing regular eating and sleeping patterns could be a potential strategy to reduce the tendency for late-night snacking on UPFs. Maintaining a consistent daily eating and sleep schedule can help regulate hunger and cravings [76], possibly making individuals less likely to turn to convenient but unhealthy UPF snacks, especially in the evenings. Adherence to a structured eating pattern, with nutritious whole foods at designated mealtimes, can help individuals feel more satisfied and less prone to impulsive late-night indulgences in UPF options. Similarly, ensuring adequate and quality sleep can play a

Strategies to reduce UPFs consumption

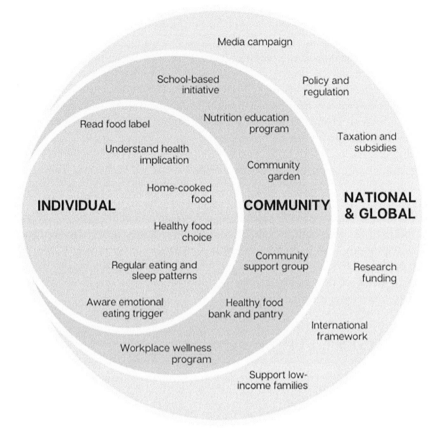

Fig. 15.1 Strategies to reduce UPF consumption at individual, community, national and global levels

crucial role in managing appetite hormones and reducing the urge for late-night snacking. By embedding these healthy lifestyle habits, individuals can build resilience against the temptation of UPFs and make more-mindful, healthier choices throughout the day.

Beyond individual-level interventions, community-based strategies can also play roles in reducing UPF consumption. Increasing the availability and accessibility of whole, minimally processed foods in local communities, such as through the establishment of farmers markets, community gardens, or healthy food banks and pantries, can make healthier options more convenient and affordable for the community or residents [79]. Moreover, school-based initiatives can be applied to reduce UPF consumption among children and adolescents. A randomized controlled trial study on children reported that children who participated in school-based gardening and nutrition education had a reduced intake of UPFs compared to the control group [80]. Hence, schools can be an important setting for fostering healthy eating habits.

Simultaneously, initiatives at the national level are required to create a conducive environment for reducing UPF consumption. Governments need to restrict the marketing and advertising of UPFs, particularly to vulnerable populations like children, which could help shift social norms and reduce the influence of these products on consumer behavior. Another approach is to incentivize the development and accessibility of less-processed, healthier alternatives. Simultaneously, reducing subsidies on the ingredients used in UPFs and redirecting those resources toward the production and distribution of whole, minimally processed foods can help make healthier options more affordable and accessible. Such measures can help make nutritious alternatives more competitive and more accessible to a broader range of consumers.

Conclusion

Addressing the challenge of UPF consumption requires a multipronged approach that spans the individual, community, and national levels. Empowering individuals with education and support for healthier lifestyle habits; fostering community-based initiatives that improve access to whole, minimally processed foods; and implementing comprehensive policy interventions at the national level will require coordinated, collaborative efforts from government agencies, the food industry, and public health stakeholders in developing and implementing a holistic approach aimed at cultivating a more sustainable, equitable, and health-promoting food system. This will collectively contribute to reducing the burden of UPF consumption and its associated health consequences.

Further Practice

1. Which of the following strategies is used to reduce late-night UPF intake?

   A. Watching movies
   B. Reading books
   C. Drinking water
   D. Consistent daily eating
   E. Intermittent fasting

2. Which of the following is an example of a minimally processed food?

   A. Canned vegetables
   B. Biscuits
   C. Bread
   D. Smoked meat
   E. Nuts

3. Ultra-processed foods are prepared by using ingredients not commonly used at home.

   True/false

4. Processed foods have no added sugar/salt, for health purposes.

   True/false

5. Which classification system is used for categorizing food according to its processing techniques?

   A. Owa
   B. NOVA
   C. Dove
   D. Rowa
   E. TOVA

6. Ultra-processed foods are usually high in fiber but low in essential nutrients.

   True/false

7. Which of the following components is used as a food colorant in ultra-processed food?

   A. Vitamin C
   B. Sodium
   C. Titanium dioxide
   D. Potassium
   E. Vitamin B

8. The high concentration of caffeine in ultra-processed food may disrupt the sleep–wake cycle.

   True/false

9. Which if the following is *not* a characteristic of ultra-processed food?

   A. Tasteful
   B. Convenient
   C. Highly profitable
   D. Shelf-stable
   E. Healthy

10. Olive oil and butter are classified as_____.

    A. Processed food
    B. Ultra-processed food
    C. Processed culinary ingredients
    D. Fast food
    E. Unprocessed food

11. Products low in fat or sugar must be labeled as _____.

    A. Light
    B. Heavy
    C. Unhealthy
    D. Healthy
    E. Essential

12. Ultra-processed food may cause cancer because they contain _____.

    A. Nuts
    B. Carcinogens
    C. Vitamins
    D. Minerals
    E. Meat

13. Which of the following refers to the imbalance of gut microbiota that may result from the consumption of UPFs and is linked to an increased risk of cancer?

    A. Dysbiosis
    B. Inflammation
    C. Cytokine
    D. Carcinogenesis
    E. Apoptosis

14. Which of the following is an example of an artificial additive added to ultra-processed food?

    A. Protein
    B. Artificial sweetener
    C. Carbohydrate
    D. Fat
    E. Fiber

15. Ultra-processed food can increase food craving.

True/false

Answer Key

1. D, 2. E, 3. True, 4. False, 5. B, 6. False; 7. C; 8. True; 9. E; 10. C; 11. A; 12. B, 13. A, 14. B, 15. True

References

1. Monteiro CA, Cannon G, Levy RB, Moubarac JC, Louzada ML, Rauber F, et al. Ultra-processed foods: what they are and how to identify them. Public Health Nutr. 2019;22(5):936–41.
2. Meneguelli TS, Juvanhol LL, da Silva Leite A, Bressan J, Hermsdorff HHM. Minimally processed versus processed and ultra-processed food in individuals at cardiometabolic risk. Br Food J. 2021;124(3):1–22.

3. Beslay M, Srour B, Méjean C, Allès B, Fiolet T, Debras C, Chazelas E, Deschasaux M, Wendeu-Foyet MG, Hercberg S, et al. Ultra-processed food intake in association with BMI change and risk of overweight and obesity: a prospective analysis of the French Nutri Net-Santé cohort. PLoS Med. 2020;17:e1003256.

4. Cordova R, Viallon V, Fontvieille E, Peruchet-Noray L, Jansana A, Wagner KH, Kyrø C, Tjønneland A, Katzke V, Bajracharya R, Schulze MB, Masala G, Sieri S, Panico S, Ricceri F, Tumino R, Boer JMA, Verschuren WMM, van der Schouw YT, Jakszyn P, et al. Consumption of ultra-processed foods and risk of multimorbidity of cancer and cardiometabolic diseases: a multinational cohort study. Lancet Reg Health Eur. 2023;35:100771.

5. Lane MM, Gamage E, Du S, Ashtree DN, McGuinness AJ, Gauci S, Baker P, Lawrence M, Rebholz CM, Srour B, Touvier M, Jacka FN, O'Neil A, Segasby T, Marx W. Ultra-processed food exposure and adverse health outcomes: umbrella review of epidemiological meta-analyses. BMJ (Clin Res ed). 2024;384:e077310.

6. Monteiro CA, Levy RB, Claro RM, Castro IR, Cannon G. A new classification of foods based on the extent and purpose of their processing. Cad Saude Publica. 2010;26(11):2039–49.

7. Monteiro CA, Cannon G, Levy R, Moubarac JC, Jaime P, Martins AP, Canella D, Louzada M, Parra D. NOVA. The star shines bright. World Nutr. 2016;7(1–3):28–38.

8. Monteiro CA, Cannon G, Lawrence M, Costa Louzada M, Pereira Machado P. Ultra-processed foods, diet quality, and health using the NOVA classification system. Rome: FAO; 2019b.

9. Scrinis G, Monteiro C. From ultra-processed foods to ultra-processed dietary patterns. Nature food. 2022;3(9):671–3.

10. Srour B, Kordahi MC, Bonazzi E, Deschasaux-Tanguy M, Touvier M, Chassaing B. Ultra-processed foods and human health: from epidemiological evidence to mechanistic insights. Lancet Gastroenterol Hepatol. 2022;7:1128–40.

11. Martínez Leo EE, Peñafiel AM, Hernández Escalante VM, Cabrera Araujo ZM. Ultra-processed diet, systemic oxidative stress, and breach of immunologic tolerance. Nutrition. 2021;91–92:111419.

12. Tristan Asensi M, Napoletano A, Sofi F, Dinu M. Low-grade inflammation and ultra-processed foods consumption: a review. Nutrients. 2023;15:1546.

13. Rauber F, da Costa Louzada ML, Steele EM, Millett C, Monteiro CA, Levy RB. Ultra-processed food consumption and chronic non-communicable diseases-related dietary nutrient profile in the UK (2008–2014). Nutrients. 2018;10:587.

14. Pérez-Escamilla R, Obbagy JE, Altman JM, Essery EV, McGrane MM, Wong YP, Spahn JM, Williams CL. Dietary energy density and body weight in adults and children: a systematic review. J Acad Nutr Diet. 2012;112:671–84.

15. Canella DS, Levy RB, Martins AP, Claro RM, Moubarac JC, Baraldi LG, Cannon G, Monteiro CA. Ultra-processed food products and obesity in Brazilian households (2008–2009). PLoS One. 2014;9:e92752.

16. Lam MCL, Adams J. Association between home food preparation skills and behaviour, and consumption of ultra-processed foods: cross-sectional analysis of the UK National Diet and nutrition survey (2008–2009). Int J Behav Nutr Phys Act. 2017;14:68.

17. Robinson E, Almiron-Roig E, Rutters F, de Graaf C, Forde CG, Tudur Smith C, Nolan SJ, Jebb SA. A systematic review and meta-analysis examining the effect of eating rate on energy intake and hunger. Am J Clin Nutr. 2014;100:123–51.

18. Schulte EM, Avena NM, Gearhardt AN. Which foods may be addictive? The roles of processing, fat content, and glycemic load. PLoS One. 2015;10:e0117959.

19. Carter A, Hendrikse J, Lee N, Yücel M, Verdejo-Garcia A, Andrews ZB, Hall W. The neurobiology of "food addiction" and its implications for obesity treatment and policy. Annu Rev Nutr. 2016;36:105–28.

20. Lustig RH. Ultraprocessed food: addictive, toxic, and ready for regulation. Nutrients. 2020;12(11):3401.

21. Louzada ML, Baraldi LG, Steele EM, Martins AP, Canella DS, Moubarac JC, et al. Consumption of ultra-processed foods and obesity in Brazilian adolescents and adults. Prev Med. 2015;81:9–15.

22. Pereira N, Naufel MF, Ribeiro EB, Tufik S, Hachul H. Influence of dietary sources of melatonin on sleep quality: a review. J Food Sci. 2020;85:5–13.
23. Rico-Campà A, Martínez-González MA, Alvarez-Alvarez I, et al. Association between consumption of ultra-processed foods and all-cause mortality: SUN prospective cohort study. BMJ. 2019;365:l1949.
24. Hall KD, Ayuketah A, Brychta R, et al. Ultra-processed diets cause excess calorie intake and weight gain: an inpatient randomized controlled trial of ad libitum food intake. Cell Metab. 2019;30:67–77.e3.
25. Filippini T, Malavolti M, Whelton PK, Vinceti M. Sodium intake and risk of hypertension: a systematic review and dose–response meta-analysis of observational cohort studies. Curr Hypertens Rep. 2022;24(5):133–44.
26. Chen Z, Khandpur N, Desjardins C, et al. Ultra-processed food consumption and risk of type 2 diabetes: three large prospective U.S. cohort studies. Diabetes Care. 2023;46:1335–44.
27. El-Ezaby MM, Abd-El Hamide N-AH, El-Maksoud MAE, Shaheen EM, Embashi MMR. Effect of some food additives on lipid profile, kidney function and liver function of adult male albino rats. J Bas Environ Sci. 2018;5:52–9.
28. Chassaing B, Koren O, Goodrich JK, Poole AC, Srinivasan S, Ley RE, Gewirtz AT. Dietary emulsifiers impact the mouse gut microbiota promoting colitis and metabolic syndrome. Nature. 2015;519:92–6.
29. Bird SR, Hawley JA. Update on the effects of physical activity on insulin sensitivity in humans. BMJ Open Sport Exerc Med. 2017;2:e000143.
30. Kazemi A, Barati-Boldaji R, Soltani S, Mohammadipoor N, Esmaeilinezhad Z, Clark CCT, et al. Intake of various food groups and risk of breast cancer: a systematic review and dose-response meta-analysis of prospective studies. Adv Nutr. 2021;12:809–49.
31. De Nucci S, Zupo R, Castellana F, Sila A, Triggiani V, Lisco G, et al. Public health response to the SARS-CoV-2 pandemic: concern about ultra-processed food consumption. Food Secur. 2022;11:950.
32. Kelly B, Jacoby E. Public health nutrition special issue on ultra-processed foods. Public Health Nutr. 2018;21(1–4):10.
33. Lian Y, Wang GP, Chen GQ, Chen HN, Zhang GY. Association between ultra-processed foods and risk of cancer: a systematic review and meta-analysis. Front Nutr. 2023;10:1175994.
34. Li D, Hao X, Li J, Wu Z, Chen S, Lin J, et al. Dose-response relation between dietary inflammatory index and human cancer risk: evidence from 44 epidemiologic studies involving 1,082,092 participants. Am J Clin Nutr. 2018;107:371–88.
35. Morze J, Danielewicz A, Przybyłowicz K, Zeng H, Hoffmann G, Schwingshackl L. An updated systematic review and meta-analysis on adherence to mediterranean diet and risk of cancer. Eur J Nutr. 2021;60:1561–86.
36. Farvid MS, Sidahmed E, Spence ND, Mante Angua K, Rosner BA, Barnett JB. Consumption of red meat and processed meat and cancer incidence: a systematic review and meta-analysis of prospective studies. Eur J Epidemiol. 2021;36:937–51.
37. Svendsen C, Vogel U, Andersen E, et al. Polycyclic aromatic hydrocarbons in meat and meat products and their association with PAH-metabolizing genes and genotypes. Food Chem Toxicol. 2021;148:111942.
38. Carrascal J, Barco A, Amiano P, et al. Heterocyclic aromatic amines in meat and meat products: a systematic review. Food Chem Toxicol. 2021;152:112159.
39. Fernandes AE, Rosa PWL, Melo ME, Martins RCR, Santin FGO, Moura A, et al. Differences in the gut microbiota of women according to ultra-processed food consumption. Nutr Metab Cardiovasc Dis. 2023;33:84–9.
40. Edalati S, Bagherzadeh F, Asghari Jafarabadi M, Ebrahimi-Mamaghani M. Higher ultra-processed food intake is associated with higher DNA damage in healthy adolescents. Br J Nutr. 2021;125:568–76.

41. Lane MM, Lotfaliany M, Forbes M, Loughman A, Rocks T, O'Neil A, et al. Higher ultra-processed food consumption is associated with greater high-sensitivity C-reactive protein concentration in adults: cross-sectional results from the Melbourne collaborative cohort study. Nutrients. 2022;14:3309.

42. Buckley JP, Kim H, Wong E, Rebholz CM. Ultra-processed food consumption and exposure to phthalates and bisphenols in the US National Health and nutrition examination survey, 2013–2014. Environ Int. 2019;131:105057.

43. Cuevas-Sierra A, Milagro FI, Aranaz P, Martínez JA, Riezu-Boj JI. Gut microbiota differences according to ultra-processed food consumption in a Spanish population. Nutrients. 2021;13:2710.

44. Wiss DA, LaFata EM. Ultra-processed foods and mental health: where do eating disorders fit into the puzzle? Nutrients. 2024;16(12):1955.

45. Choudhary AK, Lee YY. Neurophysiological symptoms and aspartame: what is the connection? Nutr Neurosci. 2018;21:306–16.

46. Quines CB, Rosa SG, Da Rocha JT, Gai BM, Bortolatto CF, Duarte MMMF, Nogueira CW. Monosodium glutamate, a food additive, induces depressive-like and anxiogenic-like behaviors in young rats. Life Sci. 2014;107:27–31.

47. Grissa I, Guezguez S, Ezzi L, Chakroun S, Sallem A, Kerkeni E, Elghoul J, El Mir L, Mehdi M, Cheikh HB, et al. The effect of titanium dioxide nanoparticles on neuroinflammation response in rat brain. Environ Sci Pollut Res Int. 2016;23:20205–13.

48. Yuan N, Chen Y, Xia Y, Dai J, Liu C. Inflammation-related biomarkers in major psychiatric disorders: a cross-disorder assessment of reproducibility and specificity in 43 meta-analyses. Transl Psychiatry. 2019;9:233.

49. Yau YHC, Potenza MN. Stress and eating behaviors. Minerva Endocrinol. 2013;38:255–67.

50. Gerritsen S, Egli V, Roy R, Haszard J, Backer CD, Teunissen L, Cuykx I, Decorte P, Pabian SP, Van Royen K, et al. Seven weeks of home-cooked meals: changes to new Zealanders' grocery shopping, cooking and eating during the COVID-19 lockdown. J R Soc N Zealand. 2021;51(Suppl 1):S4–S22.

51. Dehghan M, Mente A, Rangarajan S, Mohan V, Swaminathan S, Avezum A, Lear SA, Rosengren A, Poirier P, Lanas F, Lopez-Jaramillo P, Soman B, Wang C, Orlandini A, Mohammadifard N, AlHabib KF, Chifamba J, Yusufali AH, Iqbal R, Khatib R, et al. Ultra-processed foods and mortality: analysis from the prospective urban and rural Epidemiology study. Am J Clin Nutr. 2023;117(1):55–63.

52. Taneri PE, Wehrli F, Roa-Díaz ZM, Itodo OA, Salvador D, Raeisi-Dehkordi H, Bally L, Minder B, Kiefte-de Jong JC, Laine JE, Bano A, Glisic M, Muka T. Association between ultra-processed food intake and all-cause mortality: a systematic review and meta-analysis. Am J Epidemiol. 2022;191(7):1323–35.

53. Schnabel L, Kesse-Guyot E, Allès B, Touvier M, Srour B, Hercberg S, et al. Association between Ultraprocessed food consumption and risk of mortality among middle-aged adults in France. JAMA Intern Med. 2019;179(4):490.

54. Suksatan W, Moradi S, Naeini F, Bagheri R, Mohammadi H, Talebi S, Mehrabani S, Hojjati Kermani MA, Suzuki K. Ultra-processed food consumption and adult mortality risk: a systematic review and dose-response meta-analysis of 207,291 participants. Nutrients. 2021;14(1):174.

55. Sansano M, Heredia A, Peinado I, Andrés A. Dietary acrylamide: what happens during digestion. Food Chem. 2017;237:58–64.

56. Zinöcker MK, Lindseth IA. The Western diet-microbiome-host interaction and its role in metabolic disease. Nutrients. 2018;10(3):365.

57. Pagliai G, Dinu M, Madarena MP, Bonaccio M, Iacoviello L, Sofi F. Consumption of ultra-processed foods and health status: a systematic review and meta-analysis. Br J Nutr. 2021;125(3):308–18.

58. Menezes-Júnior LAA, Andrade ACS, Coletro HN, Mendonça RD, Menezes MC, Machado-Coelho GLL, Meireles AL. Food consumption according to the level of processing and sleep quality during the COVID-19 pandemic. Clin Nutr ESPEN. 2022;49:348–56.
59. Duquenne P, Capperella J, Fezeu LK, Srour B, Benasi G, Hercberg S, Touvier M, Andreeva VA, St-Onge MP. The association between ultra-processed food consumption and chronic insomnia in the NutriNet-Santé Study. J Acad Nutr Diet. 2024;124(9):1109–17.
60. Sousa RDS, Bragança MLBM, Oliveira BR, Coelho CCNDS, Silva AAMD. Association between the degree of processing of consumed foods and sleep quality in adolescents. Nutrients. 2020;12(2):462.
61. Delpino FM, Figueiredo LM, Flores TR, Silveira EA, Silva Dos Santos F, Werneck AO, Louzada MLDC, Arcêncio RA, Nunes BP. Intake of ultra-processed foods and sleep-related outcomes: a systematic review and meta-analysis. Nutrition. 2023;106:111908.
62. Andreeva VA, Perez-Jimenez J, St-Onge MP. A systematic review of the bidirectional association between consumption of ultra-processed food and sleep parameters among adults. Curr Obes Rep. 2023;12:439–52.
63. Huang RC. The discoveries of molecular mechanisms for the circadian rhythm: the 2017 Nobel prize in physiology or medicine. Biom J. 2018;41(1):5–8.
64. Aoyama S, Shibata S. The role of circadian rhythms in muscular and osseous physiology and their regulation by nutrition and exercise. Front Neurosci. 2017;11:63. https://doi.org/10.3389/fnins.2017.00063.
65. Wolfson AR, Montgomery-Downs HE. The Oxford handbook of infant, child and adolescent sleep and behavior. New York: Oxford University Press; 2013.
66. Zisapel N. New perspectives on the role of melatonin in human sleep, circadian rhythms and their regulation. Br J Pharmacol. 2018;175(16):3190–9.
67. Ferracioli-Oda E, Qawasmi A, Bloch MH. Meta-analysis: melatonin for the treatment of primary sleep disorders. PLoS One. 2013;8(5):e63773.
68. Zuraikat FM, Wood RA, Barragán R, St-Onge MP. Sleep and diet: mounting evidence of a cyclical relationship. Annu Rev Nutr. 2021;41:309–32.
69. Polianovskaia A, Jonelis M, Cheung J. The impact of plant-rich diets on sleep: a mini-review. Front Nutr. 2024;11:1239580.
70. Boege HL, Bhatti MZ, St-Onge MP. Circadian rhythms and meal timing: impact on energy balance and body weight. Curr Opin Biotechnol. 2021;70:1–6.
71. Lopez-Minguez J, Saxena R, Bandín C, Scheer FA, Garaulet M. Late dinner impairs glucose tolerance in MTNR1B risk allele carriers: a randomized, cross-over study. Clin Nutr. 2018;37(4):1133–40.
72. Bonaccio M, Ruggiero E, Di Castelnuovo A, Martínez CF, Esposito S, Costanzo S, Cerletti C, Donati MB, de Gaetano G, Iacoviello L, On behalf of the INHES Study Investigators. Association between late-eating pattern and higher consumption of ultra-processed food among Italian adults: findings from the INHES study, vol. 15. Nutrients; 2023. p. 1497.
73. Detopoulou P, Dedes V, Syka D, Tzirogiannis K, Panoutsopoulos GI. Relation of minimally processed foods and ultra-processed foods with the Mediterranean diet score, time-related meal patterns and waist circumference: results from a cross-sectional study in university students. Int J Environ Res Public Health. 2023;20:2806.
74. Zhong L, Han X, Li M, Gao S. Modifiable dietary factors in adolescent sleep: a systematic review and meta-analysis. Sleep Med. 2024;115:100–8.
75. Clark I, Landolt HP. Coffee, caffeine, and sleep: a systematic review of epidemiological studies and randomized controlled trials. Sleep Med Rev. 2017;31:70–8.
76. St-Onge MP, Ard J, Baskin ML, Chiuve SE, Johnson HM, Kris-Etherton P, Varady K. American Heart Association Obesity Committee of the Council on lifestyle and Cardiometabolic health; council on cardiovascular disease in the young; council on clinical cardiology; and stroke council. Meal timing and frequency: implications for cardiovascular disease prevention: a scientific statement from the American Heart Association. Circulation. 2017;135(9):e96–e121.

77. Papatriantafyllou E, Efthymiou D, Zoumbaneas E, Popescu CA, Vassilopoulou E. Sleep deprivation: effects on weight loss and weight loss maintenance. Nutrients. 2022;14(8):1549.
78. Bolhuis D, Mosca AC, Pellegrini N. Consumer awareness of the degree of industrial food processing and the association with healthiness—a pilot study. Nutrients. 2022;14(20):4438. https://doi.org/10.3390/nu14204438. PMID: 36297121; PMCID: PMC9610034
79. Sato PM, Ulian MD, da Silva Oliveira MS, Cardoso MA, Wells J, Devakumar D, Lourenço BH, Scagliusi FB. Signs and strategies to deal with food insecurity and consumption of ultra-processed foods among Amazonian mothers. Glob Public Health. 2020;15(8):1130–43.
80. Jeans MR, Landry MJ, Vandyousefi S, Hudson EA, Burgermaster M, Bray MS, Chandra J, Davis JN. Effects of a school-based gardening, cooking, and nutrition cluster randomized controlled trial on unprocessed and ultra-processed food consumption. J Nutr. 2023;153(7):2073–84.

Unraveling the Impact and Benefits of Chrononutrition and Circadian Rhythms on Health

16

Aliyar Cyrus Fouladkhah and Minoo Bagheri

Learning Objectives

After completing this chapter, you will be able to

- Introduce chrononutrition and circadian rhythms
- Discuss the importance of evidence-based decision-making in the interpretation of chrononutrition literature for making community-based and precision nutrition dietary recommendations
- Discuss the impact of chrononutrition on health promotion
- Evaluate the impact of chrononutrition on the prevention of obesity and noncommunicable diseases
- Evaluate the impact of chrononutrition on mental and athletic performance
- Discuss the knowledge gaps in and the need for additional evidence for developing and implementing chrononutrition-based best practices and dietary recommendations

A. C. Fouladkhah (✉)
Public Health Microbiology Laboratory, Tennessee State University, Nashville, TN, USA

Public Health Microbiology Foundation, Franklin, TN, USA
e-mail: aliyar.fouladkhah@aya.yale.edu

M. Bagheri
Department of Biomedical Informatics, Precision Nutrition Laboratory, Vanderbilt University Medical Center, Nashville, TN, USA
e-mail: minoo.bagheri@vumc.org

© The Author(s), under exclusive license to Springer Nature Switzerland AG 2025
A. K. Mitra, D. Vanoh (eds.), *Essentials of Clinical and Public Health Nutrition*, Nutrition and Health, https://doi.org/10.1007/978-3-031-95373-6_16

Introduction: Chrononutrition and Evidence-Based Decision-Making

Throughout evolution and on the basis of the earth's rotation, various organisms have developed an internal circadian clock for adapting to the external environment for day-to-day activities. For humans, external environmental factors, such as cycles of light and darkness, can thus affect the circadian system such that it generates rhythms in bodily activities and functions that affect various aspects of life, such as overall metabolism, the immune system, and the sleeping cycle [1]. Based on this concept, chrononutrition encompasses the scientific procedures that study the interaction of "the internal biological clock" (the circadian body rhythm) with food intake, metabolism, and meal timing. Specifically, chrononutrition studies the impact of circadian body rhythm regularity, frequency, and timing for food intake and their impacts on obesity and other noncommunicable diseases [2]. This is a rapidly emerging field in nutrition, and compared to many other topics in health and nutrition, a considerable knowledge gaps persists. According to the National Heart, Lung, and Blood Institute (NHLBI) of the US National Institute of Health (NIH), investigations into how circadian rhythms affect nutrition and health have been gaining importance and momentum in recent years [3]. An important early study in this emerging field of research and practice was an epidemiological study conducted on obese people, which concluded that those with unusual eating times (such as lunch after 3 pm) can experience disruption in their circadian system, leading to unhealthy outcomes such as difficulty in losing weight. These significant differences were observed after adjusting for confounding factors such as the level of appetite hormones, the intake and expenditure of energy, age, and the duration of sleep [3, 4]. A clinical trial similarly showed the importance of chrononutrition on health, where the study evaluated the glycemic control of individuals with daytime and nighttime eating. The researchers observed that nighttime eating impaired tolerance to glucose, whereas limiting meals to daytime prevented this impairment [3, 5]. Based on these important early studies and an array of recently completed projects, in addition to genotype-based research, the use of chrononutrition in public health practices has shown promising potential for improving health and preventing noncommunicable diseases (Fig. 16.1). This could be crucial in the context of precision medicine and precision nutrition, where recommendations and advice are provided while considering individuals' genes, lifestyles, and environments [6–8].

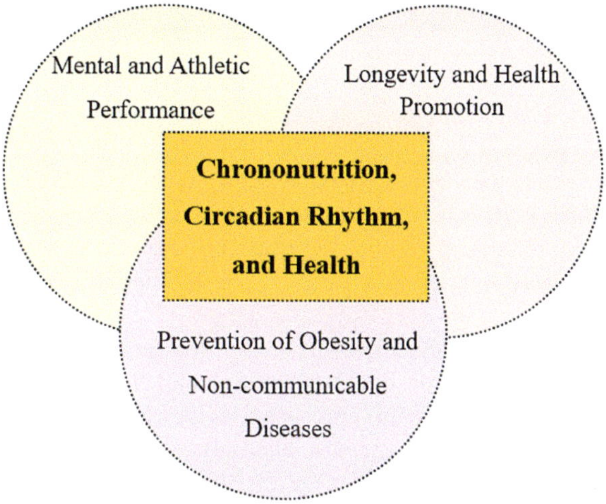

Fig. 16.1 Impact of chrononutrition and circadian rhythms on health: (i) preventing obesity and noncommunicable diseases, (ii) promoting overall health, and (iii) improving mental and athletic performance

---

Box 16.1 Evidence-based decisions on interpreting chrononutrition literature
Chrononutrition is a novel and emerging research and practice area. To draw conclusions and thus make dietary recommendations at the population level and in the context of precision nutrition, the knowledge gaps in this area would need to be addressed by various adequately powered and well-designed observational and randomized studies. Evidence-based conclusions could then be drawn and implemented after carrying out a careful examination of the literature by well-constructed systematic reviews and/or meta-analyses. To draw evidence-based conclusions from the chrononutrition literature, careful technical aspects have to be considered, including the use of validated inclusion and exclusion criteria to select high-quality and reputable studies, consideration of important topics such as publication bias and the *winner's curse*, and use of advanced analytical tools such as sensitivity analyses. Relying on these approaches allows an evidence-based review of the chrononutrition literature to overcome the challenges associated with decision-making based on a limited number of studies and/or relying on traditional literature reviews.

As discussed earlier, chrononutrition is a novel and emerging research and practice area. To draw conclusions and thus make dietary recommendations at the population level and in the context of precision nutrition, the knowledge gaps in this area would need to be addressed by various adequately powered and well-designed observational and randomized studies. Evidence-based conclusions could then be drawn and implemented after carrying out a careful examination of the literature by well-constructed systematic reviews and/or meta-analyses [9]. To draw evidence-based conclusions from the chrononutrition literature, careful technical aspects have to be considered, including the use of validated inclusion and exclusion criteria to select high-quality and reputable studies, conisderation of important topics such as publication bias and the *winner's curse*, and use of advanced analytical tools such as sensitivity analyses. Relying on these approaches allows an evidence-based review of the chrononutrition literature to overcome the challenges associated with decision-making based on a limited number of studies and/or relying on traditional literature reviews [9].

This book chapter discusses only overviews of the recent chrononutrition literature and its potential impact on health promotion and the prevention of noncommunicable diseases. The information presented in the chapter, thus, is introductory in nature and is for educational purposes, and only a limited number of recent and important studies are discussed. Before putting this information into practice at the population level or in the context of precision nutrition, knowledge gaps in this area should be addressed by adequately powered and big-data epidemiological studies and well-designed randomized trials. Therefore, in important federal nutrition guidelines such as the US Department of Agriculture's Dietary Guidelines for Americans for 2020–2025, the topics of chrononutrition and circadian rhythms have not yet been discussed in great detail [10].

Chrononutrition for Health Promotion

Studying the impact of chrononutritional habits on health promotion is a difficult task due to the limited availability of clinical trials and observational studies in this area and the complexities of studying circadian rhythms and dietary intake patterns on various aspects of health in diverse populations. However, many recent studies have shown the beneficial impacts of chrononutrition-related recommendations on improving various aspects of health. Some of these studies have discussed the impact of dietary compounds such as polyphenolics and caffeine on regulating the circadian clock [11], and others have studied the impact of chrononutritional habits on specific health outcomes, such as cardiometabolic health [12], maintaining muscle health [13], and systematic inflammation and oxidative stress [14]. Some studies have expressed the need for adjusting chrononutrition-based recommendations for health promotion according to one's chronotype and genetics, further emphasizing the potentially important role of circadian rhythms and food intake time in the field of precision nutrition [15].

Because disruptions in circadian rhythm could negatively impact one's health, some recent studies have explored the role of bioactive compounds in the regulation and correction of circadian disorders. These studies considered the impact of a single nutrient/food compound, such as caffeine, polyphenolic compound, or palmitate [16]. Other studies took a more holistic approach by evaluating the impact of real-life dietary choices and dietary patterns in the context of chrononutrition and health. As an example, the impact of the Mediterranean diet and chrononutrition have been studied on promoting cardiometabolic health [17] and sleep quality [18].

Overall, many recent studies have illustrated the importance of chrononutritional habits on health, indicating the need for more clinical and epidemiological studies in this area. These studies have expressed that not only the quantity and quality of food consumption but also the timing of dietary intake as it relates to the circadian rhythm are crucial for maintaining and promoting various aspects of health [19–21].

Chrononutrition and Preventing Obesity and Noncommunicable Diseases

Among various topics associated with the circadian rhythm and chrononutrition, their impact on the prevention and management of chronic and noncommunicable diseases such as obesity and type 2 diabetes have perhaps been investigated the most in scientific literature. A recent study, as an example, evaluated the food diary of more than 21,000 individuals and concluded that chrononutritional behaviors, including food intake late in the day, were significantly associated with weight gain, obesity, and high body mass index (BMI) in the tested population [22]. In harmony with this study, in a cross-sectional population-based epidemiological study with more than 2000 subjects, the authors concluded that consuming the largest meals earlier in the day, taking most calories during midday meals, and consuming more meals every day could have a pronounced impact on treating obesity and overweight [23]. A recent review study similarly concluded that in addition to traditional dietary factors, "when to eat"—that is, meal timing and chrononutritional behaviors—has important and appreciable impacts on weight management and glucometabolic control [24].

Similarly, the impact of meal timing and chrononutrition on blood glucose control and the management of type 2 diabetes have been extensively investigated in recent studies. As an example, an epidemiological study with 227 participants with type 2 diabetes concluded that the consumption of calorie-dense meals later in the day could cause desynchronization in one's circadian rhythms and subsequently lead to poor blood glucose levels in participants [25]. By summarizing several epidemiological research publications, a recent review similarly determined that certain strategies, such as increasing the fat and protein content of night meals, consuming low-glycemic-index foods earlier in the day, the timing of protein and fat intake co-ingested with carbohydrates, and the order of food presentation (consuming vegetables first, followed by protein and carbohydrate), can have positive impacts on improving postprandial glycaemia for healthy individuals and those with type 2 diabetes [26].

In harmony with these findings, a recent review paper concluded that limiting meals to two to three times in a typical day, limiting meal intake to less than 10 h per day, and waiting 3–4 h after meals for snacking are some of the other chrononutritional behaviors that could help in glycemic control of type 2 diabetes patients [27].

Chrononutrition and the circadian rhythm have also been discussed as factors impacting cardiovascular health. Chrononutrition as a lifestyle intervention has also been shown to affect hypertension as well as renal and vascular functions. Thus, chrononutrition-based interventions have been proposed as potential recommendations, in addition to traditional diet therapy, to mitigate blood pressure in susceptible individuals. The chrononutritional interventions are deemed to be of particular importance for those with disruption in their circadian rhythm due to occupation or underlying health complications and diseases [28]. One recent study discussed some potential underlying mechanisms associated with the health benefits of intermittent fasting and the proper timing of dietary intake for individuals with cardiovascular diseases. However, the study concluded that more randomized studies are urgently needed in this area to be able to develop and implement evidence based information in this emerging and important area [29].

Other studies have shown the impact of chrononutrition on gut microbiota by discussing various communication pathways between the microbiota and the circadian rhythms of the hosts [30]. This interaction shows that disruption in one's circadian rhythms could lead to negative health consequences for the host due to alteration in gut microbiota, with the potential of leading to more-concerning health complications, such as various gastrointestinal cancers and irritable bowel disease [30]. Other studies have similarly shown that complex interactions between food intake, circadian rhythms, and gut microbiota could have important implications for a host, including the impact on various aspects of metabolism and the immune system [31]. These interactions and complexities could be of great importance for the implementation of chrononutrition-based dietary recommendations in the context of precision nutrition [32].

Importantly, the implementation of chrononutrition-based practices currently faces a major challenge due to knowledge gaps and the limited number of studies conducted in this area. However, the existing literature highlights the promise of this emerging and important field of research and practices as an important complement to traditional dietary guidelines.

Chrononutrition and Mental and Athletic Performance

The timing of dietary intake, particularly the intake of macronutrients, could meaningfully impact sleep quality and quantity and, thus, could impact both cognitive and athletic performance [33]. Sleep initiation, continuity, and duration could additionally impact recovery after athletic performances [34]. Sleeping, which is affected by chrononutrition, could impact the endocrine system, immune system, and metabolic cost of the walking state, thus directly impacting athletic recovery and performance [35, 36]. New studies have also reported the impact of chrononutrition on the muscle health of older individuals by studying chrononutritional habits and their impact on muscle health, mobility, and aging. In one study, researchers first adjusted for various confounding factors, such as energy, protein and fiber intake, participants' weight and height, their levels of physical activity, their education, their marital status, their age, their race, and their self-reported health status. Among more than 800 adults older than 70 years of age, researchers observed that chrononutritional habits, including "later last meal intake time," "earlier first intake time," and "longer eating window," were associated with better muscle mass and performance [37]. A recently published review study additionally acknowledged the impact of circadian rhythms on athletic performance. The study, however, expressed the need for more data in this area to better evaluate the dynamic relationship between circadian rhythms and muscle performance and recovery [38]. One study also showed that in addition to chrononutritional habits, the relationship between the time of conducting exercise and the timing of dietary intake could be important in athletic performance [39]. Other chrononutrition-related practices, such as intermittent fasting, have been shown to have a potential impact on athletic performance, including an impact on reducing systematic inflammation. However, more studies in this area are needed to make valid, evidence-based decisions [40]. One recently published review study also suggested the potential impact of time-restricted feeding on cognitive health and disorders. However, this study also acknowledged the need for more studies in the future to better evaluate chrononutritional habits and mental health and performance [41]. In harmony with these studies, another study further discussed the impact of the chrononutrition-related microbiome and dietary strategies on cognitive health diseases [42]. Overall, in many of the recent studies, the great impact of the circadian rhythm and chrononutritional behaviors was demonstrated on athletic performance and recovery, the muscle health of older individuals, and cognitive performance and mental health. Future research studies in this area are needed to better evaluate underlying mechanisms and to make valid, evidence-based recommendations at the population level and in the context of precision medicine.

Box 16.2 Health Impact of Chrononutrition
Given that this is a relatively new and novel area of research and practice, inherently studying the impact of chrononutritional habits on health is a difficult task due to the availability of limited clinical trials and observational studies in this area and the complexities of studying circadian rhythms and dietary intake patterns on various aspects of health in diverse populations. However, many recent studies have shown the beneficial impacts of chrononutrition-related recommendations on improving various aspects of health. The current literature illustrates the appreciable impact of chrononutrition and the circadian rhythm on mental and athletic performance, on the prevention of obesity and other noncommunicable diseases, and on overall health promotion, such as quality and quantity of sleep. More adequately powered clinical trials as well as large and diverse epidemiological studies on diverse populations and in various geographical regions could certainly provide valuable cornerstones for further evidence-based decision-making derived from the chrononutrition literature.

Chrononutrition Knowledge Gaps and Research Opportunities

Better evaluations of chrononutrition literature could lead to the emergence of new and exciting interventions in the field of nutrition for dietary recommendations both at the population level and in the context of precision nutrition. However, major knowledge gaps currently exist in this new and emerging area of nutrition research and practice. Due to challenges associated with cost and funding availability and concerns associated with clinical equipoise, a limited number of randomized studies are currently available to study the impact of chrononutrition and health. More adequately powered clinical studies completed on diverse populations and in various geographical regions could certainly provide a valuable cornerstone for further evidence-based decision-making derived from chrononutrition literature. Similarly, large and diverse epidemiological studies could complement clinical trials and thus provide additional needed evidence. Control over various variables as confounders in these observational studies is one of the greatest challenges to ensure the external validity of epidemiology-based chrononutrition research. Specifically, some individuals might have different chronotypes; that is, they tend to differ in whether they have a morning metabolism or an evening metabolism. Confounders such as age, sex, race, past habits, environmental exposures, the level of appetite hormones, exercise, and exposure to light and outdoor environments could all be important considerations in designing valid and impactful epidemiological studies in the future [3, 9].

In addition to such studies, studying the mechanisms of action is critical as well in the context of nutrition and molecular epidemiology. For example, better evaluations of the underlying mechanism of differences in the metabolism of nutrients consumed later relative to those consumed earlier in a day could lead to the design of more-impactful randomized and epidemiological studies in this field. Understanding specific biomarkers, genes, and the cultural and psychological factors associated with chrononutrition will also assist in reaching a more in-depth understanding of this emerging and exciting field of research and practice. Publishing more case reports associated with the impact of chrononutrition on health by practitioners in the field could also be a valuable resource to better evaluate the true impact of chrononutrition on individuals' well-being and population health.

The implementation of chrononutrition-based practices could be crucial for teaching curricula in nutrition sciences. A recent study, as an example, indicated that more than 96% of students enrolled in a human nutrition and dietetics program expressed positive feedback when practical sessions about the application of chrononutrition and dietetics were incorporated as part of their teaching curriculum [43]. When chrononutrition education was used in a trial on improving the health of students, positives results were obtained. In a study of students with more than 500 participants, 8.9%, 7.0%, and 84.1% of students reported a morning chronotype, an evening chronotype, and an intermediate chronotype, respectively. After receiving nutrition education, all chronotypes showed lower body weight and waist circumferences relative to those without receiving nutrition education [44].

Chapter Summary and Conclusions

Chrononutrition is an emerging and important topic associated with health promotion, the prevention of chronic diseases, and improving athletic and cognitive performance. However, important knowledge gaps impede ensuring that the conclusions drawn from chrononutrition are valid and evidence-based. These knowledge gaps could be addressed by conducting adequately powered traditional and big-data epidemiological studies as well as well-designed randomized and clinical trials. Upon the availability of additional observational and randomized evidence and the carrying out of well-constructed systematic reviews and/or meta-analyses, more-accurate chrononutrition-based dietary recommendations could be drawn and implemented for use at the population level and in the context of precision nutrition. The current literature contains an abundance of studies hinting at the beneficial impacts of chrononutrition on promoting a healthy lifestyle, preventing obesity and noncommunicable diseases, and mental and athletic performance. Further research and meta-analyses in this area could ultimately lead to the adaptation of comprehensive chrononutrition-based dietary guidelines for general and special populations for preventing diseases, promoting health, and potentially slowing the progress of some noncommunicable diseases.

Further Practice

1. What is the definition of chrononutrition?
    A. Interaction between the sleep–wake cycle and kidney function
    B. Interaction between sleep and the immune system
    C. Interaction between circadian body rhythms and food intake, metabolism, and meal timing
    D. Interaction between circadian body rhythms and brain function
    E. Interaction between circadian body rhythms and mood

2. Disruption to the circadian rhythm may alter gut microbiota.

    • True/false

3. Athletic performance is affected by the timing of exercise and the timing of dietary intake.

    • True/false

4. Disruption to the circadian rhythm will not affect gastrointestinal health.

    • True/false

5. Poor blood glucose control is due to the consumption of a calorie-dense meal later in the day.

    • True/false

6. Weight gain is *not* due to unusual eating times.

   - True/false

7. Chrononutrition is associated with cardiometabolic health.

   - True/false

8. Inflammation and oxidative stress can be reduced by proper sleep timing and meal timing.

   - True/false

9. Age, sex, race, and past habits are some confounders of chrononutrition.

   - True/false

10. What are chrononutrition and circadian rhythms?
11. What is the importance of evidence-based decision-making in the interpretation of chrononutrition literature for making community-based and precision nutrition dietary recommendations?
12. What are some of the impacts of chrononutrition on health promotion?
13. What are the main impacts of chrononutrition on the prevention of obesity and noncommunicable diseases?
14. How could chrononutrition impact mental and athletic performance?
15. What are some of the knowledge gaps and research opportunities associated with chrononutrition-based dietary recommendations and practices?

Answer Key

1. C, 2. True, 3. True, 4. False, 5. True, 6. False, 7. True, 8. True, 9. True.

10. Throughout evolution and based on the earth's rotation, various organisms have developed an internal circadian clock for adapting to the external environment for day-to-day activities. For humans, external environmental factors such as cycles of light and darkness, can thus affect the circadian system such that it generates rhythms in bodily activities and functions affecting various aspects of life such as overall metabolism, the immune system, and the sleeping cycle. Based on this concept, chrononutrition encompasses the scientific procedures that study the interaction of "the internal biological clock" (the circadian body rhythm) with food intake, metabolism, and meal timing. Specifically, chrononutrition studies the impact of circadian body rhythm regularity, frequency, and timing for food intake and their impact on obesity and other noncommunicable diseases.

11. chrononutrition is a novel and emerging research and practice area. To draw conclusions and thus make dietary recommendations at the population level and in the context of precision nutrition, the knowledge gaps in this area would need to be addressed by various adequately powered and well-designed observational and randomized studies. Evidence-based conclu-

sions could then be drawn and implemented after carrying out a careful examination of the literature by well-constructed systematic reviews and/or meta-analyses. To draw evidence-based conclusions from the chrononutrition literature, careful technical aspects have to be considered, including the use of validated inclusion and exclusion criteria to select high-quality and reputable studies, consideration of important topics such as publication bias and the *winner's curse*, and utilization of advanced analytical tools such as sensitivity analyses.

12. chrononutrition-related recommendations on improving various aspects of health. Some of these studies have discussed the impact of dietary compounds such as polyphenolics and caffeine on regulating the circadian clock, and others have studied the impact of chrononutritional habits on specific health outcomes, such as cardiometabolic health, maintaining muscle health, and systematic inflammation and oxidative stress. Some studies have expressed the need for adjusting chrononutrition-based recommendations for health promotion according to one's chronotype and genetics, further emphasizing the potentially important role of circadian rhythms and food intake time in the field of precision nutrition.

13. Among various topics associated with the circadian rhythm and chrononutrition, their impact on the prevention and management of chronic and noncommunicable diseases such as obesity and type 2 diabetes have perhaps been investigated the most in scientific literature. Among many other topics, chrononutrition and the circadian rhythm have also been discussed as factors impacting cardiovascular health, gut microbiota, and various aspects of metabolism and the immune system.

14. In many recent studies, the great impact of the circadian rhythm and chrononutritional behaviors was demonstrated on athletic performance and recovery, the muscle health of older individuals, and cognitive performance and mental health. Future research studies in this area are needed to better evaluate underlying mechanisms and to make valid, evidence-based recommendations at the population level and in the context of precision medicine.

15. Better evaluations of chrononutrition could lead to the emergence of new and exciting interventions in the field of nutrition for dietary recommendations both at the population level and in the context of precision nutrition. However, major knowledge gaps currently exist in this new and emerging area of nutrition research and practice. Due to challenges associated with cost and funding availability and concerns associated with clinical equipoise, a limited number of randomized studies are currently available to study the impact of chrononutrition and health. More adequately powered clinical studies completed on diverse populations and in various geographical regions could certainly provide a valuable cornerstone for further evidence-based decision-making derived from chrononutrition literature. Similarly, large and diverse epidemiological studies could complement clinical trials and thus provide additional needed evidence.

References

1. Ahluwalia MK. Chrononutrition—when we eat is of the essence in tackling obesity. Nutrients. 2022;14(23):5080.
2. Abdi T, Andreou E, Papageorgiou A, Heraclides A, Philippou E. Personality, chrono-nutrition and cardiometabolic health: a narrative review of the evidence. Adv Nutr. 2000;11:1201–10.
3. The U.S. National Institute of Health (NIH), National Heart, Lung, and Blood Institute. 2023. Chrononutrition: timing of meals matters for your health. Accessed 5 July 2024. Available at: https://www.nhlbi.nih.gov/news/2023/chrononutrition-timing-meals-matters-your-health
4. Lopez-Minguez J, Gómez-Abellán P, Garaulet M. Timing of breakfast, lunch, and dinner. Effects on obesity and metabolic risk. Nutrients. 2019;11(11):2624.
5. Chellappa SL, Qian J, Vujovic N, Morris CJ, Nedeltcheva A, Nguyen H, Rahman N, Heng SW, Kelly L, Kerlin-Monteiro K, Srivastav S. Daytime eating prevents internal circadian misalignment and glucose intolerance in night work. Sci Adv. 2021;7(49):eabg9910.
6. Petzschner FH. Practical challenges for precision medicine. Science. 2024;383(6679):149–50.
7. Ulusoy-Gezer HG, Rakıcıoğlu N. The future of obesity management through precision nutrition: putting the individual at the center. Current Nutrition Reports; 2024. p. 1–23.
8. Bagheri M, Bombin A, Shi M, Murthy VL, Shah R, Mosley JD, Ferguson JF. Genotype-based "virtual" metabolomics in a clinical biobank identifies novel metabolite-disease associations. Front Genet. 2024;15:1392622.
9. Fouladkhah AC, Bagheri M. Systematic review and meta-analysis: evidence-based decision-making in public health. Stat Appr Epidemiol. 2024:257–73.
10. U.S. Department of Agriculture and U.S. Department of Health and Human Services. Dietary Guidelines for Americans, 2020–2025. 9th Edition.
11. Takahashi M, Tahara Y. Timing of food/nutrient intake and its health benefits chrono-nutrition (SY (T1) 4). J Nutr Sci Vitaminol. 2022;68(Supplement):S2–4.
12. Katsi V, Papakonstantinou IP, Soulaidopoulos S, Katsiki N, Tsioufis K. Chrononutrition in cardiometabolic health. J Clin Med. 2022;11(2):296.
13. Farsijani S, Mao Z, Cawthon P, Kritchevsky S, Glynn N, Toledo F, Newman A. The relationship between chrono-nutrition behaviors and muscle health in older adults. Innov Aging. 2023;7(S1):379.
14. Garrido M, Terron MP, Rodriguez AB. Chrononutrition against oxidative stress in aging. Oxidative Med Cell Longev. 2013;2013(1):729804.
15. Eberli NS, Colas L, Gimalac A. Chrononutrition in traditional European medicine—ideal meal timing for cardiometabolic health promotion. J Integrative Medicine. 2024;
16. Dufoo-Hurtado E, Wall-Medrano A, Campos-Vega R. Naturally-derived chronobiotics in chrononutrition. Trends Food Sci Technol. 2020;95:173–82.
17. Yilmaz SK, Yangılar F. Evaluation of the relationship between chronotype, adherence to the Mediterranean diet, and cardiometabolic health in adults. Revista Española de Nutrición Humana y Dietética. 2022;26(4):338–47.
18. Naja F, Hasan H, Khadem SH, Buanq MA, Al-Mulla HK, Aljassmi AK, Faris ME. Adherence to the Mediterranean diet and its association with sleep quality and chronotype among youth: a cross-sectional study. Front Nutr. 2022;8:805955.
19. Adafer R, Messaadi W, Meddahi M, Patey A, Haderbache A, Bayen S, Messaadi N. Food timing, circadian rhythm and chrononutrition: a systematic review of time-restricted eating's effects on human health. Nutrients. 2020;12(12):3770.
20. Mentzelou M, Papadopoulou SK, Psara E, Voulgaridou G, Pavlidou E, Androutsos O, Giaginis C. Chrononutrition in the prevention and management of metabolic disorders: a literature review. Nutrients. 2024;16(5):722.
21. Chen Y. Effect of chrono-nutrition–based dietary intervention on metabolic disease. Precision Nutrition. 2024;3(2):e00076.
22. Crispim CA, Rinaldi AE, Azeredo CM, Skene DJ, Moreno CR. Is time of eating associated with BMI and obesity? A population-based study. Eur J Nutr. 2024;63(2):527–37.

23. Longo-Silva G, de Oliveira Lima M, Pedrosa AKP, Serenini R, de Menezes Marinho P, de Menezes RCE. Association of largest meal timing and eating frequency with body mass index and obesity. Clinic Nutr ESPEN. 2024;60:179–86.
24. Verde L, Di Lorenzo T, Savastano S, Colao A, Barrea L, Muscogiuri G. Chrononutrition in type 2 diabetes mellitus and obesity: a narrative review. Diabetes Metab Res Rev. 2024;40(2):e3778.
25. Chandorkar SS, Mehta NS, Rathod NM. Chrono-nutrition and its association with chronotype and blood glucose control among people with type 2 diabetes. Diabetes. 2023;
26. Henry CJ, Kaur B, Quek RYC. Chrononutrition in the management of diabetes. Nutr Diabetes. 2020;10(1):6.
27. Gómez-Ruiz RP, Cabello-Hernández AI, Gómez-Pérez FJ, Gómez-Sámano MÁ. Meal frequency strategies for the management of type 2 diabetes subjects: a systematic review. PLoS One. 2024;19(2):e0298531.
28. Bohmke NJ, Dixon DL, Kirkman DL. Chrono-nutrition for hypertension. Diabetes Metab Res Rev. 2024;40(1):e3760.
29. Billingsley HE. The effect of time of eating on cardiometabolic risk in primary and secondary prevention of cardiovascular disease. Diabetes Metab Res Rev. 2024;40(2):e3633.
30. Lotti S, Dinu M, Colombini B, Amedei A, Sofi F. Circadian rhythms, gut microbiota, and diet: possible implications for health. Nutr Metab Cardiovasc Dis. 2023;33(8):1490–500.
31. de Oliveira Melo NC, Cuevas-Sierra A, Souto VF, Martínez JA. Biological rhythms, chrono-nutrition, and gut microbiota: epigenomics insights for precision nutrition and metabolic health. Biomol Ther. 2024;14(5):559.
32. Ordovás J. The use of chrono nutrition in precision nutrition. In: Precision nutrition. Academic Press; 2024. p. 43–60.
33. Ayala V, Martínez-Bebia M, Latorre JA, Gimenez-Blasi N, Jimenez-Casquet MJ, Conde-Pipo J, Bach-Faig A, Mariscal-Arcas M. Influence of circadian rhythms on sports performance. Chronobiol Int. 2021;38(11):1522–36.
34. Vitošević B. The circadian clock and human athletic performance. Bull Nat Sci Res. 2017;7(1)
35. Doherty R, Madigan S, Warrington G, Ellis J. Sleep and nutrition interactions: implications for athletes. Nutrients. 2019;11(4):822.
36. Doherty R. Sleep, nutrition, and recovery in athletes. University of Northumbria at Newcastle (United Kingdom); 2021.
37. Mao Z, Cawthon PM, Kritchevsky SB, Toledo FG, Esser KA, Erickson ML, Newman AB, Farsijani S. The association between chrononutrition behaviors and muscle health among older adults: the study of muscle, mobility and aging. Aging Cell. 2024;23(6):e14059.
38. Pradhan S, Parganiha A, Agashe CD, Pati AK. Circadian rhythm in sportspersons and athletic performance: a mini review. Chronobiol Int. 2024;41(2):137–81.
39. Kim HK, Radak Z, Takahashi M, Inami T, Shibata S. Chrono-exercise: time-of-day-dependent physiological responses to exercise. Sports Med Health Sci. 2023;5(1):50–8.
40. Mandal S, Simmons N, Awan S, Chamari K, Ahmed I. Intermittent fasting: eating by the clock for health and exercise performance. BMJ Open Sport Exerc Med. 2022;8(1):e001206.
41. Currenti W, Godos J, Castellano S, Mogavero MP, Ferri R, Caraci F, Grosso G, Galvano F. Time-restricted feeding and mental health: a review of possible mechanisms on affective and cognitive disorders. Int J Food Sci Nutr. 2021;72(6):723–33.
42. Codoñer-Franch P, Gombert M, Martínez-Raga J, Cenit MC. Circadian disruption and mental health: the chronotherapeutic potential of microbiome-based and dietary strategies. Int J Mol Sci. 2023;24(8):7579.
43. Izquierdo-Pulido M, Zerón-Rugerio MF, Cambras T. Chrononutrition: a new strategy for human nutrition and dietetics students. Can J Diet Pract Res. 2024;85(3):264–5.
44. Kabalı S, Çelik MN, Öner N. Associations of nutrition education with diet quality indexes and chronotype: a cross-sectional study. Int J Environ Health Res. 2024:1–13.

Cancer Prevention Using Nutrimetabolomics and Nutriproteomics

Mogana Das Murtey ⓘ, Mohammad Jahidul Islam ⓘ, and Divya Vanoh ⓘ

Learning Objectives

After completing this chapter, you will be able to

- Understand the principles and methodologies of analytical techniques in metabolomics
- Identify the role of proteins and peptides derived from various food sources in chemoprevention
- Apply knowledge of anticancer plant proteins and peptides
- Interpret the significance of proteomic technology in identifying and characterizing the ingredients and biomarkers related to cancer prevention

M. D. Murtey (✉)
School of Dental Sciences, Health Campus, Universiti Sains Malaysia,
Kubang Kerian, Kelantan, Malaysia
e-mail: moganadasmurtey@usm.my

M. J. Islam
Department of Pharmacology, Faculty of Basic Science and Para Clinical Science,
Bangbandhu Sheikh Mujib Medical University (BSMMU), Dhaka, Bangladesh
e-mail: jahidul_islam@bsmmu.edu.bd

D. Vanoh
Dietetics Programme, School of Health Sciences, Universiti Sains Malaysia,
Kubang Kerian, Kelantan, Malaysia
e-mail: divyavanoh@usm.my

© The Author(s), under exclusive license to Springer Nature
Switzerland AG 2025
A. K. Mitra, D. Vanoh (eds.), *Essentials of Clinical and Public Health Nutrition*,
Nutrition and Health, https://doi.org/10.1007/978-3-031-95373-6_17

Introduction

Cancer, one of the leading causes of mortality worldwide, remains a formidable challenge in public health. Although significant progress has been achieved thanks to traditional cancer treatment methods, the pursuit of preventive measures remains imperative [1]. In recent times, the expanding domains of metabolomics and proteomics have surfaced as potent instruments for deciphering the complex interplay between diet and preventing cancer. This introduction lays the groundwork for comprehending how the integration of these disciplines with nutrimetabolomics and nutriproteomics presents fresh perspectives on the molecular pathways involved in cancer prevention via dietary approaches [2]. Metabolomics is the investigation of endogenous and exogenous metabolites (< 1000 Da molecules) in biological specimens, which provides information on nutritional deficiency, metabolic imbalance, and the composition of the gut microbiome. Besides that, metabolomic analysis quantifies the pathways associated with the metabolism of macronutrients, mitochondrial function, microbiota, and biomarkers of oxidative stress [3]. An assessment of metabolites via metabolomics analysis has shown the physiological status of an individual as a result of drug treatment, environmental factors, dietary habits, lifestyles, and genetic influences. Metabolomics is complementary to transcriptomics, proteomics, and genomics and is related to the interactions between DNA, mRNA, and protein [4]. Another emerging concept in the field of metabolomics is nutrimetabolomics, or nutritional metabolomics. The application of metabolomics in the field of nutritional sciences enables the discovery of novel biomarkers related to dietary intake and further elucidates the association between food compounds and diseases or clinical phenotypes [5, 6]. Meanwhile, proteomics, the systematic analysis of proteins within a given sample, offers unparalleled insights into the functional implications of cellular processes. By deciphering the complex interplay of protein–protein interactions and post-translational modifications, proteomic technologies shed light on the molecular mechanisms underlying cancer initiation, progression, and responses to treatment [7]. Likewise, nutriproteomics utilizes proteomic technologies to investigate the wide range of proteins and peptides sourced from food and their impact on health and illness. By clarifying the bioactive elements in food, nutriproteomics provides an understanding of how dietary proteins and peptides contribute to preventing cancer, thereby facilitating the creation of precise dietary interventions for cancer prevention [8].

The emergence of nutrimetabolomics and nutriproteomics represents a paradigm shift in our approach to cancer prevention. These interdisciplinary methods offer prospects not only for understanding how bioactive food components function but also for discovering new avenues for preventing cancer by utilizing the molecular foundations of dietary interventions. This chapter sets the stage for exploring the multidimensional role of nutrimetabolomics and nutriproteomics in harnessing the potential of dietary interventions for cancer prevention.

Analytical Techniques in Metabolomics

Analytical techniques play pivotal roles in metabolomics, facilitating the identification, quantification, and characterization of the metabolites in complex biological samples. Gas chromatography–mass spectrometry(GC-MS), liquid chromatography–mass spectrometry, nuclear magnetic resonance spectroscopy, and capillary electrophoresis–mass spectrometry are among the key techniques employed in metabolomics research, each offering unique advantages and applications [9]. Continued advancements in analytical instrumentation and methods are poised to further enhance the capabilities of metabolomics in elucidating the complexities of cellular metabolism and its implications in health and disease [10].

Gas Chromatography–Mass Spectrometry (GC-MS)

Gas chromatography–mass spectrometry (GC-MS) is a widely utilized analytical technique in metabolomics due to its high sensitivity, reproducibility, and ability to analyze a wide range of metabolites. In GC-MS, metabolites are separated according to their volatility and affinity for the stationary phase in the gas chromatography column, followed by detection and identification using mass spectrometry. This technique is particularly effective for volatile and thermally stable metabolites, making it suitable for the analysis of primary metabolites such as amino acids, organic acids, and sugars [11]. Gas chromatography–mass spectrometry (GC-MS) plays a crucial role in metabolomic studies focused on cancer prevention by enabling the comprehensive analysis of metabolic profiles associated with dietary interventions and their impact on cancer development. Through GC-MS, researchers can identify and quantify a diverse array of metabolites in biological samples, providing insights into the metabolic alterations induced by specific dietary components or interventions [12].

By comparing the metabolomic profiles of cancer patients and those of healthy individuals or by assessing changes in metabolite levels following dietary modifications, GC-MS facilitates the identification of potential biomarkers for cancer risk assessment and the evaluation of the efficacy of dietary interventions in cancer prevention. Furthermore, GC-MS allows for the elucidation of the metabolic pathways implicated in cancer development, offering mechanistic insights into how dietary factors influence cancer initiation, progression, and responses to treatment [13].

Liquid Chromatography–Mass Spectrometry (LC-MS)

Liquid chromatography–mass spectrometry (LC-MS) is an analytical technique in metabolomics that offers high sensitivity and selectivity for a diverse range of metabolites. In LC-MS, metabolites are separated according to their interactions with the liquid chromatography column, followed by ionization and detection using mass spectrometry [14]. LC-MS is well suited for the analysis of polar and nonvolatile metabolites, including secondary metabolites such as flavonoids, alkaloids, and lipids. Furthermore, advancements in LC-MS instrumentation, such as high-resolution mass spectrometry and hyphenated techniques, have expanded its capabilities for metabolite identification and structural elucidation [15]. LC-MS enables researchers to probe the intricate metabolic profiles associated with dietary interventions and their potential impact on cancer risk. By separating and identifying a wide range of metabolites, including bioactive compounds derived from dietary sources, LC-MS facilitates the elucidation of the metabolic pathways implicated in cancer development and progression. By conducting a comparative analysis of metabolomic profiles between cancer patients and healthy individuals, as well as before and after dietary interventions, LC-MS allows for the identification of metabolic signatures indicative of cancer risk or responses to preventive measures [16].

Capillary Electrophoresis–Mass Spectrometry (CE-MS)

Capillary electrophoresis–mass spectrometry (CE-MS) is a powerful analytical technique for the separation and characterization of charged metabolites. In CE-MS, metabolites are separated according to their charge-to-size ratio in a capillary electrophoresis system, followed by detection and identification using mass spectrometry. CE-MS offers high resolution and sensitivity for the analysis of polar and ionic metabolites, making it suitable for applications such as the analysis of neurotransmitters, amino acids, and organic acids in biological samples [17].

CE-MS has emerged as a promising analytical technique in the realm of cancer prevention research, offering a precise and sensitive analysis of metabolites with distinct advantages in studying the impact of dietary interventions on the metabolic pathways relevant to cancer development. By characterizing the metabolomic signatures of individuals undergoing dietary interventions or at varying stages of cancer susceptibility, CE-MS facilitates the identification of biomarkers indicative of cancer risk or responses to preventive measures [18]. Additionally, CE-MS contributes to the discovery of bioactive compounds derived from dietary sources that possess anticancer properties, providing insights into their mechanisms of action and paving the way for the development of targeted dietary strategies for cancer prevention [19].

Nuclear Magnetic Resonance (NMR) Spectroscopy

Nuclear magnetic resonance (NMR) spectroscopy is a nondestructive analytical technique that provides valuable information on the structure and dynamics of metabolites. In NMR spectroscopy, metabolites are subjected to a strong magnetic field, causing nuclei with a magnetic moment to absorb and emit radiofrequency radiation. By analyzing the chemical shifts and coupling patterns of NMR signals, metabolites can be identified and quantified in complex biological samples. NMR spectroscopy is particularly advantageous in the analysis of intact molecules and the determination of metabolic fluxes in metabolic pathways [20]. NMR spectroscopy enables the identification and quantification of metabolites present in complex biological matrices, providing insights into the metabolic alterations associated with cancer development and progression. By comparing the metabolomic profiles of individuals undergoing dietary interventions or at varying stages of cancer susceptibility, NMR spectroscopy facilitates the identification of biomarkers indicative of cancer risk or responses to preventive measures. Furthermore, NMR spectroscopy aids in the discovery of bioactive compounds derived from dietary sources that exhibit anticancer properties, shedding light on their mechanisms of action and informing the development of targeted dietary strategies for cancer prevention [21].

There are similarities and differences between NMR spectroscopy and mass spectrometry (MS). Both of these methods are precise and can identify a wide group of small molecules from a small sample (10–400 µl). NMR is a precise, nondestructive method that can be conducted by using small samples, but it is less sensitive than MS. On the other hand, MS is a more sample-destructive, more time-consuming, and less destructible method [22]. The analysis using both of these methods can be either targeted or untargeted. Targeted analysis is a hypothesis-driven method of identifying a group of known metabolites, whereas untargeted analysis explores unknown metabolites or discovers novel biomarkers or pathways associated with diseases [23]. Different biological samples, such as those of blood, urine, and saliva, can be used for metabolomics analysis. However, sample preparation and handling must be carried out under sterile environmental conditions to produce good results.

Nutrimetabolomics Application in Cancer

Cancer prevalence is increasing worldwide, and the pathology is closely associated with multiple factors. Nutrition-related factors, such as alcohol consumption, an unhealthy diet rich in saturated fat, and a lack of fiber, and the accumulation of adipose tissue are some of the risk factors of cancer. On the other hand, protective dietary factors against cancer include the intake of various foods, namely vegetables, dairy foods, carotenoids, and fiber-rich foods [24]. Understanding the impact of metabolites from ingested food on metabolism will help to better understand the underlying mechanism related to increased or decreased cancer risk and the discovery of novel biomarkers.

Alteration in metabolic function is the key event in tumorigenesis. Diet is an important source of biologically active compounds that act as free radical scavengers and that protect against cancer-causing active electrophiles [25]. Metabolites obtained from the diet have been curated in several online databases, such as the

Kyoto Encyclopedia of Genes and Genomes (KEGG) for human metabolic pathways, the Madison Metabolomics Consortium Database (MMCD), and the Metlin database. Diet-related metabolite analysis in the Supplementation Vitamines et Mineraux Antioxydants (SUVIMAX) study conducted on 200 women with breast cancer demonstrated low levels of plasma piperine and high concentrations of acetyltributylcitrate (ATBC), pregnene-diol sulfate, and 2-amino-4-cyanobutanoic acid [26].

Box 17.1 Nutritional Drivers of Tumorigenesis

The impact of certain dietary factors on tumorigenesis is profound. Factors such as a high intake of processed meats, a high intake of sugary beverages, and a high intake of saturated fats have been linked to an increased risk of cancer initiation and progression. Conversely, diets rich in fruits, vegetables, whole grains, and lean proteins are associated with lower cancer risk. The interplay between nutrients and metabolic pathways within the body influences cell proliferation, DNA repair mechanisms, inflammation, and oxidative stress. Furthermore, dietary components can alter gut microbiota composition, which in turn influences immune function and inflammation, further shaping the tumor microenvironment.

Piperine is an alkaloid commonly found in pepper species, where the highest content is found in black pepper (Piper nigrum L). The piperine present in black pepper contributes to black pepper's strong aroma and its various pharmacological properties, such as anti-inflammatory, antimutagenic, and cancer-preventive effects [27]. Piperine has been found to inhibit the mutagenicity caused by food mutagens that cause mutation to DNA, such as aflatoxin, 3-amino-1-methyl-5H-pyridol [4,3-b]indole (Trp-P-2), 2-amino-3-methylimidazo [4,5-f] quinolone (IQ), and 2-amino-3,8-dimethylimidazo [4,5-f] quinoxaline (MeIQx) [27, 28]. On the other hand, the potential anticancer properties of piperine have been exhibited in various cancers by inducing apoptosis in the HRT-18 human rectal adenocarcinoma cells and by inhibiting the development of colorectal cancer cells by suppressing the activities of tumor necrosis alpha and mTORC1 in human intestinal epithelial cells [29]. In lung cancer cell line (A549), piperine causes increased activity in the Caspase-3 and Caspase-9 pathways and stimulates apoptosis via the inhibition of the cell cycle phase of G2/M [30]. Thus, the addition of pepper to daily meals can reduce the risk of cancer when other confounding factors, such as smoking, a sedentary lifestyle, and undesirable food choices, have been controlled.

Another metabolite that can increase the risk of cancer in acetyltributylcitrate, commonly known as ATBC. ATBC is a plasticizer used for packaging food items such as cheese, wrapped cake, microwaved soup, biscuits, and skimmed milk. During the heating process, ATBC will leak into the food or liquid. Hot beverages should not be drunk from a plastic cup or container. Coffee or tea that is drunk from a plastic cup will be contaminated by the foreign particles present in the plastic cup. In addition, the presence of protein liquid, such as milk in coffee, will further accelerate the transfer of ATBC into the coffee [31]. Furthermore, alcohol should be avoided to prevent cancer. Alcohol stimulates the rise in hormones such as estrone sulfate and dehydroepiandrosterone, which may accelerate breast tumor growth [32].

In addition, the Prostate, Lung, Colorectal and Ovarian (PLCO) Cancer Screening Trial Cohort investigated diet-related metabolites in the blood serum of 621 post-menopausal invasive breast cancer cases and 621 matched control cases. The findings from this study revealed that three metabolites were significantly related to increased overall breast cancer risk, namely the caprate present in butter, dessert-related γ-carboxyethyl hydrochroman (γ-CEHC), and alcohol-related 4-androsten-3 β,17β-diol-monosulfate. Besides that, another 19 metabolites were reported to be associated with estrogen receptor (ER)-positive (ER+), which were present in butter, alcohol, margarine, fried food, vitamin E, and fat-containing dessert [33]. In this rat race world, cooking has been a tedious task due to time constraints. People are seeking simple ways to prepare appetizing food and one such way is frying. Deep-fried foods cooked at high temperatures will form a carcinogenic compound known as acrylamide, which is commonly found in French fries and potato chips [34]. Besides that, butter, fried food, and fat-containing dessert have a high amount of saturated fatty acid, which may increase the risk of cancer. Meanwhile, margarine-containing foods are high in trans fatty acid, which also increases the risk of cancer [35].

A study on diet-related metabolites has provided information about the types of food that must be limited in our daily diet to prevent cancer. A key strategy for cancer prevention is to adopt a healthy lifestyle by preparing healthy home-cooked food while limiting the use of unsaturated oil, sugar, and red meat and increasing the consumption of vegetables and fruits. Healthy cooking methods such as baking, blanching, steaming, and roasting can replace deep-frying, which may cause health-harming structural changes in the oil used. Nutritional metabolomics is an essential approach to understanding cancer etiology and could pave the way for establishing new theories about the fundamental role of diet in cancer prevention.

Role of Protein and Peptides Extracted from Food in Chemoprevention

Proteins play an essential role in any biological process in the human body. A large and highly dynamic network of proteins expressed in a person's genome is known as the proteome. The human proteome is made up of 20,000–25,000 genes [36]. Relevant abundance and protein structure can affect the physiological nature of a cell or tissue and determines its form. The aim of proteomics is to identify the entire collection of proteins expressed in a given organism, tissue, or organ at any given time. Qualitative proteomics is the study of post-translational modifications in proteins that can absorb various environmental materials [37]. Comparative proteomics studies concentrate on this heterogeneity, whereas proteomics compares the quantitative (or differential) abundance of particular proteins in various environments. In contrast to the static genome, internally variable and context-dependent functional proteomics are proteomes. Functional interactions between proteins and other macromolecules are studied extensively in modern molecular biology [38].

Dietary nutrients or ingredients can be viewed as "signals," which can be obtained by replicating material or by using "nutrient sensors," which responds to the signals. Transcription factors modify the DNA replication of a specific gene in response to the nutrition signal, changing the pattern of genes and thus the protein expression nutrition response. Certain diets influence gene expression patterns, protein expression patterns, and produce metabolism. Such nutrients or ingredients are referred to as diet signatures [39]. There are two ways in which dietary components interact with proteins: After expression or translation, proteins, small molecular-protein interactions, and protein structures undergo three-dimensional changes. Nutritional science may benefit from protcomic techniques to develop disease biomarkers and functional methods for determining causes and effects in living systems. Dietary or behavioral modifications are used to intervene and assess patients' well-being. When nutriproteomics is combined with other fields (nutrigenomics and nutrimetabolomics), it can help evaluate human health, explain the impact of diet on human metabolism, and establish tailored dietary guidelines for disease prevention in individuals [40].

Anticancer Plant Proteins and Peptides

Plant proteins and peptides with cytotoxic activity against cancer cells have been discovered in recent years. They could be viable alternatives to new cancer treatments. The next part of the discussion will focus on anticarcinogenic proteins and peptides [41].

Plant-Derived Lectin

Plant-derived lectins are proteins or nonimmune glycoproteins found in the seeds, roots, stalks, and leaves of plants. Leptins are classified as carbohydrate-binding proteins on the basis of their ability to bind carbohydrates [42]. Leptins are divided into 12 classes; interestingly, proteins within the legume lectin domain are among them, and they've been researched extensively for their effects on a variety of diseases, including cancer. Lectins have been shown in several studies to have mitogenic, antiproliferative, antitumor [43], antiviral, and immune-stimulating properties [44]. Mistletoe lectins have gotten more attention because of their antiproliferative properties against a variety of cancer cell lines. Their ability to bind sugar, ability to induce apoptosis through caspase-dependent and caspase-independent pathways, cell-cycle-arresting ability [45], autophagy, neo-angiogenesis, and metastasis inhibition potential are all stimulated, via immunomodulatory activities, by stimulating tumor-related macrophages to increase nitric oxide production and induce cytotoxicity against tumor cells, which appears to play an important role in the assessment of cancer cell selective toxicity [46]. In addition, mistletoe lectins interact with sugar chains or additive receptors on the cell surface. Proof of the antiproliferative activity of different lectins on various cancer cell lines is available for acute human lymphoblastic leukemia, hepatocarcinoma, gingival fibroblasts, melanoma, glioblastoma U87, ovarian cancer SKOV3, and colon cancer [33].

Milk-Derived Anticancer Proteins and Peptides

Lactoferrin is a protein that has many physiological functions, including antimicrobial and immunomodulatory properties, which contribute to its chemopreventive effects. Lactoferrin is a milk-derived anticancer peptide that has been shown to be effective against a number of cancer cell lines, including breast, colon, fibrosarcoma, leukemia, nasal, and ovarian cancer cells [47]. However, in that study, lymphocytes, fibroblasts, endothelial cells, and epithelial cells were not affected. Lactophericin has been shown to regulate gene expression in a way that inhibits angiogenesis, interrupts the cell cycle, and induces apoptosis. Lactoferrin therapy inhibits the cell cycle in the G1/S transition, preventing the growth of breast cancer in MDA-MB-231 cells. Lactoferrin also causes a rise in SMAD-2 nuclear deposits in Henrietta Lacks (HeLa) cells [48]. The suppression of the Akt signaling pathway in nasopharyngeal carcinoma cells has been confirmed. In tumor-bearing rats, oral administration of recombinant human lactoferrin significantly decreased squamous cell carcinoma in the head and neck. Interleukin (IL)-8 and natural killer cell activation on one hand and the formation of CD8 + T-cells on another are two potential modes of action for this enzyme. In transgenic rats, oral administration of bovine lactoferrin resulted in a substantial reduction in lung cancer tumor development and levels of tumor necrosis factor reduction (TNF)-6, IL-4, IL-6, and IL-10 [49].

Anticancer Properties of Egg Proteins and Peptides

The protein content of egg whites is high (11%). Ovalbumin is the most abundant protein (54%). The next most common proteins were ovotransferrin (12%), ovomucoid (11%), lysozyme (3.5%), and ovomukin (1.2%) [50]. Furthermore, although lipids make up the majority of the yolk (31–35%), the yolk also contains lipovitellins (36%), levitins (38%), phosphatin (8%), and low-density lipoproteins (17%). Lysozyme is a protein with anticancer properties that has been studied extensively [51]. Oral administration of this protein has been shown to inhibit the formation of the structure in multiple-tumor development. Colorectal cancer was reduced in rats treated with hydrolyzed egg yolk protein, according to some reports, by inhibiting tumor cell proliferation. These defensive effects may be attributed to the protein phosphatidylserine's powerful antioxidant properties and the phospho-oligopeptides that it creates [52].

Ingredients and Biomarkers Containing Proteins and Peptides

Proteins play a central role in all biological processes in humans. Proteomics is a powerful tool for elucidating molecular events like nutrition because it can categorize and enumerate bioactive proteins and peptides and can shed light on their effects at the protein/peptide level (biomarkers) and thus address nutritional bioefficacy issues [53].

Box 17.2 Biomarker Discovery and Detection Strategies
A biomarker is a measurable predictor of a specific biology related to the risk of contracting a disease or the stage of a disease. Different methods for recognizing and tracking molecular biomarkers' activities in disease conditions or disease progression have been studied because molecular biomarkers can take a variety of forms. Finding biomarkers and drug targets is made easier with affinity purification, activity-based profiling, the microarray strategy, and global proteomic methods [54].

Proteomic Technology

In the primary nutrition process, quantitative and functional proteomic methods are used to classify, measure, and test proteins expressed under the stimulus of dietary nutrition (or protein profiling, as in Fig. 17.1) [55]. Quantitative proteomics is concerned with the parameters or measurements of a protein sample. However, functional proteomics can be used to examine post-translational changes in proteins, their alignment and clarification (interaction/complexity) for target molecules, and protein functionality [56]. Protein profiles have become simpler and more versatile thanks to advances in biological compound isolation, mass spectrometry, bioinformatic equipment, protein comparisons, genome sequencing, and partial proteomic sequences of tissues and cells. Immunochemical methods are often used to identify and characterize proteins, but their availability and specificity are restricted [51].

Conclusion

The integration of nutrimetabolomics and nutriproteomics has significantly advanced the understanding of the important relationship between diet and cancer prevention. These approaches allow for the discovery of novel biomarkers and

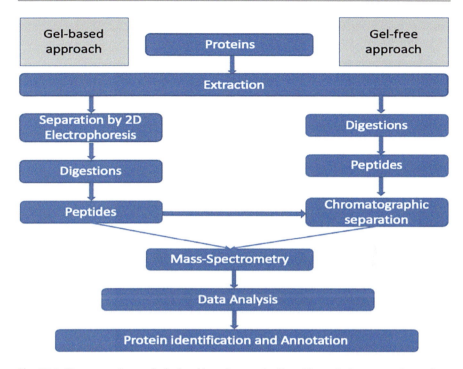

Fig. 17.1 Target proteins can be isolated by using standard/specific methods, separated on gels or columns by using either a gel-based or gel-free process, digested into peptides with enzymes (trypsin), and analyzed by using mass spectrometric instruments. Reference protein databases can also be used to classify and quantify them.

therapeutic targets, facilitating early detection, monitoring, and the development of personalized dietary interventions. Researchers can identify key nutrients and nutraceuticals that modulate pathways related to inflammation, oxidative stress, and tumorigenesis by analyzing the molecular responses to bioactive food components. This knowledge paves the way for preventive strategies that intervene before disease onset or support recovery during early stages. In summary, nutrimetabolomics and nutriproteomics provide essential tools for decoding the preventive power of food, establishing new paradigms for cancer prevention in molecular nutrition.

Further Practice

1. Which analytical technique is commonly used in nutrimetabolomics to identify biomarkers of dietary exposure?

   A. Gas chromatography–mass spectrometry (GC-MS)
   B. Liquid chromatography–mass spectrometry (LC-MS)
   C. Nuclear magnetic resonance (NMR) spectroscopy
   D. High-performance liquid chromatography (HPLC)

2. What type of profiles can plasma proteomics provide to predict individual future health risks?

   A. Metabolic profiles
   B. Proteomic profiles
   C. Lipid profiles
   D. Genetic profiles

3. What is the focus of advancements in carbohydrate metabolomics discussed in this chapter?

   A. Techniques for protein analysis
   B. The current state of lipidomics
   C. Evolving methods in metabolomics
   D. Applications of NMR spectroscopy

4. What is the focus of sample preparation discussed in this chapter for gas chromatography–mass spectrometry (GC-MS)?

   A. Animal tissue
   B. Human blood samples
   C. Plant tissue
   D. Synthetic compounds

5. What is the typical sample volume required for analyzing small molecules in metabolomics?

   A. 1–5 ml
   B. 10–400 µl
   C. 500–1000 µl
   D. 2–5 ml

6. Which societal value discussed in this chapter is associated with nutriproteomics and proteogenomics?

   A. Personalized medicine
   B. Environmental conservation
   C. Agricultural sustainability
   D. Technological innovation

7. What type of metabolites is well suited for analysis using liquid chromatography–mass spectrometry (LC-MS)?

   A. Volatile metabolites
   B. Nonpolar metabolites
   C. Nonvolatile metabolites
   D. Secondary metabolites

8. Capillary electrophoresis–mass spectrometry (CE-MS) offers high separation and characterization for which of the following?

   A. Nonpolar metabolites
   B. Volatile metabolites
   C. Charged metabolites
   D. Secondary metabolites

9. What does nuclear magnetic resonance (NMR) spectroscopy enable researchers to identify and quantify in complex biological samples?

   A. Intact molecules
   B. Volatile metabolites
   C. Charged metabolites
   D. Secondary metabolites

10. What is the primary advantage of liquid chromatography–mass spectrometry (LC-MS) in metabolomic research?

   A. Its high sensitivity
   B. Its nondestructive analysis
   C. Its ability to separate intact molecules
   D. Its characterization of volatile metabolites

11. How can nutrimetabolomics contribute to understanding the association between food compounds and diseases?

   A. By analyzing DNA sequences
   B. By studying protein–protein interactions
   C. By elucidating novel biomarkers related to dietary intake
   D. By focusing on RNA expression patterns

12. What is the aim of proteomics in relation to proteins expressed in a given organism?

   A. To identify only a small subset of proteins
   B. To study DNA sequences
   C. To determine the entire collection of proteins expressed at a given time
   D. To focus on a single protein at a time

13. How can proteomic technology be used to identify target proteins for analysis?

   A. By using immunochemical methods exclusively
   B. By isolating proteins by using specific methods and analyzing them with mass spectrometry
   C. By relying solely on genome sequencing
   D. By studying protein–protein interactions

14. How can proteomics shed light on the molecular mechanisms underlying cancer initiation?

    A. By analyzing DNA sequences
    B. By studying protein–protein interactions and modifications
    C. By focusing on RNA expression patterns
    D. By examining metabolite levels

15. How can dietary nutrients or ingredients influence gene expression patterns and protein expression patterns?

    A. By directly modifying DNA sequences
    B. By altering the structure of proteins
    C. By interacting with transcription factors
    D. By inhibiting protein synthesis

Answer Key

1. A, 2. B, 3. C, 4. C, 5. B, 6. A, 7. D, 8. C, 9. A, 10. A, 11. C, 12. C, 13. B, 14. B, 15. C

References

1. Siegel RL, Miller KD, Wagle NS, Jemal A. Cancer statistics, 2023. CA Cancer J Clin. 2023;73(1):17–48.
2. Suri GS, Kaur G, Carbone GM, Shinde D. Metabolomics in oncology. Cancer Rep. 2023;6(3):e1795.
3. Tsoukalas D, Fragoulakis V, Sarandi E, Docea AO, Papakonstaninou E, Tsilimidos G, et al. Targeted metabolomic analysis of serum fatty acids for the prediction of autoimmune diseases. Front Mol Biosci. 2019;6:120.
4. Unión-Caballero A, Meroño T, Zamora-Ros R, Rostgaard-Hansen AL, Miñarro A, Sánchez-Pla A, et al. Metabolome biomarkers linking dietary fibre intake with cardiometabolic effects: results from the Danish diet, cancer and health-next generations MAX study. Food Funct. 2024;15(3):1643–54.
5. Dessì A, Cesare Marincola F, Masili A, Gazzolo D, Fanos V. Clinical metabolomics and nutrition: the new frontier in neonatology and pediatrics. BioMed Research International; 2014.
6. Garcia-Aloy M, Llorach R, Urpi-Sarda M, Tulipani S, Salas-Salvadó J, Martínez-González MA, et al. Nutrimetabolomics fingerprinting to identify biomarkers of bread exposure in a free-living population from the PREDIMED study cohort. Metabolomics. 2015;11:155–65.
7. You J, Guo Y, Zhang Y, Kang JJ, Wang LB, Feng JF, et al. Plasma proteomic profiles predict individual future health risk. Nat Commun. 2023;14(1):7817.
8. Costello E, Goodrich JA, Patterson WB, Walker DI, Chen J, Baumert BO, et al. Proteomic and Metabolomic signatures of diet quality in young adults. Nutrients. 2024;16(3):429.
9. Kathuria D, Thakur S, Singh N. Advances of metabolomic in exploring phenolic compounds diversity in cereal and their health implications. Int J Food Sci Technol. 2024;59:4213.
10. Singh R, Fatima E, Thakur L, Singh S, Ratan C, Kumar N. Advancements in CHO metabolomics: techniques, current state and evolving methodologies. Front Bioeng Biotechnol. 2024;12:1347138.

11. Manickavasagam G, Saaid M, Lim V. Exploring stingless bee honey from selected regions of peninsular Malaysia through gas chromatography–mass spectrometry–based untargeted metabolomics. J Food Sci. 2024;89(2):1058–72.

12. Dagar R, Gautam A, Priscilla K, Sharma V, Gupta P, Kumar R. Sample preparation from plant tissue for Gas Chromatography–Mass Spectrometry (GC-MS) we. In: Plant functional genomics: methods and protocols, vol. 2. New York: Springer; 2024. p. 19–37.

13. Sahoo BC, Singh S, Sahoo S, Kar B. Comparative metabolomics of high and low essential oil yielding landraces of Betelvine (Piper betle L.) by two-dimensional gas chromatography time-of-flight mass spectrometry (GC× GC TOFMS). Anal Lett. 2024;57(5):694–710.

14. Wen S, Tu X, Zang Q, Zhu Y, Li L, Zhang R, Abliz Z. Liquid chromatography–mass spectrometry-based metabolomics and fluxomics reveals the metabolic alterations in glioma U87MG multicellular tumor spheroids versus two-dimensional cell cultures. Rapid Commun Mass Spectrom. 2024;38(2):e9670.

15. Doğan HO. Metabolomics: a review of liquid chromatography mass spectrometry-based methods and clinical applications. Turk J Biochem. 2024;1:1.

16. Jimoh MO, Jimoh MA, Kerebba N, Bakare OO, Senjobi CT, Saheed SA, et al. Liquid chromatography–mass spectrometry and xCELLigence real time cell analyzer revealed anticancer and antioxidant metabolites in Trianthema portulacastrum L. (Aizoaceae). Phytomedicine Plus. 2024;4(2):100550.

17. Li Y, Miao S, Tan J, Zhang Q, Chen DDY. Capillary electrophoresis: a three-year literature review, vol. 96. Analytical Chemistry; 2024. p. 7799.

18. Frantzi M, Morillo AC, Lendinez G, Blanca-Pedregosa A, Lopez Ruiz D, Parada J, et al. Validation of a urine-based proteomics test to predict clinically significant prostate cancer: complementing MRI pathway. medRxiv, 2024–04; 2024.

19. Am A, Faccio ME, Pinvidic M, Reygue E, Doan BT, Lescot C, et al. A methodological approach by capillary electrophoresis coupled to mass spectrometry via electrospray interface for the characterization of short synthetic peptides towards the conception of self-assembled nanotheranostic agents. J Chromatogr A. 2024;1713:464496.

20. Khalil A, Kashif M. Nuclear magnetic resonance spectroscopy for quantitative analysis: a review for its application in the chemical, pharmaceutical and medicinal domains. Crit Rev Anal Chem. 2023;53(5):997–1011.

21. Rafalskiy VV, Zyubin AY, Moiseeva EM, Kupriyanova GS, Mershiev IG, Kryukova NO, et al. Application of vibrational spectroscopy and nuclear magnetic resonance methods for drugs pharmacokinetics research. Drug Metab Personal Ther. 2023;38(1):3–13.

22. Tzoulaki I, Ebbels TM, Valdes A, Elliott P, Ioannidis JP. Design and analysis of metabolomics studies in epidemiologic research: a primer on-omic technologies. Am J Epidemiol. 2014;180(2):129–39.

23. Nicholson JK, Holmes E, Kinross JM, Darzi AW, Takats Z, Lindon JC. Metabolic phenotyping in clinical and surgical environments. Nature. 2012;491(7424):384–92.

24. Key TJ, Bradbury KE, Perez-Cornago A, Sinha R, Tsilidis KK, Tsugane S. Diet, nutrition, and cancer risk: what do we know and what is the way forward? BMJ. 2020;368:m511.

25. Michels K. Current opportunities to catalyze research in nutrition and cancer prevention—an interdisciplinary perspective. BMC Med. 2019;17(1):148.

26. Lécuyer L, Dalle C, Lefèvre-Arbogast S, Micheau P, Lyan B, Rossary A, et al. Diet-related metabolomic signature of long-term breast cancer risk using penalized regression: an exploratory study in the SU. VI. MAX cohort. Cancer Epidemiol Biomarkers Prev. 2020;29(2):396–405.

27. Stojanović-Radić Z, Pejčić M, Dimitrijević M, Aleksić AV, Anil Kumar N, Salehi B, et al. Piperine-a major principle of black pepper: a review of its bioactivity and studies. Appl Sci. 2019;9(20):4270.

28. Kumar A, Sasmal D, Sharma N. Immunomodulatory role of piperine in deltamethrin induced thymic apoptosis and altered immune functions. Environ Toxicol Pharmacol. 2015;39(2):504–14.

29. Kaur H, He B, Zhang C, Rodriguez E, Hage DS, Moreau R. Piperine potentiates curcumin-mediated repression of mTORC1 signaling in human intestinal epithelial cells: implications for the inhibition of protein synthesis and TNFα signaling. J Nutr Biochem. 2018;57:276–86.
30. Lin Y, Xu J, Liao H, Li L, Pan L. Piperine induces apoptosis of lung cancer A549 cells via p53-dependent mitochondrial signaling pathway. Tumour Biol. 2014;35:3305–10.
31. Nara K, Nishiyama K, Natsugari H, Takeshita A, Takahashi H. Leaching of the plasticizer, acetyl tributyl citrate: (ATBC) from plastic kitchen wrap. J Health Sci. 2009;55(2):281–4.
32. Coronado GD, Beasley J, Livaudais J. Alcohol consumption and the risk of breast cancer. Salud Publica Mex. 2011;53(5):440–7.
33. Sauer S, Luge T. Nutriproteomics: facts, concepts, and perspectives. Proteomics. 2015;15(5–6):997–1013.
34. Sun Y, Liu B, Snetselaar LG, Robinson JG, Wallace RB, Peterson LL, Bao W. Association of fried food consumption with all cause, cardiovascular, and cancer mortality: prospective cohort study. BMJ. 2019;364:k5420.
35. Bojková B, Winklewski PJ, Wszedybyl-Winklewska M. Dietary fat and cancer—which is good, which is bad, and the body of evidence. Int J Mol Sci. 2020;21(11):4114.
36. Barnes S, Kim H. Nutriproteomics: identifying the molecular targets of nutritive and non-nutritive components of the diet. BMB Rep. 2004;37(1):59–74.
37. Bergen WG. Contribution of research with farm animals to protein metabolism concepts: A historical Perspective1. J Nutr. 2007;137(3):706–10.
38. Bragazzi NL. Situating nutri-ethics at the junction of nutrigenomics and nutriproteomics in postgenomics medicine. Curr Pharm Personal Med. 2013;11(2):162–6.
39. Ganesh V, Hettiarachchy NS. Nutriproteomics: A promising tool to link diet and diseases in nutritional research. Biochim Biophys Acta Proteins Proteomics. 2012;1824(10):1107–17.
40. Ha BG, Yonezawa T, Son MJ, Woo JT, Ohba S, Chung UI, Yagasaki K. Antidiabetic effect of nepodin, a component of Rumex roots, and its modes of action in vitro and in vivo. Biofactors. 2014;40(4):436–47.
41. Lee SE, Schulze KJ, Cole RN, Wu LS, Yager JD, Groopman J, et al. Biological systems of vitamin K: a plasma nutriproteomics study of subclinical vitamin K deficiency in 500 Nepalese children. OMICS. 2016;20(4):214–23.
42. Mol P, Kannegundla U, Dey G, Gopalakrishnan L, Dammalli M, Kumar M, et al. Bovine milk comparative proteome analysis from early, mid, and late lactation in the cattle breed, Malnad Gidda (Bos indicus). OMICS. 2018;22(3):223–35.
43. Yau T, Dan X, Ng CCW, Ng TB. Lectins with potential for anti-cancer therapy. Molecules. 2015;20(3):3791–810.
44. Ozdemir V, Armengaud J, Dubé L, Aziz RK, Knoppers BM. Nutriproteomics and proteogenomics: cultivating two novel hybrid fields of personalized medicine with added societal value. Curr Pharm Person Med. 2010;8(4):240.
45. Gondim AC, Romero-Canelon I, Sousa EH, Blindauer CA, Butler JS, Romero MJ, et al. The potent anti-cancer activity of Dioclea lasiocarpa lectin. J Inorg Biochem. 2017;175:179–89.
46. Özdemir V, Kolker E. Precision nutrition 4.0: a big data and ethics foresight analysis—convergence of agrigenomics, nutrigenomics, nutriproteomics, and nutrimetabolomics. OMICS. 2016;20(2):69–75.
47. Schweigert FJ. Nutritional proteomics: methods and concepts for research in nutritional science. Ann Nutr Metab. 2007;51(2):99–107.
48. Schweigert FJ, Gericke B, Wolfram W, Kaisers U, Dudenhausen JW. Peptide and protein profiles in serum and follicular fluid of women undergoing IVF. Hum Reprod. 2006;21(11):2960–8.
49. Sellami M, Bragazzi NL. Nutrigenomics and breast cancer: state-of-art, future perspectives and insights for prevention. Nutrients. 2020;12(2):512.
50. Sénéchal S, Kussmann M. Nutriproteomics: technologies and applications for identification and quantification of biomarkers and ingredients. Proc Nutr Soc. 2011;70(3):351–64.
51. Sharanova NE, Vasil'ev AV. Postgenomic properties of natural micronutrients. Bull Exp Biol Med. 2018;166:107–17.

52. Vasil'ev AV, Sharanova NE. Nutrimetabolomics—a new stage of biochemistry of nutrition. The role of nutriproteomic analysis. Vopr Pitan. 2013;82(5):4–9.
53. Yonezawa T, Hasegawa SI, Asai M, Ninomiya T, Sasaki T, Cha BY, et al. Harmine, a β-carboline alkaloid, inhibits osteoclast differentiation and bone resorption in vitro and in vivo. Eur J Pharmacol. 2011a;650(2–3):511–8.
54. Yonezawa T, Lee JW, Hibino A, Asai M, Hojo H, Cha BY, et al. Harmine promotes osteo-blast differentiation through bone morphogenetic protein signaling. Biochem Biophys Res Commun. 2011b;409(2):260–5.
55. Yonezawa T, Mase N, Sasaki H, Teruya T, Hasegawa SI, Cha BY, et al. Biselyngbyaside, iso-lated from marine cyanobacteria, inhibits osteoclastogenesis and induces apoptosis in mature osteoclasts. J Cell Biochem. 2012;113(2):440–8.
56. Zhang X, Yap Y, Wei D, Chen G, Chen F. Novel omics technologies in nutrition research. Biotechnol Adv. 2008;26(2):169–76.

Perioperative Nutrition Management Through Enhanced Recovery After Surgery (ERAS) Protocols and Immunonutrition

18

Anna Dysart ⓘ

Learning Objectives

After completing this chapter, you will be able to

- Outline the importance of nutrition in the perioperative period
- Describe the enhanced recovery after surgery (ERAS) protocols
- Suggest preoperative nutrition optimization
- Introduce new research in the areas of immunonutrition
- Describe postoperative nutrition strategies

Introduction: Enhanced Recovery After Surgery

Current Evidence Base

The concept of improving surgical recovery times through multimodal and interactive collaboration between different medical disciplines was first put forth in the 1990s by Henrik Kehlet [1, 2]. The ERAS study group, which later formed the ERAS Society, was started in 2001 and continues to "develop perioperative care and to improve recovery through research, education, audit and implementation of evidence-based practice" [3]. An important component of ERAS is nutrition, given that research has established that malnutrition, or the inadequate intake of nutrients [2],

A. Dysart (✉)
Western Carolina University, Cullowhee, NC, USA
e-mail: sdysart@email.wcu.edu

has a deleterious effect on postoperative surgical outcomes [1, 2, 4–7]. Nutritional guidelines for ERAS are included in the meta-analysis and systematic reviews that make up the basis for the consensus guidelines put forth by the ERAS Society. A large component of the success of ERAS protocols is following the guidelines and protocols as precisely as possible [8]. Studies have shown that increased adherence to the interdisciplinary nature of the ERAS protocols allows for improved postoperative patient outcomes [8].

Differences in surgery location, anesthesia types and amount, the invasiveness of the procedure (i.e., laparoscopic or open surgery), the intravenous fluids given, and the nutrition support given have all been shown to impact outcomes [9]. Currently, the ERAS Society has guidelines and consensus reports for 23 types of surgery, including bariatric surgery, colorectal surgery, gastrectomy, liver surgery, and esophagectomy [10]. The common nutritional aspects of the guidelines are summarized in Table 18.1. Some guidelines have different nutrition-related guidelines, like emergency laparotomies, which are discussed at the end of this chapter.

Historical Guidelines on Nutrition and Surgery

Traditional nutritional preparation before surgery includes fasting from midnight the night before the surgery [4, 5]. Fasting was thought to decrease the risk for developing aspiration pneumonia, which is increased due to the effects of anesthesia [5, 11]. No differentiation was made between liquids and solids in these recommendations, and although consuming solid foods has continued to be shown in the evidence to have an increased risk of aspiration due to the relaxation of the laryngeal reflex, the consumption of clear liquids has become part of the more liberal guidelines put into effect in more-recent years [5]. Although traditional clear liquids, such as tea, water, and juices are included in newer guidelines, more-advanced clear liquids that are specifically designed to promote postoperative recovery are a large part of newer enhanced recovery after surgery (ERAS) guidelines.

Table 18.1 Nutrition-related ERAS guidelines based on surgical type

	Immunonutrition and nutrition support	Preoperative carbohydrate loading	Clear fluid intake up to 2 hours after surgery	Prophylactic prevention of postoperative nausea and vomiting	Allow oral intake soon after surgery
Head and neck cancers	Immunonutrition is controversial and not yet recommended Preoperative enteral nutrition only in malnourished patients	Weak evidence of benefit	Recommended	Recommended	
Gastrectomies	Recommended when patients are malnourished	Recommended	Recommended	Recommended	Recommended
Bariatric surgery		Weak evidence of benefit	Recommended	Recommended	Recommended
Colonic resection		Recommended	Recommended	Recommended	Recommended
Cardiac surgery	Recommended when patients are malnourished	Recommended	Recommended		Recommended
Liver surgery	Immunonutrition is controversial and not yet recommended Recommended when patients are malnourished	Recommended	Recommended	Recommended	Recommended

ERAS and Nutrition

Baseline Status

Nutritional status prior to surgery has been shown to have large impacts on postsurgical outcomes [2, 4, 7, 12, 13]. Surgery puts the body into a hypermetabolic-catabolic state due to the necessary postoperative wound healing [13]. When the body is in this state, gluconeogenesis is active and the muscle is catabolized to provide amino acids [9, 13]. In patients who are malnourished prior to surgery, an increased risk of complications, longer hospital stays, a higher risk of infections, and an increase in mortality rates have been shown [2, 12–15]. As shown in Fig. 18.1, nutritional inputs, such as baseline nutritional status and fasting, are in a balancing act with the outputs of surgery.

A patient may be malnourished or undernourished prior to surgery for a variety of reasons. When looking at the global population, malnutrition has decreased overall in recent years, though it remains high in many areas of the world [16]. Individuals who have a lower sociodemographic index are more likely to experience malnutrition. Children and elderly people are also at a higher risk of malnutrition. Elderly people frequently become malnourished with hospitalization, with decreases in appetite and intestinal absorption playing a role in further malnourishment [16].

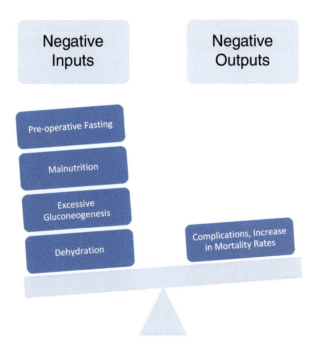

Fig. 18.1 Complications that may stem from baseline nutritional status and changes to metabolism based on surgery

Other diseases also play a role in malnutrition, with patients who have cancer, gastrointestinal disease, and dysphagia also experiencing higher rates of malnutrition [2, 12, 17, 18]. Hydration status is also of concern in patients undergoing surgery, where resuscitation and corrections to any underlying imbalances are paramount [19].

Additionally, blood glucose levels prior to surgery have been shown to have an impact on complications postoperatively [9]. When a patient has high blood glucose levels prior to surgery, future complications such as poor outcomes, wound complications [20], and increased mortality [21, 22] have been observed [9]. This holds true for both patients with a diagnosis of diabetes and those without [9] as well as for both patients with a healthy body mass index (BMI) and those with an obese BMI [23]. Studies have shown that insulin sensitivity is decreased postsurgery in patients [9, 23] and may be connected to the traditional prolonged period of fasting prior to surgery [23]. Control over preoperative blood glucose levels may be obtained through continuous intravenous insulin infusion or through subcutaneous insulin dosing depending on the anticipated length of the surgery [9].

To control blood glucose levels in patients with type 2 diabetes prior to surgery, prolonged fasting should be avoided and the usage of antidiabetic pharmacotherapy should be continued until the day prior to surgery [9]. Insulin therapy should also be continued. More research needs to be conducted on the many types of oral diabetic medications before guidance can be given on each medication. In patients with type 1 diabetes, care should be taken to prevent hypoglycemia, and insulin dosages should be adjusted on the basis of the patient's fasting state [9].

General Preoperative Nutrition

Although patients who are malnourished or undernourished are at an increased risk of complications and poorer outcomes after surgery, even patients who have acceptable nutrition levels prior to surgery have been shown to have decreased nutritional status after surgery [9, 24]. The catabolic reaction of the body postsurgery results in increased needs for macro- and micronutrients to promote wound healing [2, 9]. The stress of surgery results in cortisol being released, triggering increased hepatic glucose production, the breakdown of protein, and gluconeogenesis [9, 23]. Carbohydrate drinks have been shown to postoperatively decrease insulin resistance [25, 26], lessen postoperative nitrogen loss [26, 27], maintain lean body mass [26, 28], and lessen impairment of muscle function [8, 28].

Not all preoperative carbohydrate drinks are created equally, with research showing that drinks higher in carbohydrate (125 mg/ml of carbohydrate (CHO) or a total of approximately 175–200 g of CHO preoperatively) have more benefits when studying whole body protein balance and insulin sensitivity [26]. Insulin resistance postsurgery has been established as a characteristic of postoperative metabolism [26], with a growing body of evidence recommending perioperatively optimizing carbohydrate and protein consumption to mitigate insulin resistance and catabolism

[11]. Protein intake before surgery in the form of free amino acids is recommended to mitigate negative protein balance. Branched-chain amino acids can be utilized as a fuel source, and essential amino acids can be helpful in supporting protein synthesis and wound healing [11].

> **Box 18.1: How Registered Dietitian-nutritionists Can Show Their Value**
> Reducing the length of stay for hospital patients can result in lower costs for both the patient and the hospital. By providing optimal nutrition support and nutrition guidance during the perioperative period, registered dietitians can benefit the patient physically and financially. Registered dietitian-nutritionists should take notes on the patients that they implement ERAS protocols with, monitoring the rate of complications, the length of hospital stays, and the costs associated with nutrition supplements and nutrition support. When advocating for additional registered dietitian-nutritionist staff or advocating against budget cuts to the nutrition department, having the data is important to show how nutrition and registered dietitian-nutritionists can impact outcomes. These data can also be used when negotiating new supplement and nutrition support contracts for the hospital.

Upper Gastrointestinal Surgeries

ERAS guidelines were released in 2016 for patients with head and neck cancers who undergo surgical interventions in the upper gastrointestinal tract and in the mouth [18]. Patients that have head and neck cancers that require surgical intervention are frequently undernourished due to their disease state prior to surgery. Many have dysphagia and other difficulties chewing and swallowing their foods and drinks, which reflects their nutritional status. This population is at risk of refeeding syndrome, so extra care should be taken when starting preoperative nutrition through oral or nutrition support routes. Preoperative nutrition for malnourished patients is strongly recommended. Using types of enteral formulas containing additional concentrations of arginine, glutamine, omega-3 fatty acids, and/or ribonucleic acids, frequently referred to as immunonutriton, is controversial in this population [18].

Preoperative carbohydrate loading with carbohydrate-rich drinks has worked in many other patient populations to decrease the length of hospital stays and reduce risks of complications [18]. The official ERAS Society guidelines report low confidence in preoperative carbohydrate-rich drink usage in this population, citing the lack of randomized controlled trials in this population. Clear fluid intake up to 2 h until anesthesia is recommended. Postoperatively, patients are encouraged to eat an oral diet as soon as tolerable. In discussion with the interdisciplinary team, prognosis for oral nutritional adequacy should be evaluated both prior to and after surgery to determine the need for a nasoenteric or gastrostomy feeding tube. The need for nutrition support will vary depending on the patient's baseline nutritional status, the site of surgery within the head and neck, and the postoperative recovery timeline. Vomiting is concerning after head and neck surgeries and can result in wound dehiscence, fistula, and poor outcomes. All patients should be given intra- and postoperative antiemetic and antinausea medications prophylactically and as needed [18].

For patients undergoing gastrectomy, preoperative nutrition support via enteral feedings is recommended only as required in malnourished patients [15]. Patients who do not have malnutrition do not reap any benefit from preoperative nutrition support. Patients who are malnourished may benefit from oral nutrition supplementation if they are able to tolerate it. Parenteral nutrition may be used if the gastrointestinal tract is not working. Immunonutrition has been shown to have benefits for some abdominal surgeries, though no consensus existed among the limited randomized control trials completed at the time of the gastrectomy ERAS guidelines' release for it to be recommended in gastrectomy patients [15].

Prior to gastrectomy, evidence has shown that alcohol misusers should abstain from alcohol use for 1 month to improve outcomes [15]. In general, postoperative morbidity is increased in alcohol misusers [29]. Oral bowel preparation is not recommended preoperatively because it has been shown to not have any benefits and because it might lead to dehydration and fluid imbalances [15]. Evidence is lacking for carbohydrate loading in the gastrectomy patient group, but the current ERAS guidelines still strongly recommend limited fasting and the usage of clear carbohydrate drinks up until 2 h presurgery. This recommendation also supports the goal of reducing postoperative insulin resistance and maintaining euglycemia [15].

Historically, patients undergoing total gastrectomy were not allowed to eat for several days following the procedure [15]. These patients are at high risk of malnutrition and cachexia. Due to the risk of malnutrition, ERAS protocols recommend that these patients be allowed to eat at will postoperatively from day 1 following surgery. The interdisciplinary team will closely monitor the progression of intake and recommend that patients slowly increase intake. If a gastrectomy patient is unable to consume 60% of their estimated nutritional requirements 6 days postsurgery, then strong evidence indicates that the interdisciplinary team should intervene with oral nutrition supplements or nutrition support as appropriate. Postoperative nausea and vomiting should be mitigated with the use of prophylactic antinausea and antiemetic medications [15].

Bariatric Surgery

Bariatric surgery is a term for the surgical intervention for severe obesity that encompasses sleeve gastrectomies, gastric bypass, and gastric banding [30]. Patients who have a BMI $\geq$ 40 kg/m^2 or BMI $\geq$ 35 kg/m^2 with a comorbidity qualify for bariatric surgery. Additionally, per the recommendations of the Diabetes Surgery Summit, individuals with a BMI $\geq$ 30 kg/m^2 with type 2 diabetes and inadequately controlled blood glucose levels should be considered candidates for bariatric surgery. Recommendations for ERAS procedures during bariatric surgeries were first published in 2016 and then updated in 2022. General education and counseling and specific nutrition education and counseling prior to bariatric surgeries are highly recommended. This helps the patients to be prepared for the life-long changes that result from this surgery. While evidence is inconclusive on the full benefits of pre-operative education, in this and other populations, the ERAS guidelines continue to recommend preoperative education as a step of informed consent [30].

Patients are recommended to abstain from alcohol for 1–2 years prior to surgery if they have had prior overconsumption [30]. In the immediate 2–4-week preoperative period, patients should also follow a very low-calorie diet (VLCD) (800 kcal/day). Following the VLCD will allow for preoperative weight loss, a reduction in liver volume, and a reduction in postoperative complications. Inconclusive evidence also points to greater postoperative weight loss for patients who participate in the VLCD prior to bariatric surgery. Within the bariatric surgery patient population, evidence remains low for using preoperative carbohydrate-loading drinks. Patients with severe obesity should follow the recommendations for other gastrointestinal surgeries for food and drink before surgery; no solid food 6 h prior to surgery and clear liquids allowed until 2 h prior to surgery [30].

Postoperative nausea and vomiting may be increased in this patient population because the gastric size has been decreased [30]. Multimodal prevention, such as a combination of avoiding opioids and giving antiemetics, for nausea and vomiting should be used intra- and postoperatively. Maintaining fluid balance is challenging in the obese population because fluid compartments and body composition are different than those in other populations. Intravenous fluids should be administered judiciously and with the goal of avoiding fluid restriction or fluid overload. Both fluid states can lead to worse postoperative outcomes [30].

Postoperatively, patients should progress to oral nutritional intake within a few hours postsurgery [30]. A registered dietitian-nutritionist should be consulted to advise on the progression of the diet and protein intake. Based on the procedure type, protein recommendations range from 1–2.1 g/kg of ideal body weight, with hypoabsorptive procedures like the biliopancreatic diversion with duodenal switch being on the higher side of protein requirements. There is a very high risk that patients will experience multiple vitamin and mineral deficiencies after having a bariatric surgery. These include iron, folate, zinc, copper, selenium, and vitamins B_{12}, A, D, E, and K. Patients should undergo biochemical monitoring and have discussions with their registered dietitian-nutritionist and healthcare team to plan for the supplementing vitamins and minerals that they are missing [30].

Lower Gastrointestinal Surgeries

In agreement with the guidelines and recommendations for upper gastrointestinal surgeries, preoperative oral bowel preparation is not recommended for lower gastrointestinal surgeries or for colonic resections in specific [4]. Oral bowel preparation can cause dehydration in this patient population and increase the risk of anastomotic leak while not providing any benefits [4]. Carbohydrate drinks given preoperatively to colon and rectal surgical patients reduce risk of postoperative symptoms of nausea, vomiting, pain, diarrhea, and dizziness and the risk of wound dehiscence [8]. Additionally, patients given clear liquid carbohydrate drinks following an ERAS protocol are less likely to be thirsty, hungry, or experience anxiety [4, 8].

Giving a preoperative carbohydrate drink of 12.5 g of carbohydrates per 100 ml to colorectal surgical patients is also significantly associated with a decreased risk of fluid overload and the subsequent complications of fluid overload, which may include cardiorespiratory complications [8]. Fluid overload in colorectal surgical patients may happen due to increased amounts of intravenous fluids administered perioperatively [8], with some patients receiving as much as 13 liters of intravenous fluids during the surgery and postsurgical period [4]. Each additional liter of intravenous fluid increases the risk of complications and delayed discharge following surgery [8]. Additionally, excessive intravenous fluids can delay normal gastrointestinal function [4]. Therefore, the goal in colonic resection surgeries is to maintain fluid balance [4].

To promote fluid balance, decrease the length of stay, and decrease infection risk, patients should be allowed to resume oral fluids 2 h postoperatively and oral food 4 h postoperatively [4]. Similar to upper gastrointestinal surgeries, care should be taken to screen for and identify patients with or at risk of malnutrition. These patients should be encouraged to use oral nutrition supplements to improve baseline nutritional status prior to surgery. All patients benefit from oral nutritional supplements after surgery until normal oral intake is sufficient to meet their nutritional needs. Nasogastric intubation for decompression following lower gastrointestinal surgery is also not recommended [4].

Cardiac Surgeries

ERAS guidelines for cardiac surgeries were released in 2019 by the ERAS Cardiac Society [31]. Prior to cardiac surgery, hemoglobin A_{1c} levels and albumin levels should be measured as a method to assess risk. Higher hemoglobin A_{1c} and lower albumin levels suggest a greater surgical risk. Patients who are malnourished, and those with serum albumin levels less than 3.0 g/dl, should be given 7–10 days of oral nutritional supplements to bring their baseline status up to an acceptable level [31].

For cardiac patients who are able, prehabilitation and patient engagement can be beneficial to promote better outcomes, increased patient knowledge, and decreased patient anxiety [31]. These prehabilitation efforts might include physical activity, social support, and nutrition optimization. Preoperative exercise in specific can improve insulin sensitivity and lean body mass ratios. Additionally, any anemia should be corrected prior to surgery. Patients experiencing anemia from chronic disease, vitamin B_{12} deficiency, iron deficiency, and other causes should be evaluated. Anemia is associated with poor postsurgical outcomes [31]. Alcohol misuse in the preoperative period has been associated with infections, bleeding, and longer hospital stays [29]. For individuals who misuse alcohol, a 1-month preoperative abstinence from alcohol has been shown to decrease postoperative risks [29, 31].

In the immediate time frame prior to cardiac surgery, clear, nonalcoholic liquids can be given to patients up to 2 h before surgery [31]. Including clear carbohydrate liquids in the preoperative liquid intake can be beneficial for postoperative glucose control, insulin function, and improved cardiac function following cardiac surgeries. Continued studies should be conducted in cardiac surgical patients to further clarify the amounts and types of carbohydrate beverages and the exact mechanisms of action for any benefits seen [31].

Box 18.2: Implementing ERAS Protocols Takes a Team
When implementing ERAS protocols, the entire interdisciplinary team should work together. For example, when working with patients undergoing liver surgery, a nurse might conduct the recommended preoperative counseling. A registered dietitian-nutritionist and a physical therapist might work together on the prehabilitation phase. The surgeon will conduct a minimally invasive laparoscopic liver resection. And nurses, physicians, and registered dietitian-nutritionists will work together with the patient to promote glycemic control postoperatively. All team members must be ready to work together because ERAS protocols are most effective when all guidelines are followed.

Liver Surgeries

Guidelines for ERAS in liver surgeries were first released in 2016 and subsequently updated in 2023 [32]. Prehabilitation 4–6 weeks before surgery should encompass physical exercises, nutritional interventions, and/or anxiety-reduction exercises for the most-at-risk population. Those who complete prehabilitation tend toward having better outcomes postoperatively, though this is not definitive in the literature. During a similar timeline of 4–8 weeks prior to surgery, those who are heavy alcohol drinkers should be counseled about alcohol cessation to lower the risks of postoperative complications. If hepatic surgery patients are found to have malnutrition, delaying surgery to optimize their nutritional status may be appropriate. Optimizing nutritional status should be achieved through enteral nutrition whenever possible because parenteral nutrition has additional risk factors [32].

Although optimizing nutrition is recommended, the use of immunonutrition in this patient population lacks evidence [32]. Omega-3 supplementation to promote a reduction in inflammation has been associated with improved liver function; however, results have been mixed. Some biomarkers have been improved in patients supplemented with various immunonutrition formulas. However, most trials done with immunonutrition in human patients undergoing liver surgery have been of poor quality. The official ERAS guidelines for liver surgery do not recommend immunonutrition in hepatic surgery [32].

In hepatic surgery patients, solid fasting for 6 h prior to surgery and liquid fasting for 2 h prior to surgery is recommended [32]. Liquids taken prior to surgery should include carbohydrate-loading drinks, which reduce insulin resistance, anxiety, nausea, vomiting, and the length of hospital stays. Also, some limited evidence has shown that including an amino acid snack in addition to the carbohydrate loading in the preoperative time period improves nutritional status [32].

Postsurgically, the use of prophylactic nasogastric tubes should be avoided [32]. These tubes may cause an extended hospital stay and a delay in return to an oral diet. An oral diet should be resumed early in the postoperative timeline to decrease the time to first bowel movement. Nausea and vomiting should be prophylactically treated to promote intake and patient comfort. Any nutrient deficiencies found should be corrected. For individuals not meeting their needs on an oral diet, enteral nutrition is preferred to parenteral nutrition. Parenteral nutrition has been associated with worse outcomes for the length of hospital stay, bowel movements, and serum albumin levels. Insulin therapy to maintain normoglycemia should be put in place. Fluid therapy should be goal directed to optimize outcomes and cardiac output. Postoperative weight monitoring can assist in managing fluid status [32].

Emergency Laparotomy

Guidelines for perioperative care in emergency laparotomies were published in 2021, and follow-up guidelines for intra- and postoperative care were published in 2023 [19, 33]. As already discussed, correcting hydration imbalances is important in the emergency surgery population because hypovolemia can impact circulation. Having optimal fluid balance pre- and postoperatively has been shown to reduce the length of hospital stays and decrease mortality rates [19, 34–36]. Screening and monitoring for sepsis, along with early control of sepsis, is important [19]. Additionally, the ERAS protocol for emergency laparotomies recommends completing 11 of the 12 ERAS items for planned, elective surgeries [19]. Table 18.2

Table 18.2 Nutrition-related ERAS emergency laparotomy guidelines for the preoperative phase

Broad item	Level of evidence	Recommendation grade
Age-related evaluation of frailty and cognitive assessment	Low (physician should be a geriatric expert) to high (all patients over 65 should be assessed for frailty)	Strong
Preoperative glucose and electrolyte management	Moderate	Weak
Preoperative carbohydrate loading	Not recommended	
Preoperative nasogastric intubation	Moderate	Strong
Patient and family education and shared decision-making	Low	Strong

describes the nutrition-related ERAS recommendations for emergency laparotomies.

Preoperative glucose and electrolyte management are important to maintain homeostasis and potentially decrease complications [9, 19]. Approximately 20–40% of general surgery patients experience perioperative hyperglycemia, with approximately 12–30% of those patients not having a diagnosis of diabetes [9]. Hyperglycemia during the preoperative stage can lead to excess levels of reactive oxygen species, free fatty acids, and inflammatory mediators [9]. This in turn can lead to cellular damage and immune dysfunctions. Administering insulin to correct hyperglycemia leads to decreased complications while in the hospital and decreased mortality [9]. Although professional medical societies agree that hyperglycemia should be controlled perioperatively, the glucose targets vary from 140 mg/dl to 200 mg/dl [9]. The guidelines for emergency laparotomies put forth by the ERAS Society target blood glucose levels at 144–180 mg/dl with control maintained through sliding scale insulin [19]. The evidence for these guidelines is moderately strong, with variance between studies and societal guidelines, and concern over the risk of hypoglycemia and the detriments therein [19].

Electrolyte imbalances can occur in patients who are undergoing emergency laparotomies due to the loss of body fluids and fluid shifts within the body [19]. Electrolyte imbalances, including hypomagnesemia, hypokalemia, and hypophosphatemia, may lead to cardiac dysrhythmias and atrial fibrillation. Magnesium, potassium, and phosphorus should be given intravenously as appropriate per hospital policy to maintain electrolyte balance [19].

Within most ERAS protocols, preoperative carbohydrate loading with a clear liquid carbohydrate drink is suggested [2, 4, 18, 19]. Within emergency laparotomies, evidence is lacking on whether preoperative carbohydrate loading is helpful or appropriate [19]. Carbohydrate loading in this population could lead to increased blood glucose levels without any mitigating effect on insulin sensitivity after surgery (as seen in other surgical populations). Additionally, the guidelines state that moderate evidence has shown that for this patient population, preoperatively using nasogastric tubes to control gastric distention and gastric contents is beneficial for lowering the risk of aspiration [19].

Immunonutrition

Introduction to Immunonutrition

Immunonutrition, sometimes also referred to as immune-enhancing formulas or immune-modulating formulas, is the use of a combination of nutrients, including arginine, glutamine, nucleotides or RNA, omega-3 fatty acids, antioxidants, and polyunsaturated long-chain fatty acids, to support nutritional status in critically ill and surgical patients [6, 7, 37–43]. The common components of immunonutrition are immune-modulating components, antioxidants, and anti-inflammatories [6, 41]. Surgery increases systemic inflammation and results in changes in proinflammatory cytokines and acute-phase proteins [41]. Omega-3 fatty acids have been shown to have anti-inflammatory effects by reducing tissue inflammation through an increase in eicosapentaenoic acid and docosahexaenoic acid in cell membrane phospholipids [41]. Arginine is an essential amino acid for wound healing [38], and arginine levels are decreased in those with surgical trauma [41]. L-arginine improves macrophage function and lymphocyte responsiveness, increasing resistance to infection [41]. Glutamine can become conditionally essential during stress or infection, as seen in surgical patients [44]. RNA can promote T-cell response [38] and modulate inflammation, which has a positive effect on inflammation-related side effects [45].

Due to the differences in systemic response to surgery and chronic diseases like cancer, immunonutrition protocols frequently focus on some, but not all, of the frequently used immunonutrition components. Surgical formulations frequently have higher levels of amino acids and some omega-3 fatty acids, whereas formulations for cancer patients have lower amino acid content and higher levels of omega-3 fatty acids [43]. This variability in formulation and the variability in timing of initiating immunonutrition can hinder forming a consensus on the benefits of and best practices for immunonutrition.

Some common enteral immunonutrition formula types include the IMPACT formula from Nestlé [40, 46] and the use of formulas with supplemental eicosapentaenoic acid [40]. The IMPACT formula has 4.7 g of L-arginine, 0.45 g of dietary nucleotides, and 1.23 g of omega-3 fatty acids [46]. The Abbott formulary also has an "Ensure Surgery Immunonutrition Shake" that contains 4.2 g of arginine and 1.1 g of omega-3 fatty acids [47]. Both Nestlé and Abbott offer oral and enteral nutrition formulations of their immunonutrition products.

Immunonutrition in Practice

In patients undergoing elective surgery, immunonutrition has shown lower infection rates, wound complications, and a decreased length of stay [38, 41]. Immunonutrition with glutamine, arginine, and omega-3 fatty acids will shorten hospital stays and decrease infection rates in patients undergoing pancreaticoduodenectomies [44]. These patients are frequently undernourished or malnourished prior to surgery, and immunonutrition can help give the immune system support when given perioperatively [44]. Immunonutrition given prior to oncological surgery results in decreased inflammatory markers and decreased infections postoperatively, with the best effects being seen in patients who receive immunonutrition preoperatively [43]. However, as stated earlier in this chapter, further research needs to be conducted on patients with head and neck cancer before immunonutrition can be recommended in that patient population specifically [43].

In patients undergoing abdominal surgery, the postoperative supplementation of arginine, glutamine, and omega-3 fatty acids has been shown to decrease the length of hospital stays and morbidity [45]. Perioperatively using formulas with RNA, arginine, and omega-3 fatty acids is superior to the standard approach, but not as effective as using arginine, glutamine, and omega-3 fatty acids. Some protocols recommend using a combination of immunonutrition formulas to reap the best benefits [45]. Enteral immunonutrition has also shown benefits for trauma surgery patients through the use of nasogastric, nasoduodenal, or jejunostomy tubes [38]. In the critically ill, nonsurgical patient population, immunonutrition has shown to be less promising. It has no effect on mortality, infections, or the length of hospital stays in critically ill patients [37, 42].

The standard enteral immunonutrition dosage is 25 kcal/kg/day [7], and it has been shown to reduce rates of respiratory tract infections [39]. Immunonutrition formulas also come in oral nutrition support formulations, and there is inconclusive evidence on what amount per day is adequate to see benefits in infection rates, morbidity, and the length of hospital stays. Although there is no standard preoperative initiation of immunonutrition, current recommendations suggest initiating immunonutrition 5 days prior to surgery and continuing it into the postoperative period [39, 41]. Immunonutrition may also be initiated in the postoperative period to see benefits in infection rate, morbidity, and the length of hospital stays [45, 48]. The use of immunonutrition remains imprecise due to low research study quality [6, 38, 40, 41] and bias from industry-funded studies [6]. Further research on the individual components of immunonutrition and their effects on inflammation and the immune system as individual components and as combined therapies also needs to be conducted.

Postoperative Nutritional Strategies

Postoperative nutrition, insulin management [9], and mobilization [4], in addition to controlling blood glucose levels and mitigating insulin resistance through preoperative carbohydrate loading, can help to control blood glucose levels and decrease insulin resistance. Glucose control in noncritically ill surgical patients is typically achieved through subcutaneous insulin [9]. Blood glucose checks are completed every 2 hours postoperatively and rapid-acting insulin given if the patient is hyperglycemic. If the patient is hypoglycemic postoperatively, an oral glucose solution or intravenous solution will be given according to the alertness of the patient. Once patients have transitioned to the general hospital floors and have been started on an oral diet, basal insulin boluses plus correctional rapid-acting insulin regimens should be instituted. Sliding scale insulin should not be relied on as the sole source of insulin due to the risks for developing hypo- and hyperglycemia [9].

Postoperatively returning to a normal diet results in improved healing and a decreased length of stay [2, 11]. However, some patients can experience decreased appetite after surgery [11]. Nutritional supplements can assist those who have a depressed appetite by providing a more concentrated source of carbohydrates and protein. Postoperatively, patients experience muscle atrophy, where muscle tissue is catabolized to provide energy through gluconeogenesis and to maintain bodily protein synthesis [11]. Therefore, protein needs are higher in postoperative patients and should be considered along with carbohydrate intake to maximize the recovery of the surgical patient [11]. Protein intake in the postoperative period, while the patient is under metabolic stress and/or prolonged periods of physical inactivity, will result in insulin stimulation and muscle protein synthesis [49–51]. Protein recommendations vary widely in the surgical population, as they do in the general population, though they are agreed to be elevated after injury and surgery [11, 52, 53]. The recommendation is a minimum of 1.6 g/kg/day, with guidelines also ranging up to 3 g/kg/day for optimal rehabilitation for previously active individuals postsurgery [52].

Postoperative carbohydrate intake can assist in meeting calorie needs to promote healing and rehabilitation [11, 49]. Approximately 55% of total kilocalories, or 3–5 g/kg/day of carbohydrates, should be provided in the recovery period [52]. Whole-food carbohydrate sources, such as whole fruits and vegetables, are also high in micronutrients, which are beneficial for healing. Providing a high-carbohydrate diet versus a high-fat diet has been shown to be protein sparing and reduce muscle breakdown in the recovery period [52]. However, fat is an indispensable part of the recovery diet and helps with cell proliferation and providing energy. The essential fatty acids omega-3 and omega-6 are recommended postoperatively, with consideration for limiting excessive amounts of omega-6 fatty acids due to their proinflammatory nature [11, 52]. Omega-3 fatty acids are typically found in plant sources like avocadoes, olive oil, nuts, and seeds but can also be found in fatty fish. Omega-6 fatty acids are found in vegetable oils, nuts, and poultry fats, among other sources.

Conclusion

The nutritional intake of carbohydrates, protein, fluids, and immune-supporting nutrients is vital in the perioperative period. Increasing the preoperative nutritional status of patients who are malnourished through nutrition supplements or nutrition support can promote postoperative recovery. Following ERAS guidelines with an interdisciplinary team will promote better outcomes for surgical patients. The use of immunonutrition supplements and enteral formulas may promote better outcomes and a decreased length of stay for patients. Maintaining normal blood glucose levels for all patients will promote healing in patients. The perioperative nutritional status of the patient should be a focus for all members of the interdisciplinary team.

Further Practice

1. Anesthesia given during surgery can cause the laryngeal reflex to relax. Why is this a concern with oral nutrition?
   A. It can cause aspiration pneumonia.
   B. It can cause gastroesophageal reflux disease.
   C. It can cause discomfort.
   D. Oral nutrition can decrease the effectiveness of anesthesia.

2. How does nutritional status affect postoperative outcomes?

   A. Surgery puts the body into a hypermetabolic-anabolic state, and the body needs more nutrition.
   B. Surgery puts the body into a hypermetabolic-catabolic state, and the body needs more nutrition.
   C. Surgery puts the body into a hypermetabolic-anabolic state, and the body needs less nutrition.
   D. Surgery puts the body into a hypermetabolic-catabolic state, and the body needs less nutrition.

3. What types of amino acids may be supplemented prior to surgery to maintain a positive protein balance?

   A. Branched-chain amino acids
   B. Essential amino acids
   C. Nonessential amino acids
   D. Both a and b

4. Blood glucose levels are important to control in which populations prior to surgery?

   A. All populations
   B. Diabetic populations
   C. Obese populations
   D. Overweight populations

5. What are the ERAS recommendations for oral intake after gastrectomy?

   A. Oral intake is allowed 3 days after surgery.
   B. Oral intake is allowed 4 days after surgery.
   C. Oral intake is allowed 5 days after surgery.
   D. Oral intake is allowed immediately after surgery.

6. If patients are unable to meet their needs orally, what type of nutrition support is recommended?

   A. Total parenteral nutrition
   B. Peripheral parenteral nutrition
   C. Enteral nutrition
   D. Trophic enteral nutrition

7. What are the patient qualifications for bariatric surgery?

   A. Patients who have a BMI ≥ 45 kg/m^2 or BMI ≥ 30 kg/m^2 with a comorbidity qualify for bariatric surgery.
   B. Patients who have a BMI ≥ 35 kg/m^2 or BMI ≥ 30 kg/m^2 with a comorbidity qualify for bariatric surgery.

    C. Patients who have a BMI $\geq$ 50 kg/m^2 or BMI $\geq$ 45 kg/m^2 with a comorbidity qualify for bariatric surgery.

    D. Patients who have a BMI $\geq$ 40 kg/m^2 or BMI $\geq$ 35 kg/m^2 with a comorbidity qualify for bariatric surgery.

8. Bariatric patients are at risk of all of the following vitamin and mineral deficiencies except for _____.

    A. Iron
    B. Folate
    C. Vitamin B$_{12}$
    D. Vitamin C

9. What are the preoperative risks of oral bowel preparation?

    A. Oral bowel preparation can cause hyperglycemia.
    B. Oral bowel preparation can cause dehydration and increase the risk of anastomotic leak.
    C. Oral bowel preparation can cause hypoglycemia.
    D. Oral bowel preparation can cause nausea and vomiting.

10. Prehabilitation has been recommended in which patients?

    A. Malnourished patients
    B. Undernourished patients
    C. Cardiac and liver patients
    D. Emergency laparotomy patients

11. What populations should avoid alcohol?

    A. Alcohol misusers
    B. Moderate alcohol users
    C. Diabetics
    D. Cardiac surgery patients

12. What is hyperglycemia associated with in the preoperative stage?

    A. Cellular damage and immune dysfunctions
    B. Better patient outcomes
    C. Nausea and vomiting
    D. Nephropathy

13. What are the common components of immunonutrition?

    A. Arginine
    B. Glutamine
    C. Nucleotides or RNA
    D. Omega-3 fatty acids
    E. All of the above

14. Muscle tissue may be postoperatively catabolized to provide energy through gluconeogenesis and to maintain bodily protein synthesis. What is the protein intake recommendation to mitigate the loss of lean body mass?

    A. 0.8–1.0 g/kg/day
    B. 1.2–1.5 g/kg/day
    C. 1.6–3.0 g/kg/day
    D. 2.0–2.9 g/kg/day

15. Postoperative diets should be highest in which macronutrient?

    A. Carbohydrate
    B. Fat
    C. Protein

Answer Key

1. A, 2. B, 3. D, 4. A, 5. D, 6. C, 7. D, 8. D, 9. B, 10. C, 11. A, 12. A, 13. E. 14. C, 15. A

References

1. Scott MJ, Baldini G, Fearon KCH, Feldheiser A, Feldman LS, Gan TJ, et al. Enhanced recovery after surgery (ERAS) for gastrointestinal surgery, part 1: pathophysiological considerations. Acta Anaesthesiol Scand. 2015;59(10):1212–31.
2. Fayez O, Khalid A, Peterson S. Exercise and nutrition pre- and post-surgery. ACSMs Health Fit J. 2023;27(6):26–32.
3. ERAS Society [Internet]. [cited 2024 Mar 12]. History Available from: https://erassociety.org/about/history/
4. Fearon KCH, Ljungqvist O, Von Meyenfeldt M, Revhaug A, Dejong CHC, Lassen K, et al. Enhanced recovery after surgery: a consensus review of clinical care for patients undergoing colonic resection. Clin Nutr. 2005;24(3):466–77.
5. Ljungqvist O, Søreide E. Preoperative fasting. Br J Surg. 2003;90(4):400–6.
6. Probst P, Ohmann S, Klaiber U, Hüttner FJ, Billeter AT, Ulrich A, et al. Meta-analysis of immunonutrition in major abdominal surgery. Br J Surg. 2017;104(12):1594–608.
7. Cerantola Y, Hübner M, Grass F, Demartines N, Schäfer M. Immunonutrition in gastrointestinal surgery. Br J Surg. 2011;98(1):37–48.
8. Gustafsson UO, Hausel J, Thorell A, Ljungqvist O, Soop M, Nygren J, et al. Adherence to the enhanced recovery after surgery protocol and outcomes after colorectal cancer surgery. Arch Surg. 2011;146(5):571–7.
9. Duggan EW, Carlson K, Umpierrez GE. Perioperative hyperglycemia management: an update. Anesthesiology. 2017;126(3):547–60.
10. ERAS Society [Internet]. [cited 2024 Feb 23]. Guidelines. Available from: https://erassociety.org/guidelines/
11. Hirsch KR, Wolfe RR, Ferrando AA. Pre- and post-surgical nutrition for preservation of muscle mass, strength, and functionality following orthopedic surgery. Nutrients. 2021;13(5):1675.
12. Gillis C, Fenton TR, Gramlich L, Keller H, Sajobi TT, Culos-Reed SN, et al. Malnutrition modifies the response to multimodal prehabilitation: a pooled analysis of prehabilitation trials: applied physiology, nutrition & metabolism. Appl Physiol Nutr Metab. 2022;47(2):141–50.

13. Zink TM, Kent SE, Choudhary AN, Kavolus JJ. Nutrition in surgery: an orthopaedic perspective. J Bone Jt Surg. 2023;105(23):1897–906.
14. Thomas MN, Kufeldt J, Kisser U, Hornung HM, Hoffmann J, Andraschko M, et al. Effects of malnutrition on complication rates, length of hospital stay, and revenue in elective surgical patients in the G-DRG-system. Nutrition. 2016;32(2):249–54.
15. Mortensen K, Nilsson M, Slim K, Schäfer M, Mariette C, Braga M, et al. Consensus guidelines for enhanced recovery after gastrectomy. Br J Surg. 2014;101(10):1209–29.
16. Zhang X, Zhang L, Pu Y, Sun M, Zhao Y, Zhang D, et al. Global, regional, and national burden of protein–energy malnutrition: a systematic analysis for the global burden of disease study. Nutrients. 2022;14(13):2592.
17. Osland E, Yunus RM, Khan S, Memon MA. Early versus traditional postoperative feeding in patients undergoing resectional gastrointestinal surgery. J Parenter Enter Nutr. 2011;35(4):473–87.
18. Dort JC, Farwell DG, Findlay M, Huber GF, Kerr P, Shea-Budgell MA, et al. Optimal perioperative care in major head and neck cancer surgery with free flap reconstruction: a consensus review and recommendations from the enhanced recovery after surgery society. JAMA Otolaryngol Neck Surg. 2017;143(3):292–303.
19. Peden CJ, Aggarwal G, Aitken RJ, Anderson ID, Bang Foss N, Cooper Z, et al. Guidelines for perioperative care for emergency laparotomy enhanced recovery after surgery (ERAS) society recommendations: part 1—preoperative: diagnosis, rapid assessment and optimization. World J Surg. 2021;45(5):1272–90.
20. Han HS, Kang SB. Relations between long-term glycemic control and postoperative wound and infectious complications after total knee arthroplasty in type 2 diabetics. Clin Orthop Surg. 2013;5(2):118.
21. Abdelmalak BB, Knittel J, Abdelmalak JB, Dalton JE, Christiansen E, Foss J, et al. Preoperative blood glucose concentrations and postoperative outcomes after elective non-cardiac surgery: an observational study. BJA Br J Anaesth. 2014;112(1):79–88.
22. Halkos ME, Lattouf OM, Puskas JD, Kilgo P, Cooper WA, Morris CD, et al. Elevated preoperative hemoglobin A1c level is associated with reduced long-term survival after coronary artery bypass surgery. Ann Thorac Surg. 2008;86(5):1431–7.
23. Tewari N, Awad S, Duška F, Williams JP, Bennett A, Macdonald IA, et al. Postoperative inflammation and insulin resistance in relation to body composition, adiposity and carbohydrate treatment: a randomised controlled study. Clin Nutr Edinb Scotl. 2019;38(1):204–12.
24. Lalueza MP, Colomina MJ, Bagó J, Clemente S, Godet C. Analysis of nutritional parameters in idiopathic scoliosis patients after major spinal surgery. Eur J Clin Nutr. 2005;59(5):720–2.
25. Soop M, Nygren J, Myrenfors P, Thorell A, Ljungqvist O. Preoperative oral carbohydrate treatment attenuates immediate postoperative insulin resistance. Am Physiol Soc. 2001;280(4):E576–83.
26. Svanfeldt M, Thorell A, Hausel J, Soop M, Rooyackers O, Nygren J, et al. Randomized clinical trial of the effect of preoperative oral carbohydrate treatment on postoperative whole-body protein and glucose kinetics. Br J Surg. 2007;94(11):1342–50.
27. Crowe PJ, Dennison A, Royle GT. The effect of pre-operative glucose loading on postoperative nitrogen metabolism. Br J Surg. 1984;71(8):635–7.
28. Yuill KA, Richardson RA, Davidson HIM, Garden OJ, Parks RW. The administration of an oral carbohydrate-containing fluid prior to major elective upper-gastrointestinal surgery preserves skeletal muscle mass postoperatively—a randomised clinical trial. Clin Nutr. 2005;24(1):32–7.
29. Tønnesen H, Rosenberg J, Nielsen HJ, Rasmussen V, Hauge C, Pedersen IK, et al. Effect of preoperative abstinence on poor postoperative outcome in alcohol misusers: randomised controlled trial. BMJ. 1999;318(7194):1311–6.
30. Stenberg E, dos Reis Falcão LF, O'Kane M, Liem R, Pournaras DJ, Salminen P, et al. Guidelines for perioperative care in bariatric surgery: enhanced recovery after surgery (ERAS) society recommendations: a 2021 update. World J Surg. 2022;46(4):729–51.

31. Engelman DT, Ben Ali W, Williams JB, Perrault LP, Reddy VS, Arora RC, et al. Guidelines for perioperative care in cardiac surgery: enhanced recovery after surgery society recommendations. JAMA Surg. 2019;154(8):755–66.

32. Joliat GR, Kobayashi K, Hasegawa K, Thomson JE, Padbury R, Scott M, et al. Guidelines for perioperative Care for Liver Surgery: enhanced recovery after surgery (ERAS) society recommendations 2022. World J Surg. 2023;47(1):11–34.

33. Scott MJ, Aggarwal G, Aitken RJ, Anderson ID, Balfour A, Foss NB, et al. Consensus guidelines for perioperative care for emergency laparotomy enhanced recovery after surgery (ERAS) society recommendations part 2—emergency laparotomy: intra- and postoperative care. World J Surg. 2023;47(8):1850–80.

34. Møller MH, Adamsen S, Thomsen RW, Møller AM, On Behalf of the Peptic Ulcer Perforation (PULP) Trial Group. Multicentre trial of a perioperative protocol to reduce mortality in patients with peptic ulcer perforation. Br J Surg. 2011;98(6):802–10.

35. Tengberg LT, Bay-Nielsen M, Bisgaard T, Cihoric M, Lauritsen ML, Foss NB, et al. Multidisciplinary perioperative protocol in patients undergoing acute high-risk abdominal surgery. Br J Surg. 2017;104(4):463–71.

36. Sethi A, Debbarma M, Narang N, Saxena A, Mahobia M, Tomar GS. Impact of targeted preoperative optimization on clinical outcome in emergency abdominal surgeries: a prospective randomized trial. Anesth Essays Res. 2018;12(1):149–54.

37. Tan HB, Danilla S, Murray A, Serra R, El Dib R, Henderson TO, et al. Immunonutrition as an adjuvant therapy for burns. Cochrane Database Syst Rev. 2014;12:CD007174.

38. Gregori P, Franceschetti E, Basciani S, Impieri L, Zampogna B, Matano A, et al. Immunonutrition in orthopedic and traumatic patients. Nutrients. 2023;15(3):537.

39. Yu K, Zheng X, Wang G, Liu M, Li Y, Yu P, et al. Immunonutrition vs standard nutrition for cancer patients: a systematic review and meta-analysis (part 1). J Parenter Enter Nutr. 2020;44(5):742–67.

40. Mingliang W, Zhangyan K, Fangfang F, Huizhen W, Yongxiang L. Perioperative immunonutrition in esophageal cancer patients undergoing esophagectomy: the first meta-analysis of randomized clinical trials. Dis Esophagus. 2020;33(4):doz111.

41. Marik PE, Zaloga GP. Immunonutrition in high-risk surgical patients. J Parenter Enter Nutr. 2010;34(4):378–86.

42. Heyland DK, Novak F, Drover JW, Jain M, Su X, Suchner U. Should immunonutrition become routine in critically ill patients?A systematic review of the evidence. JAMA. 2001;286(8):944–53.

43. García-Malpartida K, Aragón-Valera C, Botella-Romero F, Ocón-Bretón MJ, López-Gómez JJ. Effects of immunonutrition on cancer patients undergoing surgery: a scoping review. Nutrients. 2023;15(7):1776.

44. Fan Y, Li N, Zhang J, Fu Q, Qiu Y, Chen Y. The effect of immunonutrition in patients undergoing pancreaticoduodenectomy: a systematic review and meta-analysis. BMC Cancer. 2023;23(1):351.

45. Ricci C, Serbassi F, Alberici L, Ingaldi C, Gaetani L, De Raffele E, et al. Immunonutrition in patients who underwent major abdominal surgery: a comprehensive systematic review and component network metanalysis using GRADE and CINeMA approaches. Surgery. 2023;174(6):1401–9.

46. Nestlé Medical Hub [Internet]. [cited 2024 Apr 15]. IMPACT Peptide 1.5. Available from: https://www.nestlemedicalhub.com/products/impact-peptide-15

47. Ensure Surgery Immunonutrition Shake [Internet]. [cited 2024 Apr 15]. Available from: https://abbottstore.com/adult-nutrition/ensure/ensure-surgery/ensure-surgery-immunonutritionshake/ensure-surgery-immunonutrition-shake-vanilla-8-fl-oz-bottle-case-of-15-66436.html

48. Matsui R, Sagawa M, Inaki N, Fukunaga T, Nunobe S. Impact of perioperative immunonutrition on postoperative outcomes in patients with upper gastrointestinal cancer: a systematic review and meta-analysis of randomized controlled trials. Nutrients. 2024;16(5):577.
49. Phillips SM, Paddon-Jones D, Layman DK. Optimizing adult protein intake during catabolic health conditions. Adv Nutr. 2020;11(4):S1058–69.
50. Gillis C, Carli F. Promoting perioperative metabolic and nutritional care. Anesthesiology. 2015;123(6):1455–72.
51. Paddon-Jones D. Interplay of stress and physical inactivity on muscle loss: nutritional countermeasures 12. J Nutr. 2006;136(8):2123–6.
52. Smith-Ryan AE, Hirsch KR, Saylor HE, Gould LM, Blue MNM. Nutritional considerations and strategies to facilitate injury recovery and rehabilitation. J Athl Train. 2020;55(9):918–30.
53. Tipton KD. Nutritional support for exercise-induced injuries. Sports Med. 2015;45(1):93–104.

Gastronomic Solutions: Exploring Enteral and Parenteral Nutrition for Optimal Patient Care

19

Kehinde Tom-Ayegunle

Learning Objectives

After completing this chapter, you will be able to

- Identify different types of enteral feeding methods and their appropriate applications
- Evaluate indications and contraindications for both enteral nutrition and parenteral nutrition
- Differentiate between various types of enteral feeding formulas and their specific uses
- Recognize and manage common complications associated with enteral feeding
- Calculate the nutritional requirements for patients receiving parenteral nutrition
- Apply knowledge of enteral nutrition and parenteral nutrition to develop individualized nutrition care plans
- Interpret clinical data to make informed decisions about nutrition support interventions

Introduction

Nutritional support plays a crucial role in patient care, particularly for individuals with compromised gastrointestinal function. The two primary methods of artificial nutrition delivery are enteral feeding and parenteral feeding. Although recent

K. Tom-Ayegunle (✉)
Department of Epidemiology & Biostatistics, Bloomberg School of Public Health, Johns Hopkins University, Baltimore, MD, USA
e-mail: ktomaye1@jh.edu

© The Author(s), under exclusive license to Springer Nature Switzerland AG 2025
A. K. Mitra, D. Vanoh (eds.), *Essentials of Clinical and Public Health Nutrition*, Nutrition and Health, https://doi.org/10.1007/978-3-031-95373-6_19

413

evidence supports the benefits of nutritional support, especially for severely malnourished patients [1], the optimal delivery route remains a subject of debate among
healthcare professionals. Enteral nutrition is often considered more advantageous
because it maintains gut barrier function, mimicking natural physiological processes [2–4]. This approach is typically administered through tube feeding and is
preferred due to its cost-effectiveness, lower complication rates, and superior outcomes compared to parenteral nutrition [5, 6]. In contrast, parenteral nutrition,
though sometimes necessary, tends to be costlier and might compromise gut barrier
integrity, increasing the risk of septic complications. Parenteral nutrition is an invasive therapy and serves as a vital alternative when gastrointestinal function is
severely impaired or enteral feeding is not feasible. Despite its importance in certain
clinical scenarios, it carries inherent risks that must be carefully considered [5, 6].
The choice between enteral and parenteral nutrition often depends on individual
patient factors, underlying conditions, and specific clinical circumstances.

Types of Enteral Feeding

Enteral nutrition is a critical component of medical nutrition support, with various
tube types designed to meet specific clinical needs. As outlined in Table 19.1, enteral
feeding tubes offer diverse options for providing nutritional support to patients with
different medical conditions. These tubes range from short-term solutions like

Table 19.1 Types of enteral feeding tubes and their respective applications

Enteral tube type	Insertion method	Clinical application
Nasogastric	Transnasal insertion; external measurement from nostril to ear to xiphisternum; may use stylet for stiffening	Short-term nutrition support (weeks); suitable for bolus or continuous feeding
Nasoduodenal	Administered through tube feeding and preferred due to its cost-effectiveness, lower complication rates, and superior outcomes compared to parenteral nutrition [5, 6]	Short-term feeding in patients with impaired gastric emptying or suspected proximal gastrointestinal leak; requires continuous infusion
Gastrostomy	Percutaneous placement via endoscopic, radiologic, or surgical approach	Long-term nutrition support; appropriate for patients with swallowing disorders or those requiring prolonged enteral access
Jejunostomy	Percutaneous placement via endoscopic or radiologic approach through pylorus; direct endoscopic or surgical jejunal insertion	Long-term nutrition support in patients with impaired gastric motility; necessitates continuous infusion
Gastrojejunostomy	Percutaneous placement using endoscopic, radiologic, or surgical techniques; dual-lumen design	Utilized in patients at high risk of aspiration, with impaired gastric emptying, acute pancreatitis, or proximal gastrointestinal leaks

nasogastric tubes to long-term nutritional access methods such as gastrostomy and jejunostomy tubes. The selection of an appropriate enteral feeding tube depends on multiple factors, including the patient's clinical condition, the anticipated duration of nutritional support, and specific gastrointestinal challenges.

Enteral nutrition plays a pivotal role in managing nutritional needs across different patient populations. The primary indications for enteral feeding encompass a broad spectrum of clinical conditions, including critically ill or injured patients with moderate-to-severe injuries, individuals with inflammatory bowel diseases such as Crohn's disease and ulcerative colitis, and patients at risk of malnutrition or experiencing existing nutritional deficiencies [7]. Although enteral nutrition offers substantial therapeutic benefits, a careful evaluation of its appropriateness must be carried out by considering critical contraindications. Absolute contraindications include patients with nonfunctional or severely compromised gastrointestinal tracts, complete bowel obstruction, and clinical situations where the potential risks of enteral feeding demonstrably outweigh the anticipated nutritional benefits. The decision to initiate enteral nutrition requires a comprehensive clinical assessment, balancing the potential nutritional advantages against individual patient pathophysiology, and specific medical constraints.

Box 19.1: Indications and Contraindications of Enteral Feeding
Indications:

1. Critically ill or injured patients, particularly those with moderate-to-severe injuries
2. Patients with inflammatory bowel diseases (Crohn's disease and ulcerative colitis)
3. Individuals at risk of malnutrition or with existing nutritional deficiencies
4. Patients requiring nutritional support but with functional gastrointestinal tracts

Contraindications:

1. Patients with nonfunctional or severely compromised gastrointestinal tracts
2. Cases of complete bowel obstruction
3. Situations where the risks of enteral feeding outweigh the benefits

---

Types of Enteral Feeding Formulas

Enteral nutrition encompasses a sophisticated spectrum of nutritional formulations, ranging from standard formulas to highly specialized formulas designed to address specific clinical conditions [8]. Standard enteral formulas (Table 19.2) provide a

Table 19.2 Standard enteral formula

Nutritional profile	Key features	Typical applications
Energy density: 1 kcal/ml	Comprehensive nutritional products (+)*	Appropriate for most patients requiring enteral nutrition
Protein: ~14% of total calories	Protein sources: caseins, soy proteins, lactalbumin	Some formulations suitable for oral consumption
Carbohydrates: ~60% of total calories	Carbohydrate sources: corn starch derivatives, maltodextrin, sucrose	
Lipids: ~30% of total calories	Fat sources: vegetable oils (corn, soybean, safflower)	
Micronutrients: meets daily requirements when > 1500 cal consumed	Osmolality: approximately 300 mOsm/kg	

comprehensive nutritional profile with a balanced macronutrient composition, delivering approximately 1 kcal/ml, containing 14% proteins from diverse sources like caseins and soy proteins, 60% carbohydrates primarily from corn starch derivatives and maltodextrin, and 30% lipids derived from vegetable oils, while meeting daily micronutrient requirements when consuming over 1500 cal. In contrast, specialized enteral formulas (Table 19.3) offer targeted nutritional interventions through strategic modifications, including high-energy density formulations for patients with fluid restrictions, protein-altered compositions for critically ill patients and those with malabsorption syndromes, lipid-modified designs addressing specific metabolic conditions like fat malabsorption or respiratory challenges, and advanced immunonutritional formulas enriched with specific amino acids, nucleotides, and fatty acids to support complex clinical management strategies across diverse patient populations.

Disease-Specific Enteral Feeding Formulas

The development of specialized enteral formulas has revolutionized nutritional support for patients with specific medical conditions. These formulas are designed to address the unique metabolic needs and challenges associated with certain diseases. Although standard enteral formulas are suitable for many patients, disease-specific formulas can offer significant advantages in acute situations. However, crucially, long-term use should be carefully considered, and patients should transition to standard formulas once their condition stabilizes.

Table 19.3 Specialized enteral formulas

Modification type	Characteristics	Clinical indications
High-energy-density formulations	1.5–2 kcal/ml (+)	Patients with fluid restrictions
Protein alterations	Elevated protein content (~20–25% of calories) (+)	Critically ill patients
	Protein hydrolysates (small peptides) (+)	Malabsorption syndromes
	Enhanced levels of arginine, glutamine, nucleotides, omega-3 fatty acids (+++)	Immunonutrition
	Increased branched-chain amino acids, reduced aromatic amino acids (+++)	Hepatic encephalopathy management
	Reduced protein content with high biological value	Short-term use in critically ill renal patients
Lipid modifications	Reduced fat content with partial medium-chain triglyceride (MCT) inclusion (+)	Fat malabsorption disorders
	Increased fat content (> 40% of calories) (++)	Respiratory failure with CO_2 retention (limited efficacy)
	Elevated monounsaturated fatty acid content (++)	Glycemic control in diabetes
	Increased omega-3 and decreased omega-6 fatty acids (+++)	Potential benefits in acute respiratory distress syndrome (ARDS)
Fiber supplementation	Inclusion of soy polysaccharides (+)	Improved bowel function

Renal Formulas

Patients with renal failure often require careful management of their nutritional intake due to the kidney's compromised ability to filter waste products and maintain electrolyte balance. These formulas typically contain reduced amounts of protein, phosphorus, magnesium, potassium, and sodium. They often feature a specific ratio of essential amino acids (EAAs) to nonessential amino acids (NEAAs). The theory behind this is that increased EAAs might allow for urea recycling to produce NEAAs, potentially decreasing nitrogenous waste. Clinically, short-term use (5–7 days) may benefit patients with acute renal failure, particularly those with associated hemodynamic instability who cannot undergo hemodialysis. For patients on dialysis, standard enteral formulas are recommended to prevent protein malnutrition, which can occur with the prolonged use of low-protein diets. Protein requirements should be individualized, typically ranging from 0.6 to 1.0 g of protein/kg/d, with 30 to 35 nonprotein kcal/kg/d. Studies have yielded mixed results: Although some have reported a decreased need for dialysis with specialized parenteral formulas, no significant difference in survival has been observed between patients receiving EAAs versus those receiving a combination of EAAs and NEAAs.

Hepatic Formulas

Hepatic failure alters the plasma amino acid profile, which can contribute to complications such as hepatic encephalopathy. Specialized hepatic formulas aim to address these imbalances while providing adequate nutrition. Hepatic failure typically comes with an increase in aromatic amino acids (tyrosine, methionine, and phenylalanine) and a decrease in branched-chain amino acids (valine, leucine, and isoleucine). These formulas often have a higher ratio of branched-chain amino acids to aromatic amino acids, they can alter the amino acid profile, and they may help manage hepatic encephalopathy. This may be beneficial for protein-intolerant patients, although this recommendation remains controversial. For most patients with hepatic insufficiency, standard enteral formulas are often sufficient to maintain nitrogen balance and avoid hepatic encephalopathy.

Pulmonary Formulas

Patients with pulmonary disease, especially those requiring mechanical ventilation, face unique nutritional challenges. Malnutrition can exacerbate respiratory muscle weakness and compromise immune function, whereas overfeeding can lead to increased carbon dioxide production. These formulas typically contain a higher proportion of fat (up to 55% of total calories) and a lower proportion of carbohydrates than standard formulas do. The higher fat content aims to reduce the carbon dioxide production associated with carbohydrate metabolism, potentially easing the work of breathing and decreasing the time spent on ventilator support. Due to the complexities of estimating nutritional requirements in mechanically ventilated patients, indirect calorimetry can be a valuable tool for accurate assessment, but not all patients with pulmonary disease require these specialized formulas. These formulas can be particularly beneficial in cases where standard formulas are not well tolerated or when weaning from mechanical ventilation proves challenging.

Complications of Enteral Feeding

Infection

Infection around gastrostomy sites represents one of the most frequent complications of enteral feeding procedures. The incidence of peristomal infections varies considerably, ranging from 5% to 30% [7, 9, 10], with major infections occurring in less than 2% of cases. Multiple factors contribute to infection risk, including patient-related systemic comorbidities, technical aspects such as small incisions, and nursing care issues like excessive traction between external and internal bolsters. Prophylactic administration of broad-spectrum antibiotics, particularly third-generation cephalosporins, significantly reduces infection risk during gastrostomy placement. Local *Candida* infections may develop and typically respond to topical antifungal therapy with nystatin and barrier creams, though some cases occasionally require systemic antifungal treatment. Properly stabilizing the tube and reaching the appropriate tension between external and internal bolsters during site cleaning are crucial preventive measures. Severe complications like peristomal infection progressing to peritonitis are rare, occurring in less than 1% of cases. Necrotizing fasciitis, though extremely rare, requires prompt recognition and aggressive management with intravenous antibiotics and extensive surgical debridement.

Aspiration

Aspiration is a serious concern in enterally fed patients, where varying reported frequencies are based on different definitions and patient populations. The progression from aspiration to pneumonia remains unpredictable with major risk factors, including documented prior aspiration episodes, decreased consciousness, neuromuscular disease, structural abnormalities of the aerodigestive tract, persistent vomiting, prolonged supine positioning, and consistently elevated gastric residual volumes. Minor risk factors include intermittent bolus feeding, delayed gastric emptying, poor oral hygiene, and advanced age. According to evidence, feeding tube placement at lower gastrointestinal levels, away from the pharynx, significantly reduces aspiration pneumonia risk. Other prevention strategies include maintaining head elevation between 30 and 45 degrees, monitoring gastric residuals, ensuring proper tube positioning, and implementing appropriate oral care protocols. Aspiration events can be managed via immediate gastric decompression, respiratory suctioning, and supportive care with ventilatory support as needed.

Diarrhea

Diarrhea is a common and challenging complication in enterally fed patients, where the reported incidence varies between 2% and 68% [7, 9, 10]. The clinical significance relates primarily to constant soiling with watery stool that leads to skin breakdown rather than to frequency alone. Multiple factors contribute to diarrhea development, including medication effects, formula composition, the administration rate, and infections. Medications containing sorbitol or magnesium frequently precipitate diarrhea, and antibiotic therapy can disrupt normal bowel flora, leading to *Clostridium difficile* overgrowth. Critically ill patients often demonstrate altered gastrointestinal motility and absorptive capacity, making careful feeding advancement necessary. Diarrhea can be managed by reducing administration rates and incorporating soluble fiber–containing formulas, which provide a substrate for bacterial metabolism to short-chain fatty acids, enhancing colonic water absorption.

Metabolic Complications

Metabolic disturbances frequently manifest as hyperglycemia and electrolyte abnormalities during enteral feeding. Hyperglycemia commonly occurs with high glucose-containing formulas or in diabetic patients, and it requires formula modification or insulin adjustment. Hypokalemia, particularly in the setting of metabolic alkalosis, represents the most frequent electrolyte disturbance. Refeeding syndrome, characterized by severe hypokalemia or hypophosphatemia, poses a significant risk in hypermetabolic or severely malnourished patients, potentially causing cardiac arrhythmias or respiratory depression. This complication can be prevented by giving appropriate electrolyte replacement prior to feeding advancement and avoiding overfeeding, which can exacerbate metabolic complications and impair gastrointestinal tolerance.

Buried Bumper Syndrome

Buried bumper syndrome occurs in up to 21.8% of cases [7, 9, 10], though the true incidence of incomplete burial may be higher. The condition manifests along a spectrum from simple ulceration beneath the internal bolster to complete outward erosion through the anterior abdominal wall. Excessive traction between the external and internal bolsters is the primary risk factor, causing ischemic pressure necrosis of underlying tissue. Additional contributing factors include severe malnutrition, poor wound healing, and, paradoxically, rapid nutritional improvement with significant weight gain. It can clinically present as excessive peristomal leakage, infection, resistance to infusion, abdominal pain during feeding, and tube immobility. Management approaches must be individualized, taking into account the least traumatic extraction route, whether through the stomach or the anterior abdominal wall.

Intestinal Ischemia

Enteral feeding–associated intestinal ischemia, though rare, primarily affects critically ill patients receiving intensive care. The clinical presentation typically involves a hypotensive patient on multiple vasopressor agents who develops sudden abdominal distention, increased nasogastric output, and worsening abdominal pain accompanied by blood pressure instability. Radiological findings often reveal dilated gas-filled bowel loops, with pneumatosis intestinalis or free intraperitoneal air, representing ominous signs potentially requiring emergency surgical intervention. This condition represents an ischemia-reperfusion syndrome of the mesentery, with systemic hypotension as the primary event, exacerbated by escalating vasopressor doses and hyperosmolar feeding administration during ileus.

Tube Occlusion

Tube occlusion occurs in 9–20% of cases, influenced by factors including tube length and caliber, inadequate water irrigation, continuous versus bolus infusion, medication administration, and gastric residual volume checking [7, 9, 10]. Contact between gastric acid and enteral formula frequently precipitates clog formation. This can be managed with several options, such as pancreatic enzyme concentrates mixed with bicarbonate in warm water, which has demonstrated superior efficacy compared to the efficacy of carbonated beverages. Mechanical interventions using endoscopic instruments may be necessary for resistant occlusions.

Gastrocolocutaneous Fistula

Gastrocolocutaneous fistula development can occur either immediately after a procedure or gradually over time through direct bowel puncture during the placement or erosion of an inflamed stomach into the adjacent bowel. Acute presentations include local infection and peritonitis, whereas chronic cases typically manifest with peristomal stool leakage or diarrhea. Simple tube removal with skin protection may allow spontaneous closure in uncomplicated cases, whereas surgery becomes necessary for refractory or long-standing fistulae.

Parenteral Nutrition

Parenteral nutrition (PN) serves as an essential nutritional intervention when enteral nutrition (EN) is either insufficient or contraindicated. The implementation of PN requires careful clinical assessment and adherence to evidence-based guidelines to maximize therapeutic benefits while minimizing potential complications.

Indications and Contraindications of Parenteral Nutrition

Primary Indications

Parenteral nutrition is indicated primarily in cases of intestinal failure (IF), defined as a reduction in gut function below the minimum threshold necessary for adequate nutrient absorption. The following conditions warrant consideration for PN initiation.

Gastrointestinal Tract Dysfunction The presence of anatomical or functional compromise of the gastrointestinal tract represents a primary indication for PN. This includes short bowel syndrome, high-output gastrointestinal fistulas, and severe intestinal obstruction. In cases of paralytic ileus or when prolonged bowel rest is therapeutically indicated, PN may be necessary to maintain nutritional status while allowing the gastrointestinal tract to recover.

Malabsorption and Inadequate Nutrient Intake Severe malabsorption conditions necessitate PN when enteral feeding cannot meet nutritional requirements [11]. This becomes particularly crucial when patients are unable to achieve 60% of their estimated energy requirements for more than 4–5 consecutive days or when cumulative energy deficits exceed −6000 calories or protein deficits surpass −300 g [5].

Parenteral nutrition is indicated in several specific clinical conditions, including severe abdominal sepsis, hyperemesis gravidum with inadequate oral intake, and persistent severe diarrhea unresponsive to conventional management. In these cases, PN serves as a vital bridge to maintain nutritional status until the underlying condition improves.

Absolute Contraindications

The primary absolute contraindication for parenteral nutrition (PN) is the presence of a functional and accessible gastrointestinal tract that is capable of adequate nutrient absorption. In such cases, enteral nutrition remains the preferred route of nutritional support, offering physiological benefits such as the maintenance of gut barrier function and immune system modulation.

Relative Contraindications

Hemodynamic Instability Severe cardiopulmonary compromise is a significant concern for PN administration. In patients with unstable hemodynamics, the metabolic demands and fluid volumes associated with PN may further compromise cardiovascular function; therefore, clinical stabilization should precede the initiation of comprehensive nutritional support.

Metabolic Derangements Severe electrolyte imbalances require correction prior to PN initiation. The high nutrient and mineral content of PN solutions may exacerbate existing metabolic disturbances, particularly in cases of severe acid–base disorders, significant electrolyte abnormalities, and uncontrolled hyperglycemia.

Nutritional Requirement for Parenteral Nutrition

I. *Protein and amino acid requirements*

Protein administration represents a cornerstone of parenteral nutrition (PN), delivered as sterile amino acid solutions. The baseline protein requirement for stable adults is approximately 0.8–1.0 g/kg/day, though clinical conditions frequently necessitate higher provisions. Protein-energy malnutrition demands 1.5 g/kg/day, whereas critical illness may require 1.5–2.0 g/kg/day for optimal nitrogen balance. Nitrogen balance assessment provides crucial metabolic monitoring, calculated as follows: (protein intake/6.25) – (24 h urinary urea nitrogen + 4 g). During critical illness, a mild negative balance of −2 to −4 g/d may be acceptable, whereas recovery phases should demonstrate positive nitrogen retention. Special consideration applies to renal dysfunction, where requirements vary depending on the replacement therapy: 0.6–0.8 g/kg/day without dialysis, increasing to 1.2–1.5 g/kg/day with hemodialysis, and 1.3–2.0 g/kg/day for continuous renal replacement therapy.

II. *Carbohydrate requirements*

Dextrose serves as the primary carbohydrate substrate in PN, providing 3.4–4.0 kcal/g depending on hydration status. Optimal administration requires careful attention to infusion rates, generally not exceeding 4–7 mg/kg/min to prevent hyperglycemia. Total carbohydrate provision typically comprises 50–60% of total calories, with a minimum requirement of 130 g daily in stable patients. Glucose utilization becomes impaired in several conditions, including advanced age, hepatic dysfunction, sepsis, and critical illness, and with certain medications, particularly corticosteroids and immunosuppressants, and these situations demand careful monitoring and potential dose adjustments.

III. *Lipid requirements*

Intravenous fat emulsions serve two purposes: providing essential fatty acids and reducing glucose-dependent caloric load. Standard 20% concentrations deliver 10 kcal/g, accounting for both lipid and glycerol content. Daily administration should typically not exceed 1 g/kg to prevent lipid overload syndrome.

IV. *Electrolytes, minerals, and vitamins*

(i) Sodium regulation: Parenteral sodium provision ranges from 5 to 40 mEq/day, with critical patients potentially requiring 1–2 mEq/kg/day. The total daily requirements depend on individual metabolic status, renal function, and ongoing losses.

(ii) Potassium supplementation: Standard daily potassium requirements span 40–100 mEq, with careful adjustment for renal function and medication interactions. Patients with significant gastrointestinal losses or receiving medications like amphotericin require more-aggressive replacement strategies.

(iii) Calcium and phosphorus dynamics: Calcium provision typically spans 10–20 mEq/day, with phosphorus supplementation of 20–40 mmol/day. The critical challenge lies in maintaining solubility and preventing precipitation, which requires precise molar ratios and careful mixing protocols.

(iv) Magnesium supplementation: Daily magnesium requirements fall between 8 and 16 mEq, and particular attention needs to be paid to patients undergoing cisplatin treatment or experiencing renal dysfunction.

(v) Vitamin supplementation parameters: The following two lists specify the supplementation parameters for fat-soluble vitamins and water-soluble vitamins.

Fat-soluble vitamins

- Vitamin A: 3300 IU daily
- Vitamin D: 200 IU daily
- Vitamin E: 10 IU daily
- Vitamin K: 150 µg daily

Water-soluble vitamins

- Thiamin (B1): 6 mg
- Riboflavin (B2): 3.6 mg
- Niacin (B3): 40 mg
- Pyridoxine (B6): 6 mg
- Cyanocobalamin (B12): 5 µg
- Folic acid: 600 µg
- Ascorbic acid (C): 200 mg
- Biotin: 60 µg
- Pantothenic acid: 15 mg

V. Trace elements

Trace elements function as critical enzymatic cofactors and metabolic regulators. Zinc represents a paramount consideration, with losses significantly impacting immunological and wound healing processes. Secretory diarrhea can result in substantial zinc depletion, potentially requiring 12 mg of parenteral zinc daily. Iron supplementation remains deliberately limited due to oxidative potential, typically not exceeding 1 mg daily. Iron administration requires a nuanced strategy. Despite its metabolic significance, iron is deliberately excluded from standard PN mixtures due to its oxidative potential. Parenteral iron replacement necessitates careful monitoring while paying particular attention to potential infectious risks during critical illness.

Vascular Access and Administration

Peripheral access limits osmolarity to 900 mOsm/l, restricting nutrient concentrations and total caloric delivery. Central access via peripherally inserted central catheters (PICCs) or centrally placed lines allows higher-concentration solutions. The subclavian approach generally provides optimal patient comfort and dressing maintenance. Vascular access selection is a sophisticated clinical decision involving multiple physiological and practical considerations for each approach.

Central Venous Access

1. The subclavian approach: optimal patient comfort, easiest maintenance
2. The jugular approach: reduced pneumothorax risk
3. Femoral access: strongly contraindicated due to infection risks

Catheter Material Selection

1. Silastic: lowest thrombogenic potential and ideal for long-term access
2. Polyurethane: preferred for temporary central lines
3. Polyvinyl chloride: limited contemporary applications

Peripherally Inserted Central Catheters (PICCs)

1. Permit 20–25% dextrose solutions and 4–7% amino acid concentrations
2. Reduced invasiveness compared to traditional central lines
3. Position-dependent flow characteristics
4. Limited wire-exchange capabilities

Further Practice

1. Which of the following is considered the *primary* method of nutritional support when possible?

    (a) Parenteral nutrition
    (b) Enteral nutrition
    (c) Oral feeding
    (d) Intravenous supplementation

2. A nasogastric tube is typically used for _____.

   (a) Long-term nutrition support
   (b) Short-term nutrition support (weeks)
   (c) Patients with severe malabsorption
   (d) Permanent nutritional intervention

3. Enteral nutrition is *contraindicated* in which of the following conditions?

   (a) Inflammatory bowel diseases
   (b) Complete bowel obstruction
   (c) Patients at risk of malnutrition
   (d) Critically ill patients

4. Which type of enteral formula is designed for patients with fat malabsorption disorders?

   (a) A high-energy-density formula
   (b) A lipid-modified formula with partial medium-chain triglyceride (MCT) inclusion
   (c) A protein-altered formula
   (d) A fiber-supplemented formula

5. In enterally fed patients, aspiration risk is *highest* _____.

   (a) When maintaining head elevation at 30–45 degrees
   (b) With persistent vomiting
   (c) With intermittent bolus feeding
   (d) When maintaining proper oral hygiene

6. In parenteral nutrition, what is the baseline protein requirement for stable adults?

   (a) 0.5–0.7 g/kg/day
   (b) 0.8–1.0 g/kg/day
   (c) 1.2–1.5 g/kg/day
   (d) 2.0–2.5 g/kg/day

7. Buried bumper syndrome occurs in up to _____.

   (a) 5% of cases
   (b) 10.5% of cases
   (c) 21.8% of cases
   (d) 35% of cases

8. Which condition requires a specialized hepatic enteral formula?

   (a) Renal failure
   (b) Hepatic encephalopathy
   (c) Pulmonary disease
   (d) Cardiac insufficiency

9. What is the primary absolute contraindication for parenteral nutrition?

   (a) Hemodynamic instability
   (b) Functional gastrointestinal tract
   (c) Metabolic derangements
   (d) Severe malnutrition

10. In parenteral nutrition, daily lipid administration should not exceed _____.

   (a) 0.5 g/kg
   (b) 1 g/kg
   (c) 2 g/kg
   (d) 3 g/kg

11. Pulmonary formulas typically contain _____.

   (a) Higher carbohydrate content
   (b) Higher protein content
   (c) A higher fat proportion (up to 55%)
   (d) Reduced micronutrients

12. Renal enteral formulas typically have _____.

   (a) Increased protein content
   (b) Reduced protein, phosphorus, and electrolyte contents
   (c) High sodium content
   (d) Increased potassium levels

13. What is the most frequent metabolic complication in enteral feeding?

   (a) Hypokalemia
   (b) Hyperglycemia
   (c) Hypocalcemia
   (d) Magnesium deficiency

14. What is the typical range for parenteral sodium provision?

   (a) 1–3 mEq/day
   (b) 5–40 mEq/day
   (c) 50–100 mEq/day
   (d) 150–200 mEq/day

15. Which trace element is critical in parenteral nutrition?

   (a) Iron
   (b) Copper
   (c) Zinc
   (d) Selenium

Answer Key

1. (b)
2. (b)
3. (b)
4. (b)
5. (b)
6. (b)
7. (c)
8. (b)
9. (b)
10. (b)
11. (c)
12. (b)
13. (b)
14. (b)
15. (c)

References

1. Satyanarayana R, Klein S. Clinical efficacy of perioperative nutrition support. Curr Opin Clin Nutr Metab Care. 1998;1(1):51–8. https://doi.org/10.1097/00075197-199801000-00009.
2. Silk DB, Green CJ. Perioperative nutrition: parenteral versus enteral. Curr Opin Clin Nutr Metab Care. 1998;1(1):21–7. https://doi.org/10.1097/00075197-199801000-00005.
3. Meguid MM, Campos AC, Hammond WG. Nutritional support in surgical practice: part I. Am J Surg. 1990;159(3):345–58. https://doi.org/10.1016/s0002-9610(05)81234-6.
4. Sigurdsson G. Enteral or parenteral nutrition? Pro-enteral. Acta Anaesthesiol Scand Suppl. 1997;110:143–7. https://doi.org/10.1111/j.1399-6576.1997.tb05537.
5. Braunschweig CL, Levy P, Sheean PM, Wang X. Enteral compared with parenteral nutrition: a meta-analysis. Am J Clin Nutr. 2001;74(4):534–42. https://doi.org/10.1093/ajcn/74.4.534.
6. Shenkin A, Dryburgh FJ. Parenteral nutrition. Br Med J. 1978;1(6120):1144. https://doi.org/10.1136/bmj.1.6120.1144-d.
7. DeWitt RC, Kudsk KA. Enteral nutrition. Gastroenterol Clin N Am. 1998;27(2):371–86. https://doi.org/10.1016/S0889-8553(05)70008-X.
8. Lochs H, Dejong C, Hammarqvist F, Hebuterne X, Leon-Sanz M, Schütz T, van Gemert W, van Gossum A, Valentini L, Lübke H, Bischoff S, Engelmann N, Thul P. ESPEN guidelines on enteral nutrition: gastroenterology. Clin Nutr. 2006;25(2):260–74. https://doi.org/10.1016/j.clnu.2006.01.007.
9. Iyer KR, Crawley TC. Complications of enteral access. Gastrointest Endosc Clin N Am. 2007;17(4):717–29. https://doi.org/10.1016/j.giec.2007.07.007.
10. McClave SA, Chang W-K. Complications of enteral access. Gastrointest Endosc. 2003;58(5):739–51. https://doi.org/10.1016/S0016-5107(03)02147-3.
11. Woodcock NP, Zeigler D, Palmer MD, Buckley P, Mitchell CJ, MacFie J. Enteral versus parenteral nutrition: a pragmatic study. Nutrition. 2001;17(1):1–12. https://doi.org/10.1016/S0899-9007(00)00576-1.

Index